Prescription for the Boards
USMLE Step 2

Prescription for the Boards
USMLE Step 2

Radhika Sekhri Breaden
Class of 1996
University of California, San Francisco, School of Medicine

Cheryl Denenberg
Class of 1996
University of California, San Diego, School of Medicine

Kate C. Feibusch
Class of 1996
University of California, San Francisco, School of Medicine

Stephen N. Gomperts
Medical Scientist Training Program
University of California, San Francisco, School of Medicine

Little, Brown and Company
Boston · New York · Toronto · London

Library of Congress Cataloging-in-Publication Data

Prescription for the boards : USMLE step 2 / Radhika Sekhri Breaden
    . . . [et al.]. — 1st ed.
          p.   cm.
       Includes index.
       ISBN 0-316-10626-7.
         1. Medicine—Examinations, questions, etc.   I. Breaden, Radhika Sekhri.
         [DNLM: 1. Clinical Medicine—examination questions. 2. Licensure, Medical—United States—examination questions.   WB 18.2 P933 1996]
R834.5.P67   1996
616' .0076—dc20
DNLM/DLC
for Library of Congress   95-45312
                                    CIP

Printed in the United States of America

ICP

Editorial: Evan R. Schnittman
Production Supervisor: Cate Rickard
Editorial and Production Services: Silverchair Science + Communications
Designer: Thane Kerner

Contents

Preface

Have you looked at the 20-page outline the USMLE provides as a study guide? It's overwhelming, to say the least. We all had mixed feelings about studying for the Step 2 exam. On one hand, it's a great opportunity to review medicine before residency. On the other hand, who has the time?

This book turns that overwhelming outline into a useful study tool by providing "just enough" information about each topic. As one student put it, the Step 2 is "like seeing 800 patients in two days." Therefore, our descriptions are case-based, and we have tried to limit the information to the amount expected of us at this point in our medical careers—and that's plenty! Finally, because some things just *have* to be memorized in the day or so before the exam, we've written "cram pages" full of memorizable facts. They're designed to be photocopied, personalized, and used for—what else—cramming!

This book is written *by* med students *for* med students. We see it as a work in progress, and we look forward to getting your input to shape future editions. Happy studying, and good luck on the boards!

R.S.B.
C.D.
K.C.F.
S.N.G.

Acknowledgments

This book would not have been possible without the encouragement and support of many people. We convey our deep gratitude to Patty Mintz for launching us on this journey. We also extend a very special thanks to our friends and family: Matthew Breaden and Neelam and Amita Sekhri; Brigitta Weisshuhn, Marianne Feibusch, and John Feibusch; Edward and Barbara Gomperts, Joan Autio, and Erin Gensch; and Marshall and Betty Denenberg, Laura Denenberg, and Marc Bader.

We thank our editor, Evan R. Schnittman, for his enthusiastic support and encouragement, as well as Suzanne Jeans and the rest of the staff at Little, Brown for their efforts. Many, many thanks also go to Elizabeth Willingham and the staff at Silverchair for their beautiful work.

Finally, we extend our thanks to each other for the hard work, patience, dedication, and fun. It was a wonderful (but hectic) experience. Remember Goat Rock!

"It is not often that someone comes along who is a true friend and a good writer."

—E.B. White, *Charlotte's Web*

Prescription for the Boards
USMLE Step 2

Introduction: The Inside Scoop

Another standardized test? Ugh, again?

Take heart, this one might not be so bad, and it really does give you an opportunity to review important material before internship.

This guide is written by students who have been through the ordeal and know what it's like.

Using This Book

How you use this book depends on your goals for the Step 2. Many of the students we've talked to say that simply *passing* the boards is most important to them. If you are one of these students, this book can provide a quick review of the topics you should be familiar with before taking the Step 2 exam. On the other hand, students entering highly competitive residencies, foreign medical graduates, and students who want a broad review before beginning residency will find that this book has comprehensive summaries of important topics. In addition, this book provides a guide for buying in-depth review books if more coverage of a specific subject is desired.

We hope this book will be useful in passing on the accumulated tips and strategies that medical students from across the country have shared with us. On that note, we ask that you send us your feedback about anything and everything regarding the Step 2, so that we can share the information with future fourth-year students. If you return the form we've included for this purpose (at the end of the book), your input may help shape future editions of the book. (You'll also get a $10 coupon toward other books published by Little, Brown and Company if your response is used in the next version!)

How We've Organized This Book

The United States Medical Licensing Examination (USMLE) publishes a rather overwhelming 12-page "content outline" that lists the topics covered on the exam. Our book is based loosely on this outline. For each disease listed, we include a brief description, the characteristic signs and symptoms, pertinent laboratory tests, methods of diagnosis, and brief treatment information. Information on prevention or screening is included when applicable. We've tried to incorporate information that will help you answer the many case-based questions on the exam. The outline also includes a number of "symptoms, signs, and ill-defined conditions" that don't fit well into the signs/symptoms-diagnosis-treatment model. We've defined these words and included brief differential diagnoses. Finally, we've included information about normal physiology in many chapters. Students report that a number of questions required them to decide whether a case presentation was "normal" or not. This applied particularly to obstetrics/gynecology and pediatrics. We hope the information we provide will help you to make these distinctions.

At the end of the book, we've included some "cram pages"—pages that you can rip out and use to test yourself in the days (and hours) before the exam. We encourage you to add your own "cram facts" to this list. Write to us if you'd like to share some especially helpful ones!

Description of the USMLE Step 2

The USMLE Step 2 is the second part of a three-step process to gain medical licensing in the United States. This 2-day examination is generally taken in the fourth year of medical school. It is administered once in the spring and once in the fall (Table 1). The subjects tested on the USMLE Step 2 include medicine, surgery, obstetrics and gynecology, pediatrics, psychiatry, preventive medicine, and public health. Students need to register about 3 months in advance through the National Board of Medical Examiners (NBME). Registration forms are available at medical schools or through the NBME at the following address:

USMLE
3750 Market Street
Philadelphia, PA 19104-3190
Telephone: (215) 590-9600

The USMLE Step 2 is administered in four sections over 2 days. There are approximately 180 questions in each 3-hour section. Time for lunch provides a break between the two sections each day.

Table 1.   **Dates of 1996–1997 exam administrations***

	1996		1997
Step 1	June 11–12 October 15–16	Step 1	June 10–11 October 14–15
Step 2	March 5–6 August 27–28	Step 2	March 4–5 August 26–27
Step 3	May 14–15 December 3–4	Step 3	May 13–14 December 2–3

*These dates are tentative and subject to change by the USMLE.

About 6–8 weeks after the exam, score reports arrive in the mail. The score report contains both your overall score on the Step 2 and a profile of your performance in each subject area (Fig. 1).

The front page of your score report reveals that critical four-letter word (pass or fail), your score on a scale with a mean of 200 points, and your score on an alternate scale with a mean of 82 (don't ask us why!). On the back of the score report, a topic-specific profile shows your performance in various areas. The profiles are meant for your information only and are not provided to residency programs or other institutions.

Beginning with the March 1995 administration of the exam, the NBME has raised the percentage of students who fail the Step 2. This may change the way students approach the Step 2 exam. The old adage "Study 2 weeks for Step 1, 2 days for Step 2, and bring two #2 pencils to Step 3" may no longer be true.

Test Format

Four different types of question formats are used in the USMLE Step 2. Multiple-choice, or "one best answer," is the standard question type. Generally, a brief case description is followed by four or five answer options. The vast majority of the questions on the Step 2 are in this multiple-choice format.

There are a few other ways that questions may be presented, and it's important to be familiar with them because they require different approaches.

Matching Sets

The matching set questions generally present several brief cases and ask you to select an answer for each case from a long list of options. These options are often closely related, and you must choose the *most likely* answer. More than one answer may fit the clinical scenario, but only one will be considered the "most correct." An example is provided below:

Questions 1–3. Choose the most likely virus involved in the cases presented:
(A) Herpes simplex virus *(E) Varicella-zoster virus*
(B) Cytomegalovirus *(F) Measles virus*
(C) Epstein-Barr virus *(G) Respiratory syncytial virus*
(D) Coxsackie virus *(H) Parainfluenza virus*

1. *A 20-year-old college student comes to the student health service complaining of fatigue and sore throat for the past 3 weeks. Physical findings are remarkable for a mildly erythematous oropharynx, multiple enlarged cervical nodes, and splenomegaly.*
2. *A 34-year-old man who works as a second-grade teacher complains of painful vesicles along his trunk that have been present for the past 2 days.*
3. *This virus is associated with Burkitt's lymphoma in African populations.*

(1-C, 2-E, 3-C)

US·MLE
United States
Medical
Licensing
Examination ™

UNITED STATES MEDICAL LICENSING EXAMINATION™

USMLE Step 2 is administered to students and graduates of U.S. and Canadian medical schools by the
NATIONAL BOARD OF MEDICAL EXAMINERS® (NBME®)
3750 Market Street, Philadelphia, Pennsylvania 19104-3190.
Telephone: (215) 590-9700

STEP 2 SCORE REPORT

Pass, I. William

**123 Melrose Place
Beverly Hills, CA 90210**

USMLE ID: **1-234-567-8**

Test Date: **August 1994**

The USMLE is a single examination program for all applicants for medical licensure in the United States; it replaces the Federation Licensing Examination (FLEX) and the certifying examinations of the National Board of Medical Examiners (NBME Parts I, II, and III). The program consists of three Steps designed to assess an examinee's understanding of and ability to apply concepts and principles that are important in health and disease and that constitute the basis of safe and effective patient care. **Step 2** is designed to assess whether an examinee possesses the medical knowledge and understanding of clinical science considered essential for the provision of patient care under supervision, including emphasis on health promotion and disease prevention. Results of the examination are reported to medical licensing authorities in the United States and its territories for use in granting an initial license to practice medicine. The two numeric scores shown below are equivalent; each state or territory may use either score in making licensing decisions. These scores represent your results for the administration of Step 2 on the test date shown above.

PASS	This result is based on the minimum passing score set by USMLE for Step 2. Individual licensing authorities may accept the USMLE-recommended pass/fail result or may establish a different passing score for their own jurisdictions.
200	This score is determined by your overall performance on the examination. The score scale is based on the performance of students in medical schools accredited by the Liaison Committee on Medical Education (LCME) who took the NBME comprehensive Part II examination for the first time in September 1991 and were in their final year of medical school at the time they were tested. The scale was defined to have a mean of 200 and a standard deviation of 20 for this group. Most examinees receive a score between 140 and 260. A score of 167 is set by USMLE to pass Step 2. The standard error of measurement (SEM)⁺ for this scale is five points.
82	This score is also determined by your overall performance on the examination. A score of 82 on this scale is equivalent to a score of 200 on the scale described above. A score of 75 on this scale, which is equivalent to a score of 167 on the scale described above, is set by USMLE to pass Step 2. The SEM⁺ for this scale is one point.

⁺Your score is influenced by both your general understanding of clinical science and the specific set of items selected for this Step 2 examination. The SEM provides an estimate of the range within which your scores might be expected to vary by chance if you were tested repeatedly using similar tests.

279LD429

Fig. 1.   Sample score report

INFORMATION PROVIDED FOR EXAMINEE USE ONLY

The Performance Profiles below are provided solely for the benefit of the examinee.
The USMLE will not provide or verify the Performance Profiles for any other person, organization, or agency.

USMLE STEP 2 PERFORMANCE PROFILES

PHYSICIAN TASK PROFILE	Lower Performance	Borderline Performance	Higher Performance
Health & Health Maintenance			XXXXXXXXXXX
Understanding Mechanisms of Disease		XXXXXXXXX	
Diagnosis			XXXXXXX
Principles of Management	XXXXXXXXXXXX		

ICD-9 DISEASE PROCESS PROFILE

	Lower Performance	Borderline Performance	Higher Performance
Normal Growth & Development; Principles of Care			XXXXXX*
Infectious & Parasitic Diseases			XXXXXXXXXXX
Neoplasms		XXXXXXXXXXXXX	
Immunologic Disorders			XXXXXXXXXXXXXXXX
Diseases of Blood & Blood Forming Organs		XXXXXXXXXXXXX	
Mental Disorders			XXXXXXXXXXXXX
Diseases of the Nervous System & Special Senses		XXXXXXXXXXX	
Cardiovascular Disorders	XXXXXXXXXXX		
Diseases of the Respiratory System	XXXXXXXXXXXXX		
Nutritional & Digestive Disorders			XXXXXXXXXXXXX
Gynecologic Disorders			XXXXXXXX*
Renal, Urinary & Male Reproductive Systems		XXXXXXXXXXXXXXX	
Disorders of Pregnancy, Childbirth & Puerperium		XXXXXXXXXXXXXXX	
Musculoskeletal, Skin & Connective Tissue Diseases			XXXXXXXXXXXXX
Endocrine & Metabolic Disorders		XXXXXXXXXXXXX	
Injury & Poisoning	XXXXXXXXXXXXXXXX		

DISCIPLINE PROFILE

	Lower Performance	Borderline Performance	Higher Performance
Medicine			XXXXXXX
Obstetrics & Gynecology			XXXXXXXXXXX
Pediatrics		XXXXXXXXXXX	
Preventive Medicine & Public Health			XXXXXXXXX
Psychiatry			XXXXXXXXXXX
Surgery		XXXXXXX	

The above Performance Profiles are provided to aid in self-assessment. The shaded area defines a borderline level of performance for each content area; borderline performance is comparable to a HIGH FAIL/LOW PASS on the total test.

Performance bands indicate areas of relative strength and weakness. Some bands are wider than others. The width of a performance band reflects the precision of measurement: narrower bands indicate greater precision. The band width for a given content area is the same for all examinees. An asterisk indicates that your performance band extends beyond the displayed portion of the scale.

Additional information concerning the topics covered in each content area can be found in the *USMLE Step 2 General Instructions, Content Description, and Sample Items.*

(94/95)

293JC155

With questions like these, it is vital that you do not allow the large number of choices to confuse you. Read all the choices before you make your selection. Also, remember that each answer may be used *once, more than once,* or *not at all.* In the above example, the answer to both #1 and #3 is (C) Epstein-Barr virus. We recommend that you do not cross out options after you use them to answer earlier questions. If there is a large number of options, the USMLE suggests that you try to generate your own diagnosis and then look for that answer on the option list.

Matching Sets with Multiple Answers

Matching sets with multiple answers require you to choose multiple answers for each case. An example is provided below:

(A) Iron   *(D) Fluoride*   *(G) Magnesium*
(B) Vitamin A *(E) Zinc*   *(H) Vitamin B$_{12}$*
(C) Thiamine   *(F) Vitamin D*   *(I) Folate*

1. *A 54-year-old homeless man is brought to the emergency room after a fall. His nutritional history is unclear. Lab studies reveal macrocytic anemia with low ferritin levels. (SELECT 4 SUPPLEMENTS)*
2. *A mother brings her 6-month-old male infant in for a well-baby checkup. She has been breast-feeding him since birth. His weight is in the 45th percentile for his age. (SELECT 2 SUPPLEMENTS)*

(1- A, C, H, I; 2-A, D)

Again, remember that you may use some of the answers more than once. This type of question is often used for **vitamins, drugs, diagnostic tests,** and **preventive health measures.** Always make sure that you choose the exact number of answers specified. This number will vary from question to question. You will receive credit for each correct answer. **However, if you mark more than the specified number of answers, the entire question will automatically be marked wrong.**

Pictures

Multiple-choice questions are occasionally accompanied by photos or diagrams. These are extremely difficult to predict, and many can be answered solely on the basis of the information provided in the text of the question. While we don't recommend concentrated study of the entire field of pathology, you may want to review x-rays, electrocardiograms (ECGs), fetal heart tracings, and classic physical exam findings.

Use of USMLE Scores for Resident Selection

Although the NBME has stated that the Step 2 exam is not designed for use in resident selection and may not be accurate in predicting future performance, many residency programs ignore this advice. Some programs use Step 2 scores to screen and select applicants.

Very Important		**Not Very Important**
Anesthesiology	Internal medicine	Family practice
Obstetrics/gynecology	Emergency medicine	Psychiatry
Orthopedics	Pediatrics	Pathology
Ophthalmology		
Radiology		
Surgery		

Fig. 2.   Residency programs and Step 2 score importance

Since letters of recommendation and clerkship evaluations vary so much from school to school, some programs use Step 2 scores as a nationally standardized way to evaluate the performance of each applicant. Certain specialties even require that the Step 2 exam be taken in the fall, so that they will receive the scores in time to use them as a part of your application. Residency requirements vary, so it is important to identify the requirements of programs that interest you before it is too late to register for the exam.

After reviewing the literature on resident selection and talking to other students, we have come up with a list of residencies that may find Step 2 scores important (Fig. 2). All programs differ, so take this information with a grain of salt. At the end of this chapter, we have included a bibliography of current articles on resident selection in various specialties. We suggest that you check out a couple in your favorite field—it might give you some tips that will help you during your interviews and in your application.

One book with more information about residency applications is called *Getting into a Residency: A Guide for Medical Students* by Kenneth V. Iserson (Galen Press). It describes the application process in great detail and contains lots of tips for success.

Studying for the Exam

Different students have different goals, so the amount of time students spend studying for the exam varies. An informal study of students at two top West Coast schools showed that the average time spent studying for the Step 2 was about 28 hours at one school and 62 hours at the other. The range of reported study time at both schools was quite wide—from taking it cold with no preparation (what confidence!) to about 180 hours of study time.

Obviously, the "right" amount of time to study depends on your experience, strengths, confidence, and goals. After you have registered for the Step 2, try to anticipate how much time you are willing to commit to studying. Students spend about half of their time in "leisurely study" of a few hours per week in the months before the exam. An "intense" period of study begins during the week before the exam. Think about how much time you want to spend in each of these study categories.

Our Advice

After talking to more than 100 medical students, we have put together some suggestions and tips for studying for the Step 2 exam. Here are our collective recommendations for Step 2 examinees:

- **Use the USMLE sample items.** The USMLE provides a group of 100 questions that are similar to those used on the Step 2 and may even be taken from previous administrations of the test. The questions are found with the USMLE Step 2 registration material in a booklet titled "Step 2 General Instructions, Content Description, and Sample Items." Most students agree that using these questions is the single most important way to prepare for the actual exam. Some students take the sample exam before they begin studying in order to reveal areas of weakness, while others prefer to use it toward the end to simulate the exam and establish pacing. Either way, you'll get a feel for the content, style, and speed of the test.

- **Find review books that suit your style and goals.** At the end of this chapter, we've provided the comments from fourth-year medical students about the different study books currently available. Some review books are only sample questions and explanations, others provide an overview of a topic, and still others combine the two methods. Browse through the reviews and pick the ones that sound best. But keep in mind how much time you're willing to spend studying—you don't want to waste your time and money with too many books. Review books are here to help you, not to stress you!

- **Use old notes and syllabi.** Remember studying for that killer surgery exam? Or the notes you took in OB/GYN? Dig them out and use them! Most of the students we talked to used old notes and syllabi from clinical rotations and preclinical courses. These notes have the advantage of being familiar in organization and style, which may help with memorization. If you study from old notes, be sure to use the study guideline that accompanies the Step 2 registration packet to find any topics that were overlooked in your particular syllabus. Also, avoid spending too much time on topics overemphasized by a particular instructor relative to their true medical importance.

- **Refer to more complete texts when you need detailed information.** Since all students have different experiences, interests, and weaknesses, there will be times when the overview you read in a review book is not enough for you to master a topic. Many students found it helpful to keep a "big" text, such as Harrison's or Cecil's, and a medical dictionary close at hand.

- **Don't forget to study obstetrics and gynecology, pediatrics, and surgery.** Many students make the mistaken assumption that medicine will be the predominant topic on the exam, with only a little OB/GYN, pediatrics, and other subjects mixed in. There is a large amount of material from the other fields on the exam, so make sure that you don't give them short shrift and get caught unprepared on exam day.

- **Use other helpful (and older) resources.** A number of students used some of their Step 1 books, particularly microbiology and pharmacology review books, to refamiliarize themselves with the bugs and drugs. Also, some students recommend reviewing clinical pocket handbooks (such as *The Washington Manual* or those by Ferry or Gomella). Pocket handbooks are particularly helpful in studying for the "variable" format questions by helping you remember the variety of conditions that display a particular abnormality.

- **Consider getting a few subject-specific books.** Depending on how much time you plan to spend studying, you may want to invest in a couple of the subject-specific review books for areas in which you are weakest. If it has been almost 2 years since your psychiatry rotation (or if you have no idea what public health and preventive medicine are), consider buying or borrowing books that are more thorough in these areas.
- **Study the special topics.** Other areas that students have recommended for extra attention include adult preventive health, immunization schedules, and cancer screening protocols. Also, remember to study for all the different types of questions.

Book Reviews

The following book reviews were compiled from surveys of and conversations with more than 100 medical students. We have based our ratings on a five-star scale as follows:

★★★★★   Excellent!
★★★★   Very good
★★★   Good
★★   Fair
★   Don't waste your money!

We have also provided information about the type of book (study questions, text, or both) as well as an estimate of how long it takes to get through the book. Of course, this amount of time varies greatly from student to student. The number of days provided is based on an 8-hour study day. If you can study 14 hours at a stretch, you'll be done much quicker! But if you spend fewer hours a day studying or if you tend to go through books more slowly or thoroughly than your classmates, adjust your time estimate accordingly.

We value your opinion about any of these books, as well as any suggestions you may have for books that we have missed. Please write to us on the evaluation form included at the end of this book. We would like to hear from you!

Multidisciplinary Books

National Medical Series Review for the USMLE Step 2   ★★★★

Number of days needed: 3

This book contains four sample exams, consisting of a total of 800 questions that simulate the Step 2 exam. The questions vary by subject from question to question, much as the actual exam does. The answers are given as letter answers with explanations that discuss the answers and relevant issues.

Rx: Although relatively few students were able to get a copy of this book, the general consensus was that the questions are very good and much more appropriate than the book by Catlin (see below) when compared to the actual exam. Many students liked the explained answers and felt that using this book was a very good practice and pacing tool. A few students noted some errors, but this book was considered to be very helpful overall.

Publisher: Williams & Wilkins
Publication type: Questions only
329 pages
Diagrams/Pictures: Few

ISBN: 0-683-06207-7
Year of publication: 1994
Cost: $26.95

Appleton and Lange's Review for the USMLE Step 2 *by Catlin*

★★★

Number of days needed: 5

This book consists of more than 1,200 exam-type questions divided by subject, with a comprehensive exam at the end of the book. The answers are given as letter answers with explanations that briefly discuss the topic in question.

Rₓ: Most students liked the fact that this book had hundreds of sample test questions with explained answers. However, the overall consensus was that the questions were much too difficult and picky when compared to the actual exam. Many students thought that this test review sapped confidence and was basically a waste of time. Nonetheless, some students felt that review of the explained answers was helpful and that taking sample tests was a good way to break up the monotony of studying. A number of students noted that the preventive medicine section and the surgery section were especially poor and not representative of the actual exam.

Publisher: Appleton & Lange
Publication type: Questions only
286 pages
Diagrams/Pictures: Few

ISBN: 0-8385-0226-1
Year of publication: 1993
Cost: $34.95

Appleton and Lange's Instant Review for the Step 2 *by Goldberg*

★★

Number of days needed: 6

This book is an elaboration of all topics listed in the USMLE Step 2 content outline, broken down by organ system and by diagnosis and treatment. The book has no sample test questions or explanatory diagrams.

Rₓ: Most students were pretty disappointed with this book. Although some students liked the outline format, most agreed that this book was too boring, was not detailed enough, and contained a number of errors. Students said they generally found it difficult to retain the information in this book for any length of time. As one student said, "Sketchy in some areas, overly detailed in others. I fell asleep after reading this for 5 minutes."

Publisher: Appleton & Lange
Publication type: Text only
363 pages
Diagrams/Pictures: None

ISBN: 0-8385-4038-4
Year of publication: 1993
Cost: $31.95

Clinical Science by Bollett ★★

Number of days needed: 5

This book consists of sections subdivided by specialty (e.g., medicine, pediatrics, surgery, etc.) in a narrative style, with questions at the end of each chapter. The answers provided are letter answers only.

R_x: Few students used this book. The general complaint was that it was too long and wordy. Also, some students noted that the questions often had nothing to do with the text in the chapter and had letter answers only. The book is also quite outdated (the author sometimes still refers to HIV as HTLV!). However, a few students felt that this was a kinder, gentler way to get into studying very early on.

Publisher: Year Book
Publication type: Text and questions
395 page
Diagrams/Pictures: Few

ISBN: 0-8151-1022-7
Year of publication: 1988
Cost: $36.95

National Board Exam Review Part 2 by Pieroni ★★

Number of days needed: 3

This book consists of 900 questions with explained answers and is divided by subject.

R_x: Not many students used this book. In general, its questions seemed too narrow in focus as well as outdated in format and style. However, many of the questions reflect content that is tested on the Step 2.

Publisher: Appleton & Lange
Publication type: Questions only
340 pages
Diagrams/Pictures: Many

ISBN: 0-8385-6656-1
Year of publication: 1988
Cost: $39

Preparation for the USMLE Step 2 Clinical Sciences Booklets by Maval ★★

Number of days needed: 1 per booklet

This series of booklets contains sample Step 2 questions in USMLE format. Explained answers are provided. These booklets also offer the option of mailing in your score sheet and receiving a "National Tentative Score" after 8–12 weeks. Book 6 is a double-sized booklet.

R_x: Of all sample Step 2 questions, these questions are most like "the real thing" in design, including clinical questions and radiographs. However, some of the questions are too difficult, and there are some typographical errors. The "National Tentative Score" simply compares your performance with other students who have mailed in answer sheets and is not very useful in assessing performance.

Publisher: Maval USA
Publication type: Questions only
75 pages per booklet
Diagrams/Pictures: Many

ISBN: None
Year of publication: 1995
Cost: $15–25

Rypin's Clinical Science Review *by Frolich* ★★

Number of days needed: 5

This book consists of sections subdivided by specialty (i.e., medicine, pediatrics, surgery, etc.) in a narrative style, with questions at the end of each chapter. The answers provided are letter answers only.

Rx: Generally, students did not find this book to be helpful. Students found it too long, too boring, and often too basic in its information. Many students felt that the questions were quite poor and that having letter answers only was not helpful. In general, very few students recommended buying this book.

Publisher: Lippincott
Publication type: Text and questions
415 pages
Diagrams/Pictures: None

ISBN: 0-397-51246-5
Year of publication: 1993
Cost: $37.95

Step 2 USMLE Simulated Exam *by Pretest* ★

Number of days needed: 1

This booklet contains three sets of "simulated exams" of 140 questions each. Brief explanations of the answers are included.

Rx: In general, these questions are too simple when compared to the actual exam. There are also a number of typographical errors. This book is not very useful, except as a confidence builder.

Publisher: McGraw-Hill
Publication type: Questions only
150 pages
Diagrams/Pictures: None

ISBN: 0-07-064521-3
Year of publication: 1993
Cost: $30

Medicine

Medicine *by Pretest* ★★★★

Number of days needed: 1–2

This book consists of sample Step 2 test medicine questions divided by organ system. A detailed and lengthy explanation follows each question.

Rx: The questions in this book are well-written. They appear to be targeted to the appropriate knowledge level, and many are case-based. This book is excellent for self-testing but may not be sufficient as a sole source of study if you are not strong in medicine topics.

Publisher: McGraw-Hill
Publication type: Questions only
260 pages
Diagrams/Pictures: Few

ISBN: 0-07-051989-7
Year of publication: 1994
Cost: $16.95

Medicine by *National Medical Series* ★★★

Number of days needed: 7

   This text consists of detailed outlines of each organ system and related pathology. Each chapter is followed by a few multiple-choice questions with letter answers. A short sample exam with explained answers is included at the end of the book.

   Rx: This book is well written, but it is too long for the usual Step 2 boards study schedule. If you have enough time or have used this book during clinical rotations, however, you may find it a helpful tool in getting all the concepts of medicine down clearly.

Publisher: Williams & Wilkins
Publication type: Text only
600 pages
Diagrams/Pictures: Few

ISBN: 0-683-06233-6
Year of publication: 1994
Cost: $27.00

Medical Exam Review Medicine by *Baker* ★★

Number of days needed: 2

   This text consists of 700 sample Step 2 questions with explained answers. The questions are divided by organ system, and there are a number of radiographs and diagrams.

   Rx: Few students we surveyed have used this text. The questions appear to be old-style, non–case-based questions that are no longer present on the Step 2. Also, the questions are at times too detail-oriented. However, the content of the questions appears similar to that of the Step 2.

Publisher: Appleton & Lange
Publication type: Questions only
250 pages
Diagrams/Pictures: Many

ISBN: 0-8385-5771-6
Year of publication: 1991
Cost: $19.95

Medical Secrets by *Zollo* ★★

Number of days needed: 6

   This text consists of clinical questions with lengthy answers, divided by organ system. The questions are not multiple-choice and are not in typical Step 2 format.

   Rx: This book focuses on the types of questions that are asked on rounds rather than on those following the Step 2 outline. Consequently, coverage is very sporadic, and some important topics are addressed only briefly. However, the book contains some well-done tables that are full of memorizable facts.

Publisher: Mosby-Year Book
Publication type: Questions only
550 pages
Diagrams/Pictures: Many

ISBN: 1-56053-011-1
Year of publication: 1991
Cost: $34.95

Internal Medicine by Oklahoma Notes ★

Number of days needed: 3

This book consists of an outline of all medicine topics divided by organ system. Sample questions are provided, with letter answers only.

Rx: Almost no one we surveyed recommends this book. The outlines provided are somewhat boring and difficult to read. They are also overly detailed in some areas and weak in others.

Publisher: Springer-Verlag
Publication type: Text with questions
240 pages
Diagrams/Pictures: None

ISBN: 0-387-97960-3
Year of publication: 1993
Cost: $16.95

Surgery

Surgery by Metzler ★★★

Number of days needed: 2

This book consists of 700 questions with explained answers. The questions are case-based and appear to reflect the content of the Step 2 exam.

Rx: This book has been recently updated, and seems to have been revised well. All in all, this book is a good buy for the money. However, it may not be sufficient as a sole study source if you are weak on surgery topics.

Publisher: Appleton & Lange
Publication type: Questions only
315 pages
Diagrams/Pictures: Few

ISBN: 0-8385-6195-0
Year of publication: 1995
Cost: $19.50

Surgery by Pretest ★★★

Number of days needed: 2–3

This book consists of 500 sample Step 2 surgery questions divided by subtopic. A detailed and lengthy explanation follows each question and includes references to major surgical textbooks.

Rx: The questions in this book are generally at Step 2 level and include some case-based questions. If you have the time and desire to do many sample surgery questions, this is the book for you.

Publisher: McGraw-Hill
Publication type: Questions only
324 pages
Diagrams/Pictures: Few

ISBN: 0-07-051987-0
Year of publication: 1992
Cost: $16.95

General Surgery *by Oklahoma Notes*   ★★

Number of days needed: 1–2

    This book contains an outline of most major surgery topics. There are no sample questions.

    R$_x$: This book is fairly easy to read (because it's printed in very big type) but is overly detailed in some areas and scant in others. Also, the style is pretty boring. Not completely horrible, but almost!

Publisher: Springer-Verlag	ISBN: 0-387-97958-1
Publication type: Text with questions	Year of publication: 1993
240 pages	Cost: $15.95
Diagrams/Pictures: None	

Surgery *by National Medical Series*   ★★

Number of days needed: 7

    This text consists of detailed outlines of each organ system in terms of surgical interventions. Each chapter is followed by a few multiple-choice questions and letter answers. A short sample exam with explained answers is included at the end of the book.

    R$_x$: This book is extremely thorough but also extremely long considering the subject. This test preparation is a good choice for those looking for a detailed, comprehensive text and have the time to use it.

Publisher: Williams & Wilkins	ISBN: 0-683-06270-0
Publication type: Text with questions	Year of publication: 1991
570 pages	Cost: $30
Diagrams/Pictures: Few	

Surgical Secrets *by Abernathy*   ★★

Number of days needed: 2–3

    This text consists of clinical questions with detailed answers, divided by subtopic. The questions are not multiple-choice and are not in typical Step 2 format.

    R$_x$: This book received high marks for its clinical usefulness, but it is not as good for Step 2 study. Many of the basic surgical presentations are not described; however, the book contains some good tables. It may be useful as a reference text for selected subjects but is not recommended as a sole study source.

Publisher: Mosby-Year Book	ISBN: 1-56053-013-8
Publication type: Questions only	Year of publication: 1991
330 pages	Cost: $32.95
Diagrams/Pictures: Few	

Review of Surgery *by Wapnick* ★

Number of days needed: 1

This book consists of less than 100 questions divided by subtopic. Explained answers are included.

Rx: We do not recommend this book! It is overpriced and outdated, with many old-style, K-type questions that are no longer used on the boards. Also, the questions are very picky and detailed.

Publisher: Appleton & Lange
Publication type: Questions only
150 pages
Diagrams/Pictures: None

ISBN: 0-8385-0220-2
Year of publication: 1989
Cost: $25.95

Obstetrics/Gynecology

Obstetrics & Gynecology *by Julian* ★★★

Number of days needed: 4

This book contains hundreds of sample Step 2 OB/GYN questions and explained answers, divided by subtopic. Many questions are case-based.

Rx: The updated format is very good, and the range of different subtopics is excellent. However, some of the questions may be too detailed. Also, this book is rather lengthy for general Step 2 study, unless you have the time and desire to do many OB/GYN questions.

Publisher: Appleton & Lange
Publication type: Questions only
395 pages
Diagrams/Pictures: Few

ISBN: 0-8385-0231-8
Year of publication: 1995
Cost: $29.95

Obstetrics & Gynecology *by National Medical Series* ★★★

Number of days needed: 7

This text consists of detailed outlines of all obstetrics and gynecologic topics. Each chapter is followed by a few multiple-choice questions. A short sample exam with explained answers is included at the end of the book. About half of the questions are case-based.

Rx: This book is extremely thorough but also extremely long, given the topic. It may still be a good choice for those who are looking for a detailed, comprehensive text and have the time to use it. It may also be useful during your OB/GYN rotation.

Publisher: Williams & Wilkins
Publication type: Text with questions
485 pages
Diagrams/Pictures: Few

ISBN: 0-683-06241-7
Year of publication: 1993
Cost: $27

Ob-Gyn Secrets *by Fredrickson* ★★

Number of days needed: 3

This text consists of clinical questions and explained answers, divided by subtopic. The questions are not multiple-choice and are not in typical Step 2 format.

R_x: This book focuses on the types of questions asked on rounds rather than following the Step 2 outline. As a consequence, coverage is very sporadic, and some important topics are addressed only briefly. However, the book contains some well-done tables that are full of memorizable facts. This text may be useful as a secondary resource.

Publisher: Mosby-Year Book
Publication type: Questions only
308 pages
Diagrams/Pictures: Many

ISBN: 0-932883-95-8
Year of publication: 1991
Cost: $31.95

Obstetrics & Gynecology *by Oklahoma Notes* ★★

Number of days needed: 2

This book contains an outline of most major OB/GYN topics. There are some sample questions, with letter answers only.

R_x: This book is fairly easy to read because of its large font, but it is pretty boring. It is also overly detailed in some areas and scant in others. There are a few useful tables, though.

Publisher: Springer-Verlag
Publication type: Text with questions
225 pages
Diagrams/Pictures: Few

ISBN: 0-387-94184-3
Year of publication: 1994
Cost: $16.95

Obstetrics and Gynecology *by Pretest* ★★

Number of days needed: 1–2

This book consists of 500 sample Step 2 OB/GYN questions divided by subtopic. A detailed and lengthy explanation follows each question and includes references to major textbooks.

R_x: The questions in this book seem much too picky when compared to the actual Step 2 exam. Also, there are a number of old-style, K-type questions. You may nevertheless derive some benefit from reading the answers.

Publisher: McGraw-Hill
Publication type: Questions only
230 pages
Diagrams/Pictures: Many

ISBN: 0-07-051988-9
Year of publication: 1992
Cost: $16.95

Clinical Obstetrics and Gynecology by Pretest   ★

Number of days needed: 2

This book contains more than 500 sample Step 2 OB/GYN questions divided by subtopic. Each question is accompanied by a detailed explanation and includes references to major textbooks.

R$_x$: The questions in this book are too picky when compared with the actual Step 2 exam. Also, there are few case-based questions and some old-style, K-type questions. This book is very overpriced for the number and quality of test questions.

Publisher: McGraw-Hill
Publication type: Questions only
135 pages
Diagrams/Pictures: None

ISBN: 0-07-051982-X
Year of publication: 1991
Cost: $39.95

Pediatrics

Pediatrics by Pretest   ★★★★

Number of days needed: 2

This book consists of 500 sample Step 2 pediatrics questions divided by subtopic. A detailed and lengthy explanation follows each question and includes references to major pediatric textbooks.

R$_x$: This book is a very good buy! It has been recently updated, includes many case-based questions appropriate for the Step 2, and may be very helpful considering the surprisingly large number of pediatrics questions that are usually on the exam.

Publisher: McGraw-Hill
Publication type: Questions only
250 pages
Diagrams/Pictures: Few

ISBN: 0-07-052027-5
Year of publication: 1995
Cost: $16.95

Medical Exam Review Pediatrics by Hansbarger   ★★★

Number of days needed: 2

This book contains 700 questions with explained answers, divided by subtopic. Most questions are case-based.

R$_x$: The recent revision of this text has made it fairly appropriate to the content of the Step 2. There are a good number of questions for the money.

Publisher: Appleton & Lange
Publication type: Questions only
245 pages
Diagrams/Pictures: None

ISBN: 0-8385-6223-X
Year of publication: 1995
Cost: $19.50

Pediatrics *by National Medical Series* ★★★

Number of days needed: 6–7

This text consists of detailed outlines of all pediatric topics. Questions with explained answers are included.

R$_X$: This book is extremely detailed and long, considering the subject. However, the information provided is of high quality. This text is useful if you have the time and desire to spend a week on pediatrics.

Publisher: Williams & Wilkins
Publication type: Text with questions
550 pages
Diagrams/Pictures: Few

ISBN: 0-683-06246-8
Year of publication: 1992
Cost: $27

Pediatrics *by Lorin* ★★

Number of days needed: 3

This book consists of more than 1,000 questions on pediatric topics with explained answers. Many of the questions are case-based.

R$_X$: These questions are a bit too narrow in focus when compared to the questions on the actual exam. The book is also somewhat overpriced.

Publisher: Appleton & Lange
Publication type: Questions only
220 pages
Diagrams/Pictures: None

ISBN: 0-8385-0057-9
Year of publication: 1993
Cost: $30

Pediatrics *by Oklahoma Notes* ★★

Number of days needed: 1

This book contains an outline of all major pediatric topics. There are no sample questions.

R$_X$: While the text is fairly easy to read, the style is somewhat boring. However, the authors include some interesting mnemonics and many useful tables. In general, this book is slightly better than others in the Oklahoma Notes series.

Publisher: Springer-Verlag
Publication type: Text only
250 pages
Diagrams/Pictures: None

ISBN: 0-387-97779-1
Year of publication: 1993
Cost: $16.95

Pediatric Secrets by Polin ★★

Number of days needed: 5

This text consists of clinical questions and lengthy answers, divided by organ system. The questions are not multiple choice and are not in typical Step 2 format.

R$_x$: This book focuses on the types of questions asked on rounds rather than those following the Step 2 outline. As a consequence, coverage is very sporadic. Also, this text may be too lengthy for Step 2 exam review.

Publisher: Mosby-Year Book
Publication type: Questions only
447 pages
Diagrams/Pictures: Few

ISBN: 0-932883-14-1
Year of publication: 1989
Cost: $32.95

Psychiatry

Psychiatry by Chan ★★★

Number of days needed: 2

This book contains 700 questions and explained answers, divided by subtopic. Few questions are case-based.

R$_x$: This book has been recently updated, and the content seems appropriately targeted to the Step 2 exam, although there are not very many case-based questions. This is a good, compact set of questions if you are confident in your knowledge of psychiatry.

Publisher: Appleton & Lange
Publication type: Questions only
255 pages
Diagrams/Pictures: None

ISBN: 0-8385-5780-5
Year of publication: 1995
Cost: $19.50

Psychiatry by Pretest ★★★

Number of days needed: 1–2

This book consists of 500 sample Step 2 psychiatry questions divided by subtopic. Each question is accompanied by a detailed and lengthy explanation and includes references to major psychiatric textbooks. The text has been recently updated to correspond to the newly released *Diagnostic and Statistical Manual of Mental Disorders, Fourth Edition* (DSM-IV).

R$_x$: The questions in this book are fairly applicable, including some case-based questions. However, there are probably more theoretical questions than are appropriate for the Step 2.

Publisher: McGraw-Hill
Publication type: Questions only
205 pages
Diagrams/Pictures: None

ISBN: 0-07-052064-X
Year of publication: 1995
Cost: $16.95

Review of General Psychiatry *by Goldman* ★★★

Number of days needed: 6

This book is a review text of psychiatry with no sample questions. It has been updated for the newly released DSM-IV.

R$_x$: This is a very readable, nicely designed text. Its recent revision makes it even more appealing. However, it is probably a bit too long and detailed for Step 2 studying.

Publisher: Appleton & Lange
Publication type: Text only
530 pages
Diagrams/Pictures: Few

ISBN : 0-8385-8421-7
Year of publication: 1995
Cost: $37.95

Psychiatry *by National Medical Series* ★★

Number of days needed: 4

This text consists of detailed outlines of all psychiatric topics. Questions and explained answers are included.

R$_x$: Finally, an NMS book with fewer than 350 pages! It nevertheless is a very detailed and comprehensive text. Considering the amount and level of psychiatry questions on the Step 2, this text is probably useful only to students with a great deal of time and a desire to spend 4 days studying psychiatry.

Publisher: Williams & Wilkins
Publication type: Text and questions
330 pages
Diagrams/Pictures: None

ISBN: 0-683-06264-6
Year of publication: 1990
Cost: $30

Psychiatry *by Oklahoma Notes* ★★

Number of days needed: 2

This book contains an outline of most major psychiatry topics. There are no sample questions.

R$_x$: While fairly easy to read, this book is overly detailed in some areas and scant in others. Its writing style is pretty boring. Not completely horrible, but almost!

Publisher: Springer-Verlag
Publication type: Text only
188 pages
Diagrams/Pictures: None

ISBN: 0-387-97957-3
Year of publication: 1993
Cost: $16.95

Public Health and Preventive Medicine

Preventive Medicine and Public Health
by National Medical Series   ★★

Number of days needed: 7

This detailed text outlines all important public heath and preventive medicine topics. It includes sample questions with explained answers, consisting of a mix of case-based questions and old-style, K-type questions.

R$_x$: This is a very long and detailed book that is not appropriate for normal Step 2 study, considering the few number of questions on these topics. However, it does include graphs and diagrams that may be helpful, since similar questions appear on the exam. If you are planning to do extensive study or specialization in public health or preventive medicine, this book is for you.

Publisher: Williams & Wilkins   ISBN : 0-683-06262-X
Publication type: Text with questions   Year of publication: 1992
500 pages   Cost: $25
Diagrams/Pictures: Few

Preventive Medicine and Public Health *by Pretest*   ★★

Number of days needed: 1–2

This book consists of 500 sample Step 2 public health and preventive medicine questions divided by topic. Each question is accompanied by a detailed and lengthy explanation and includes references to major textbooks.

R$_x$: The questions in this book seem too focused on details when compared to the actual Step 2 exam, and the coverage of important topics is variable. However, you may derive some benefit from reading the explained answers.

Publisher: McGraw-Hill   ISBN: 0-07-051990-0
Publication type: Questions only   Year of publication: 1992
210 pages   Cost: $16.95
Diagrams/Pictures: None

Articles about Residency Programs and Resident Selection

General Articles about Step 2 Scores

Hoffman KI. The USMLE, the NBME subject examinations, and assessment of individual academic achievement. *Acad Med* 68:740–747, 1993.

Nungester RJ. Score reporting on NBME examinations. *Acad Med* 65: 723–729, 1990.

Williams RG. Use of the NBME and USMLE examinations to evaluate medical education programs. *Acad Med* 10:748–752, 1993.

General Articles about Residency Selection

Colquitt WL. Specialty selection and success in obtaining choice of residency training among 1987 U.S. medical graduates by race-ethnicity and gender. *Acad Med* 67:660–671, 1992.

Friedman CP et al. Predictive validity of a house-officer selection process at one medical school. *Acad Med* 66:471–478, 1991.

Simmonds AC. Factors important to students in selecting a residency program. *Acad Med* 65:640–643, 1990.

Spooner CE. Help for the gatekeepers: Comment and summation on the admission process. *Acad Med* 65:183–187, 1990.

Wagoner NE. Recommendations for changing the residency selection process based on a survey of program directors. *Acad Med* 67:459–465, 1992.

Zagumny MJ. Comparing medical students' and residency directors' ratings of criteria used to select residents [letter]. *Acad Med* 67:613, 1992.

Anesthesiology

Baker JD et al. Selection of anesthesiology residents. *Acad Med* 69:161–163, 1993.

Lebovits A et al. The selection of a residency program: Prospective anesthesiologists compared to others. *Anesth Analg* 77:313–317, 1993.

Dermatology

Case SM, Swanson DB. Validity of the NBME part I and II scores for selection of residents in orthopaedic surgery, dermatology, and preventive medicine. *Acad Med* 68(Supp):S51–S56, 1993.

Lessin SR. Dermatology's resident match: It's time for a change [letter]. *Arch Dermatol* 129:1056–1057, 1993.

Emergency Medicine

Aghababian R. Selection of emergency medicine residents. *Ann Emerg Med* 22:1753–1761, 1993.

Family Practice

Galazka SS. Methods of recruiting and selecting residents for U.S. family practice residents. *Acad Med* 69:304–306, 1994.

Internal Medicine

Gayed NM. Residency directors' assessments of which selection criteria best predict the performances of foreign-born foreign medical graduates during internal medicine residencies. *Acad Med* 66:699–701, 1991.

Potts JT. Recruitment of minority physicians into careers in internal medicine. *Ann Intern Med* 116:1099–1102, 1992.

Preventive Medicine

Case SM, Swanson DB. Validity of the NBME part I and II scores for selection of residents in orthopaedic surgery, dermatology, and preventive medicine. *Acad Med* 68(Supp):S51–S56, 1993.

Radiology

Grantham JR. Radiology resident selection: Results of a survey. *Invest Radiol* 28:99–101, 1993.
O'Halloran CM. Evaluation of resident applicants by letters of recommendation: A comparison of traditional and behavior-based formats. *Invest Radiol* 28:274–277, 1993.

Surgery and Surgical Subspecialties

Calhoun KH et al. The resident selection process in otolaryngology-head and neck surgery. *Arch Otolaryngol Head Neck Surg* 116:1041–1043, 1990.
Case SM, Swanson DB. Validity of the NBME part I and II scores for selection of residents in orthopaedic surgery, dermatology, and preventive medicine. *Acad Med* 68(Supp):S51–S56, 1993.
DaRosa DA. Evaluation of a system designed to enhance the resident selection process. *Surgery* 109:715–721, 1991.
Sheldon GF. Recruitment and selection of the "best and the brightest." *Ann Thorac Surg* 55:1340–1344, 1993.

References

National Board of Medical Examiners: Report on 1995 Examinations. The National Board Examiner, Winter 1995.

Iserson K. *Getting into Residency*. Tuscon, AZ: Galen Press, 1993.

O'Donnell MJ, Obenshain SS, Erdmann JB. Background essential to the proper use of results of Step 1 and Step 2 of the USMLE. *Acad Med* 68:734–739, 1993.

National Board of Medical Examiners. 1995 *Step 2 General Instructions and Content Outline*. Philadelphia, 1995.

1

Gastroenterology

Nutritional Disorders

Obesity

Obesity is defined as body weight greater than 20% above the average weight for height, except in a very muscular person. Mild obesity is 20–40% overweight, moderate obesity is 41–100% overweight, and severe obesity is more than 100% overweight. Prevalence increases with age and is higher among black women and people of low socioeconomic status.

Obesity results from a caloric intake that is greater than expenditure, but the etiology of overeating varies. Body weight is regulated by some physiologic means, and change in the regulated level, or body weight "set point," leads to the increased intake. Many factors may contribute to the development of obesity, including genetics, social factors, metabolic and endocrine factors, psychiatric components, developmental factors, and physical activity.

Musculoskeletal complaints, irregular menstruation, sleep apnea, degenerative joint disease, and skin disorders are frequent results of obesity. Cardiovascular disease, hypertension, and diabetes are also common complications, and overall morbidity and mortality are higher in obese people. High thoracic and abdominal pressures may cause dyspnea, which is seen in the pickwickian syndrome of hypoventilation, CO_2 retention, and hypoxia. Obesity has a protective effect against osteoporosis.

The patient's body mass index (BMI) is elevated. The BMI is calculated by dividing body weight in kilograms by the height in meters squared (normal range 20–25 kg/m^2).

Weight reduction requires decreasing caloric intake and increasing energy expenditure. Behavior modification is usually necessary to maintain the weight loss. Surgery, which may be indicated for severe obesity, usually involves decreasing the patient's stomach capacity.

Anorexia Nervosa

Anorexia nervosa is a condition of extreme weight loss reulting from a severe disturbance in body image. The typical patient is a teen-age girl, often of higher socioeconomic status, who is intelligent and a perfectionist. This disorder may be mild, but it has a 10–20% mortality rate. Bulimia is a related disorder of binge eating followed by induced vomiting and laxative use.

The patient becomes increasingly cachectic and may have amenorrhea, bradycardia, low blood pressure, hypothermia, edema, and lanugo hair growth (fine hair covering the entire body, usually seen only in a fetus or premature infant). Patients remain active despite their wasted state. Depression and manipulative behavior are common. Ventricular arrhythmias can lead to sudden death. Dental decay may be present in bulimic patients due to the effects of gastric acid in the vomitus.

Loss of more than 15% of body weight in a thin patient who denies illness and has a fear of obesity.

Immediate short-term interventions (hospitalization and acute psychiatric care) are often critical to ensure the patient's safety; however, tube or intravenous (IV) feeds are rarely needed. Long-term psychiatric care and family counseling are often successful in treating this disorder.

Vitamin Deficiencies

In developed countries where a variety of foods is available, vitamin deficiencies generally result from chronic alcohol use, medication misuse, food faddism, or long-term parenteral nutrition. All are treated with vitamin replacement and maintenance.

Fat-Soluble Vitamins

- **Vitamin A** (retinol) is found in egg yolk, butter, cream, liver, and fish liver oil. It is also formed by the body from beta-carotene, which is found in yellow, orange, and leafy green vegetables. Vitamin A is a component of photoreceptor pigments in the retina and helps maintain normal epithelium. Deficiency results in **night blindness, conjunctival dryness,** and **corneal keratinization,** which may result in perforation. Other signs include dry skin and keratinization of lung, gastrointestinal (GI), and urinary epithelium. Severe deficiency predisposes to increased infections. Deficiency is noted only after liver stores are depleted.
- **Vitamin D** (calciferol) is found in yeast, fish liver oils, egg yolks, and supplemented dairy products; however, our major source of this vitamin is its formation in the skin with sun exposure. Vitamin D enhances calcium and phosphate absorption and helps maintain their appropriate levels in the blood. Vitamin D deficiency leads to **rickets** in children and **osteomalacia** in adults. X-rays show several characteristic deformities, including long-bone bowing in children and demineralization in adults.
- **Vitamin E** maintains cell membrane integrity by protecting lipids from oxidation. Vitamin E is found in vegetable oils, eggs, butter, and whole grains. Deficiency results from vitamin-insufficient infant formulas, protein-energy malnutrition, and some malabsorption syndromes with steatorrhea. **Red blood cell (RBC) hemolysis,** which may lead to anemia in infants, and **neurologic changes** are seen.
- **Vitamin K** is supplied by leafy green vegetables and is also produced by normal intestinal bacteria. It is a cofactor in the synthesis of clotting factors, so its deficiency results in **spontaneous bleeding** or prolonged oozing. Prothrombin time (PT) is increased more than partial thromboplastin time (PTT), although both may be affected. Injections of vitamin K may be given if rapid correction of the deficiency is needed.

Water-Soluble Vitamins

- **Thiamine** (vitamin B_1) contributes to carbohydrate metabolism as a coenzyme. It is found in grains, but it is removed in the production of highly polished rice. Certain conditions, including pregnancy and hyperthyroidism, increase the need for vitamin B_1 and can cause secondary deficiency. Deficiency is manifested as **beriberi**, classified as either "dry beriberi," with bilateral, symmetric peripheral neuropathy, or "wet beriberi," a cardiovascular disease of high-output heart failure. The **Wernicke-Korsakoff syndrome**, also called cerebral beriberi, results when chronic thiamine deficiency is exacerbated by acute deficiency. This condition is particularly common in alcoholics. Nystagmus, confusion, and confabulation may progress to coma and death.
- **Riboflavin** (B_2) is a component of the coenzymes flavin adenine dinucleotide (FAD) and flavin mononucleotide (FMN). Deficiency of riboflavin occurs with insufficient milk or animal protein consumption. **Cheilosis** (swollen, cracked, bright red lips) and **angular stomatitis** (fissuring at the angles of the mouth), as well as other cutaneous and ocular lesions may result.
- **Niacin** is a coenzyme in carbohydrate metabolism. Primary niacin deficiency occurs when maize (milled corn) is a diet staple, and secondary deficiency occurs with diarrhea, cirrhosis, alcoholism, and isoniazid (INH) use. Deficiency leads to **pellagra**, which is characterized by "the four Ds": diarrhea, dermatitis, dementia, and death. Symmetric cutaneous lesions, stomatitis, and glossitis (inflammation of the tongue) are typical.
- **Pyridoxine** (B_6) is active in blood, the central nervous system, and skin metabolism. It is found in many foods, so deficiency is rare but may occur due to malabsorption or increased metabolism. Manifestations include seborrheic dermatosis, peripheral neuropathy, lymphopenia, anemia, cheilosis, and glossitis. Infants may have seizures.
- **Cobalamin** (B_{12}) is important for DNA synthesis and myelin formation. It is found in meat, eggs, and milk. Once ingested, vitamin B_{12} binds to intrinsic factor from the parietal cells, and the complex is absorbed. Pernicious anemia, in which the destruction of parietal cells results in insufficient amounts of intrinsic factor, leads to vitamin B_{12} deficiency. **Megaloblastic anemia, neurologic disturbances**, and **ataxia** are the keys to diagnosis, which is confirmed by the Schilling test. Intramus-cular (IM) injections of vitamin B_{12} may be necessary.
- **Folate** is found in leafy green vegetables and citrus fruits and is used in DNA synthesis. Deficiency generally results from inadequate nutrition, seen often in the elderly, alcoholics, and the poor. **Megaloblastic anemia without neurologic changes** suggests this diagnosis.
- **Vitamin C** (ascorbic acid) is needed for the formation of collagen and the maintenance of connective tissue, bone, and teeth. Its deficiency, **scurvy**, is often due to dietary insufficiency and appears up to 1 year after the deficient state starts. Splinter hemorrhages, swollen and friable gums, myalgias, and hemarthralgias occur, followed by tooth loss, secondary infections, gangrene, and spontaneous hemorrhages.

Failure to Thrive

Organic failure to thrive (FTT) is a syndrome of poor weight gain in infants that occurs when known illnesses interfere with growth. **Nonorganic FTT** is a syndrome of growth failure due to neglect or stimulus deprivation, often considered the product of a poor "parent-child fit." Etiology may also be mixed, as in premature infants with poor growth. Weight change is a good indicator of undernutrition because it reflects a malnourished state more rapidly than height or head circumference changes do. Growth failure is usually evident by 6 months of age. Even when weight gain improves, cognitive and behavioral problems may persist.

Patients are less than 80% of their ideal weight for height. Infants often are hypervigilant and do not interact well with others.

Diet and weight are monitored carefully, but there is no diagnostic test for nonorganic FTT. Evaluation of family interaction is important, and a search for a causative underlying disorder must be undertaken.

A nutritious diet and social support services are generally all that can be provided. Foster placement is occasionally necessary.

Functional (Psychiatric) Disorders

Functional disorders involve GI symptoms with a lack of sufficient explanatory pathology. Some medical problems may be present, but functional disorders are considered primarily psychogenic. Up to 50% of referrals to gastroenterologists may involve this class of disorder. Symptoms can include dyspepsia, nausea and vomiting, globus hystericus sensation ("lump in the throat"), adult rumination (regurgitation and rechewing of small amounts of food), and psychogenic halitosis (an unfounded complaint of bad breath).

Disorders of the Mouth and Esophagus

Dental Caries

Tooth decay results when microorganisms gradually disintegrate the tooth surface, eventually affecting the pulp as well. Dietary carbohydrates, particularly sucrose, provide the substrate for bacterial production of lactic acid, which erodes the tooth enamel. Only advanced lesions produce symptoms, usually pain from eating hot, cold, or sugary foods. While the teeth are developing, usually from birth to age 13, ingestion of fluoride lends some protection against caries formation. Only about half of the U.S. population has adequate access to fluoridated water. Children should take fluoride supplements and use fluoride compounds applied directly to the teeth, such as mouth rinses and toothpaste. Dental fillings are recommended for treatment of caries.

Salivary Gland Disorders

Painful salivary glands may result from ductal stones, which are usually found in the submandibular glands. Pain with eating is common. Manipulation is often successful in removing the stone, but excision may be needed.

Painless swelling of the parotid glands occurs with mumps, sarcoidosis, cirrhosis, neoplasms, or infection. In a dehydrated person, oral bacteria are not sufficiently washed away and may ascend into the ducts, causing infection and swelling.

Tracheoesophageal Fistula

Often associated with esophageal atresia (blind pouch), tracheoesophageal fistula is a congenital deformity that involves the tract between the trachea and the esophagus.

Neonates have coughing and cyanosis during feeding and will likely develop aspiration pneumonia. If the esophagus is patent, abdominal distention may develop when air travels through the fistula to the stomach.

X-ray following nasogastric tube placement can identify esophageal atresia. Excess gas in the stomach can indicate a tracheoesophageal fistula, and bronchoscopy confirms the diagnosis.

Surgical repair is needed.

Dysphagia

Difficulty swallowing is usually caused by an impairment in esophageal transport. Pre-esophageal (or pharyngeal) sources often accompany neurologic or muscular disorders, such as dermatomyositis, myasthenia gravis, and CNS lesions. Esophageal sources generally have obstructive or motor etiologies. Obstructive disorders, such as tumors, strictures, and rings, first affect the patient's swallowing of solids; whereas motor disorders, such as achalasia, spasms, and scleroderma, affect solids and liquids equally.

Patients usually complain that "food gets stuck." Odynophagia (pain with swallowing) may be present. Nasal regurgitation or cough secondary to tracheal aspiration occurs if the lesion is pre-esophageal. Physical exam may show supraclavicular lymphadenopathy, swellings from large diverticulae, or prolonged swallowing time.

History, including whether onset involved solids, liquids, or both, is the key in diagnosing the source of dysphagia. X-rays, esophagoscopy, and esophageal manometry may be useful. Dysphagia is a different diagnosis from globus hystericus, a "lump in the throat," which is usually psychogenic.

Depends on the underlying disorder but often involves surgery.

Achalasia

Achalasia, a neurogenic motor disorder of the esophagus, involves impairment of peristalsis and lower esophageal sphincter relaxation. Etiology of the disorder is unknown. Gradual onset most commonly begins between 20 and 40 years of age. A small minority of patients presenting with achalasia have a malignancy of the gastroesophageal junction.

Dysphagia of both solids and liquids is the major complaint. Regurgitation may occur, resulting in nocturnal cough and aspiration.

Barium swallow studies show absent peristalsis. The esophagus may be greatly dilated, with a classic beak-like lower portion. If an esophagoscope cannot pass easily into the stomach, then carcinoma or stricture should be considered.

Forceful dilation is generally satisfactory to relieve the obstruction, but the procedure often must be repeated. Otherwise, myotomy (the surgical division of the involved muscle) is useful, although this may result in gastroesophageal reflux. Pulmonary complications must be managed.

Esophageal Cancer

Esophageal cancer is usually a squamous cell carcinoma. Adenocarcinoma occurs in 5–10% of cases and is usually related to Barrett's epithelium (columnar metaplasia of the lower esophageal lining). Heavy alcohol and tobacco use are major risk factors. Most patients have metastases to the lymph nodes at the time of presentation, and local extension with invasion of nearby structures is also common.

The initial symptom is dysphagia, leading to weight loss. Patients first experience difficulty swallowing solids, which gradually progresses to difficulty swallowing liquids as well. Weakness, anemia, pain, regurgitation, and aspiration are also noted. Coughing or hoarseness may be present if the laryngeal nerves are involved.

Typically, barium swallow shows a lumen narrowed by an irregular mass. Constricting bands are seen with annular lesions. Esophagoscopy with biopsy is necessary for tissue diagnosis, and a computerized tomography (CT) scan may show metastases.

Some combination of surgery, radiation, and chemotherapy. Prognosis is poor.

Infectious Esophagitis

Infection of the esophagus, which may include concurrent oral lesions, is most commonly due to *Candida* (oral thrush), herpes simplex virus (HSV), and cytomegalovirus (CMV). Infection with these agents is often seen in immunocompromised patients and diabetics, and symptoms include dysphagia and odynophagia. *Candida* is treated with antifungals. HSV and CMV are generally self-limited but can be treated with antivirals (acyclovir and ganciclovir) in immunocompromised patients.

Reflux Esophagitis

Esophageal inflammation results when low pressures at the lower esophageal sphincter allow reflux of gastric contents into the esophagus. Most cases of reflux esophagitis coexist with a hiatal hernia (see below). In addition to inflammation and ulceration, patients may develop strictures, Barrett's esophagus (columnar metaplasia sometimes leading to adenocarcinoma), bleeding, and aspiration. This condition is common in overweight patients and may be seen in infants, who present with vomiting, failure to thrive, anemia, or pulmonary symptoms.

Heartburn is described as burning pain behind the sternum that rises from the stomach toward the mouth. It generally occurs while the patient is lying flat and is relieved by sitting up, drinking fluids, and taking antacids. Patients may also experience a bitter taste in their mouth, called "water brash."

Esophagoscopy, motility studies, or a pH probe can all be used to diagnose reflux esophagitis.

The patient should elevate the head of the bed, attempt to lose weight, and change diet to decrease intake of fat, alcohol, chocolate, caffeine, and late-night snacks. If these steps are unsuccessful, medical treatment includes H_2-receptor antagonists, antacids, or a short-term trial of metoclopramide or omeprazole. A surgical procedure such as Nissen fundoplication, which wraps stomach tissue around the lower esophageal sphincter in order to tighten it, may help in severe disease.

Hiatal Hernia

Hiatal hernia is a common disorder that involves protrusion of part of the stomach above the diaphragm. A sliding hiatal hernia involves upward displacement of both the gastroesophageal junction and the stomach, while a paraesophageal hiatal hernia results when part of the stomach is pushed upward next to a normally located esophagus.

As the lower esophageal sphincter is raised, it is exposed to lower pressures in the thoracic cavity; therefore, it cannot remain closed, and gastroesophageal reflux with chest pain may occur. Most cases, however, are asymptomatic.

X-rays and barium studies show a portion of the stomach above the diaphragm.

The only therapy needed for sliding hiatal hernias is control of reflux, if present. A paraesophageal hernia can incarcerate and strangulate. This complication can be prevented by surgical reduction. Surgery is also indicated for recurrent or intractable symptoms and often involves a Nissen fundoplication.

Disorders of the Stomach and Intestine

Gastric Carcinoma

Stomach cancer is almost always adenocarcinoma, although squamous cell tumors may invade from the esophagus. There is a high incidence of gastric cancer in Japan. Gastric carcinoma can take four forms:

1. **Ulcerating carcinoma** is a penetrating, ulcer-like tumor with shallow edges, in contrast to the raised edges seen in peptic ulcer disease.
2. **Polypoid carcinoma** involves a bulky, intraluminal tumor that metastasizes late.
3. **Superficial spreading carcinoma**, also called early gastric carcinoma, is confined to the mucosa and submucosa with infrequent metastases.
4. **Linitis plastica** spreads throughout all layers of the stomach, decreasing its elasticity.

The development of stomach cancer may be related to *Helicobacter pylori* infection, and the incidence of gastric cancer decreases as the prevalence of *H. pylori* decreases. Incidence is also related to a diet of high fat and low fiber content.

The most common symptoms are abdominal heaviness, anorexia, weight loss, and, rarely, melena (black, tarry feces). Vomiting may occur, particularly if pyloric obstruction develops; the vomitus may have a "coffee-ground" appearance due to bleeding. Half of gastric carcinoma patients have a positive guaiac test, and 25% have a palpable epigastric mass. A classic sentinel node, or Virchow's node, may be found in the neck along the thoracic duct. A small percentage of gastric carcinomas metastasize to the ovary, causing ovarian masses known as Krukenberg tumors.

Carcinoembryonic antigen (CEA) levels are often elevated, especially when the tumor has spread. Hematocrit is low in many patients due to occult blood loss.

An upper GI series will show most tumors. Gastroscopy and biopsy are particularly necessary with ulcerating lesions to differentiate them from benign ulcers.

Surgical resection is the sole treatment option. Survival rates for early cancer are about 90%, but overall 5-year survival in the United States is only 12%.

Gastritis

Gastritis, inflammation of the gastric mucosa, can be acute or chronic. Chronic gastritis involves multiple punctate or aphthous ulcers and becomes increasingly common with advanced age. The etiology is varied and includes alcohol use, nonsteroidal anti-inflammatory drugs (NSAIDs), inflammatory bowel disease, and viral infection. Acute gastritis involves superficial, rapidly developing lesions and occurs with severe stress, such as major trauma, burn, head injury, or hemorrhage.

Nonerosive gastritis, caused by *H. pylori*, may involve gland atrophy or metaplasia. Complete atrophy of the fundic mucosa with loss of parietal cells can cause pernicious anemia. Metaplastic replacement of fundal tissue by antral mucosa, called antral creep, is very common in older patients and is not precancerous.

Mild dyspepsia is the presenting complaint. With acute gastritis in hospitalized patients, blood in the nasogastric aspirate is the first sign.

Endoscopy shows lesions, and scars may be visualized in cases of chronic disease.

With acute disease, vasoconstrictors, coagulation, and transfusions may be necessary. Prevention of acute gastritis with antacids or histamine blockers is common in intensive care units (ICUs), although their usefulness is yet unproved. H_2-blockers, antacids, and avoidance of troublesome foods are the best treatment options for chronic disease.

Table 1-1. Gastric ulcers versus duodenal ulcers

	Gastric ulcer	Duodenal ulcer
Frequency	25% of PUD	75% of PUD
Age	Older	Younger
Major risk factor	NSAIDs	*Helicobacter pylori*
Pain	Varies, often not relieved by eating	Improves with food, worse 2–4 hrs later
Associated disease	COPD	Liver cirrhosis, renal failure
Associated blood type	Type A	Type O

PUD = peptic ulcer disease; NSAIDs = nonsteroidal anti-inflammatory drugs; COPD = chronic obstructive pulmonary disease.

Peptic Ulcer Disease

Ulcerative corrosion of the epithelium can occur anywhere in the esophagus, stomach, or duodenum. While gastric acid is the injurious agent, *H. pylori* plays an important role in weakening the epithelium and making it susceptible to damage. In fact, only a small percentage of ulcer patients has higher than normal acid secretion. An ulcer may be complicated by bleeding, perforation, or obstruction. Peptic ulcer disease occurs most frequently in 20- to 40-year-olds and is three times more common in men than in women.

Burning or gnawing epigastric pain may be alleviated by food or antacids, depending on the location of the ulcer (Table 1-1). Nausea, vomiting, and epigastric tenderness are common. Fecal occult blood is positive in one-third of patients.

The ulcer may be seen on an upper GI series, and endoscopy confirms the diagnosis. Tissue biopsy may be evaluated for carcinoma and for the presence of *H. pylori*. Serum gastrin levels can be measured to exclude hypersecretory states such as Zollinger-Ellison syndrome (gastrinoma).

Antibiotics for *H. pylori* infection are the latest treatment option. Other medical therapy aims to decrease acid secretion with H_2-receptor antagonists or with proton pump blockers in refractory patients, and to neutralize acids as needed with antacids. To prevent recurrence, the patient may continue maintenance doses of the H_2-receptor antagonist. Surgical treatment may be needed for an intractable or bleeding ulcer, and options include either a vagotomy or an antrectomy and vagotomy.

Peritonitis

Inflammation of the peritoneum is usually due to bacterial infection. Spontaneous peritonitis is usually caused by hematogenous spread, and it tends to occur in patients with ascites from cirrhosis or nephrotic syndrome. Peritonitis may also occur after GI perforation or an invasive procedure.

Patients experience abrupt onset of fever, abdominal pain, and distention. Rebound tenderness and guarding are elicited on exam. Abdominal sounds are absent if ileus is present.

Leukocytosis is common.

Abdominal films show generalized dilation of the large and small bowel. If a perforation has occurred, air may be seen under the diaphragm. Paracentesis allows examination of the ascitic fluid, which shows a high white blood cell count with many neutrophils and organisms on Gram's stain.

IV antibiotics are always indicated. Surgery is frequently required to remove the source of infections (e.g., abscess) or correct a perforation.

Inguinal Hernias

Hernias occur when intra-abdominal tissue protrudes through the abdominal wall. Indirect inguinal hernias are congenital defects that result when the processus vaginalis fails to close after the testicle has descended into the scrotum. Direct inguinal hernias are caused by a weakness of the abdominal musculature in Hesselbach's triangle. These hernias develop in adults. The abdominal contents in a reducible hernia can be manipulated back into the abdominal cavity. This is not the case in an irreducible or incarcerated hernia.

Patients may be asymptomatic or may complain of an aching discomfort in the region. Physical exam requires digital invagination of the skin along the spermatic cord and palpation of the internal inguinal ring. An indirect hernia protrudes at this point, whereas a direct hernia will be felt medial to this ring.

Clinical inspection.

Surgical repair is necessary to prevent bowel incarceration, obstruction, and infarction.

Diverticulosis

Diverticulosis is an acquired condition of multiple "false" diverticulae in which the colonic mucosa and submucosa herniate through the muscular layer. True diverticulae involve all layers of the colon wall and are very rare. Diverticulosis is especially common in developed nations due to a low-fiber diet, resulting in increased intraluminal pressures.

Diverticulosis is generally asymptomatic. Symptoms arise from a lower GI bleed or from diverticulitis (see below).

Diverticulae are seen on barium enema or endoscopy.

Diverticulosis usually resolves spontaneously. A high-fiber diet is recommended.

Diverticulitis

Diverticulitis, a complication of diverticulosis, occurs when a diverticulum becomes infected or perforates, causing an abscess or peritonitis. Diverticulitis may be further complicated by formation of fistulas to the bladder, vagina, or skin or by the development of adhesions that cause small-bowel obstruction.

Acute lower abdominal pain, usually on the left side is accompanied by fever, chills, altered bowel habit, and bloody stools. A lower abdominal mass may be present on exam.

A plain abdominal film showing free air under the diaphragm can confirm perforation. CT scan with water-soluble contrast is the preferred method of study during an acute attack. Barium enema x-ray or colonoscopy can be used after the acute attack has resolved.

Mild cases may be managed on an outpatient basis with oral antibiotics and a clear liquid diet. Hospitalization, with nasogastric (NG) tube placement, IV antibiotics, and surgical resection, may be needed for severe disease.

Appendicitis

Inflammation of the appendix often has an identifiable cause, such as obstruction of the lumen by fecaliths or fibroid bands. As distention of the appendix and compromise of blood supply develop, gangrene and perforation become increasingly likely.

Vague periumbilic abdominal pain with nausea and vomiting are the first symptoms; pain then localizes in the right lower quadrant. Temperature is only slightly elevated if no perforation has occurred, whereas fever and increased pain indicate perforation. Pain over McBurney's point (one-third the distance from right anterior superior iliac spine to the umbilicus) is typical.

Leukocytosis with more than 75% polymorphonuclear leukocytes (PMNs) is seen in most patients.

A high index of suspicion for appendicitis is a good idea for any case of acute abdomen. Half of cases show some change on x-ray, and ultrasound or CT can be diagnostic in atypical cases. Free air under the diaphragm indicates a perforation. In men, 90% of diagnoses are true appendicitis, whereas in women, only 85% are appendicitis. The misdiagnosed cases in women are usually gynecologic disorders.

Surgical resection is mandatory.

Diarrhea

Diarrhea, an excessive volume or frequency of stool, is strictly defined as stool weight greater than 300 g per day, except when dietary fiber is very high. It is generally due to increased fecal water, with several etiologies:

1. **Osmotic diarrhea**, water retention in the lumen of the intestines, is caused by an increased amount of unabsorbed solutes in the bowel. Lactose, not absorbed in a patient with lactase deficiency, is a common culprit. Laxatives, antacids, and some sugar analogs may also be causative.
2. **Secretory diarrhea** is diagnosed when electrolytes and water are secreted rather than absorbed, secondary to bacterial toxins (cholera), viruses, bile acids, and some drugs.
3. **Malabsorption**, as in celiac sprue, can lead to osmotic diarrhea, and unabsorbed fats can also stimulate secretion.
4. **Exudative diarrhea**, secretion of plasma, blood, and mucus from the GI tract, is caused by mucosal inflammation. Bacterial infection generally causes either secretory or exudative diarrhea.
5. **Decreased transit time** from partial resection or bypass and from some drugs prevents adequate absorption. **Increased transit time** can also cause diarrhea from occasional bacterial proliferation in the small bowel.

Diarrhea itself is actually a symptom of an underlying disorder. In addition to the increased stool frequency or fluidity, complications include metabolic acidosis, hypokalemia, and dehydration, which can cause vascular collapse.

Stool volume can be measured if confirmation of diarrhea is important. Diet history, stool culture, and colonoscopy may be useful in identifying the underlying cause.

Treat the underlying disorder. Symptomatic treatment involves rehydration, anticholinergics to decrease peristalsis, a bulking agent, and codeine or paregoric. Most etiologies are discussed separately below.

Malabsorption

Malabsorption refers to a wide range of disorders of the absorption of nutrients from the small bowel. Etiologies include problems of acute abnormal epithelium (alcohol, infection), chronic abnormal epithelium (celiac sprue, tropical sprue, Whipple's disease, amyloidosis, Crohn's disease, ischemia), short-bowel syndromes (postresection, volvulus, intussusception, infarction), and impaired transport (blockage secondary to lymphoma, lymphangiectasia). Some common causes are discussed below:

- **Lactose intolerance** results from a defiency of the enzyme lactase. Lactase splits lactose into glucose and galactose, and unsplit lactose causes an osmotic diarrhea. Bacterial fermentation then produces excessive gas. Lactase deficiency is thus characterized by bloating and explosive diarrhea following milk intake. Lactase is located in the jejunal brush border, so lactase deficiency may result from diseases that alter the jejunal mucosa. This deficiency normally occurs in 75% of adults in most ethnic groups but in less than 20% of those of Northwestern European descent. Onset is between 10 and 20 years of age, and a lactose-free diet is needed for prevention of symptoms.
- **Celiac sprue** is a hereditary sensitivity to the gliadin component of gluten, a protein found in wheat, barley, and rye. Interaction of gliadin with antibodies initiates an immune reaction that causes jejunal mucosal damage. Primary symptoms are due to nutrient deficiencies and include anemia, short stature, infertility, and recurrent apthous stomatitis or dermatitis. Amenorrhea may be the first symptom in girls, but onset may be noted from infancy to adulthood. FTT, abnormal stools, and bloating are common symptoms in infants, whereas a syndrome of malabsorption and vitamin deficiency is the presentation in adults. X-ray shows dilated loops of bowel with thinned mucosal folds, and biopsy shows a flat jejunal mucosa. Patients improve on a gluten-free diet, and corticosteroids are used for refractory disease.
- **Tropical sprue**, a malabsorption syndrome of unknown etiology, is characterized by nutritional deficiencies and small-bowel mucosal abnormalities. It is an acquired disorder found primarily in the Caribbean, South India, and Southeast Asia. Multiple deficiencies occur, causing megaloblastic anemia, glossitis, diarrhea, and weight loss. Folic acid replacement and tetracycline are often curative.
- **Whipple's disease**, a rare infectious disorder of middle-aged men, affects many organs but most severely the small intestine. Abdominal pain, weight loss, diarrhea, and malabsorption may be accompanied by skin pigmentation, joint pain, anemia, cough, and

cardiac, hepatic, or neurologic symptoms. Thickened mucosal folds are seen on x-ray. Jejunal biopsy is diagnostic, with foamy macrophages containing masses of rod-shaped bacilli that stain with the periodic acid-Schiff reagent (PAS). Untreated, Whipple's disease is fatal; fortunately, several antibiotics are curative.

- **Intestinal lymphangiectasia**, a disorder of children and young adults, may involve congenital or acquired telangiectasia (masses of dilated vessels) of the intramucosal lymphatics. Massive edema of the extremities occurs in a context of diarrhea, nausea and vomiting, and abdominal pain. Jejunal biopsy is diagnostic, showing abnormal lymphatics. A low-fat diet with triglyceride supplements helps, and resection may be indicated for localized lesions.

General symptoms of malabsorption include weight loss, abdominal distention, flatulence, easy bruising (from vitamin K deficiency), and absent deep tendon reflexes. Diarrhea or steatorrhea may be present, with dehydration if the diarrhea is severe. Protein malabsorption can cause hypoproteinemic edema. Symptoms from vitamin deficiencies are common.

Microcytic anemia reflects iron deficiency, while megaloblastic anemia usually points to folic acid deficiency. Low serum ferritin generally indicates celiac disease or a postgastrectomy state because iron absorption occurs in the duodenum and upper jejunum.

The triad of weight loss, diarrhea, and anemia strongly suggests malabsorption. Direct measurement of fecal fat is a reliable test, as increased fecal fat always indicates malabsorption. The D-xylose absorption test evaluates proximal small-bowel absorption by measuring xylose excreted in the urine after an oral load. X-ray may be helpful and may show calcification indicative of chronic pancreatic disease, which can result in fat malabsorption due to deficient amounts of pancreatic lipase. Biopsy may be diagnostic.

Treat the underlying disorder, as discussed above.

Ulcerative Colitis

Ulcerative colitis, a chronic, idiopathic inflammation of the colon and rectum, has a variable course of remissions and exacerbations. Ulcerative colitis generally involves the rectum, and in half of cases it is confined solely to the rectum. Inflammation may spread proximally, up to the distal ileum in only a minority of patients. The affected colon is contiguous, without "skip lesions," which are discontinuous lesions with normal bowel in between. Ulcers and abscesses form in the mucosa and submucosa and may develop into characteristic pseudopolyps, which occur when inflammatory growths from the intestinal mucosa have a polyp-like appearance. Hemorrhage is a frequent complication, and the colon may become dilated and perforate. Patients have an increased risk of colon cancer, and other extracolonic complications are common.

Frequent complaints include rectal bleeding, tenesmus, crampy abdominal pain, and blood or mucus with diarrhea. Patients may experience fever, nausea and vomiting, weight loss, or dehydration. Common complications include anal fissures, abscesses, and fistulas.

Sigmoidoscopy shows dull, granular, friable mucosa, but biopsy of affected areas may be needed for diagnosis. Barium enemas should not be performed in acutely ill patients, but ulcerative colitis has a typical mucosal irregularity and a "lead pipe" appearance as the colon narrows, shortens, and loses its haustrations.

Sulfasalazine, steroids, or immunosuppressives are used to treat mild exacerbations and maintain periods of remission. More severe episodes require hospital admission with a nasogastric tube, parenteral nutrition, IV steroids, and antibiotics. Vigilant surveillance is needed for colon cancer, with annual colonoscopy and biopsies. Colectomy may be needed for severe or intractable disease and is curative.

Crohn's Disease

Also called regional enteritis or granulomatous colitis, Crohn's disease is a chronic and progressive inflammation of the GI tract. Its course is variable and is marked by remissions and exacerbations. Crohn's disease can cause changes anywhere along the GI tract, with lesions most frequently occurring in the distal ileum. Some patients have skip lesions. A majority of patients have granulomas in the bowel wall or mesenteric lymph nodes. Other characteristics of Crohn's disease are fissures, strictures, ulcers, and transmural involvement, as well as complications including intestinal obstruction, abscess formation, fistulas, colon cancer, and systemic manifestations.

Manifestations include diarrhea, recurrent abdominal pain, right lower quadrant abdominal mass, low-grade fever, malnutrition, weight loss, anemia, and anorectal lesions.

Proliferative and destructive changes are seen on barium study. The small bowel shows edema, ulceration, fissures, strictures, and "cobblestone" patterns. CT, magnetic resonance imaging (MRI), or ultrasound may be useful, and endoscopy is frequently needed to confirm the diagnosis.

Initially, treatment involves rest, antidiarrheal agents, and dietary changes with supplemental parenteral nutrition if disease is severe. Steroids, sulfasalazine, immunosuppressives, and antibiotics are all used with some success, and further treatment is aimed toward relief of symptoms and

Table 1-2. Ulcerative colitis and Crohn's disease

	Ulcerative colitis	Crohn's disease
Location	Continuous disease starting at the rectum and possibly including the colon and distal ileum	Entire GI tract may be involved, with multiple "skip" areas
Depth of pathology	Mucosa and submucosa	Entire bowel wall, with granulomas
Abdominal mass	Absent	Frequently present
Bloody stools	Frequently present	Usually absent
Endoscopic findings	Friable mucosa in rectal area	Aphthous ulcers and "cobblestone" pattern
Radiographic findings	"Lead pipe" colon without haustrations	"Cobblestone" pattern with small-bowel ulcerations, strictures, and fissures
Treatment	Sulfasalazine, steroids, immunosuppressives	Sulfasalazine, steroids, immunosuppressives
	Colectomy is curative	Surgery can treat complications but is not curative
Colonic complications	Perforation	Small-bowel abscesses, obstruction, and fistulas
	Hemorrhage	Perianal disease
	Toxic megacolon	Malabsorption
	Colon cancer	Toxic megacolon
		Colon cancer

complications. Surgery is necessary for complications such as obstruction and fistulas, but surgery for Crohn's disease is palliative and not curative (Table 1-2).

Ischemic Colitis

Ischemic colitis, inflammation and necrosis of the colon, is caused by vascular compromise leading to insufficient blood supply. Etiology may be atherosclerotic or embolic, and the high mortality with severe ischemic colitis reflects these underlying problems. Patients are most often elderly, or younger patients with chronic diseases such as diabetes, lupus, and sickle cell anemia. Reversible ischemic colitis heals with medical management, but irreversible cases require surgical treatment.

SIGNS & SYMPTOMS

Patients experience an abrupt onset of abdominal pain after eating, diarrhea that is often bloody, a tender abdomen, and systemic symptoms.

DIAGNOSIS

Endoscopy shows a bloody, edematous, friable mucosa and may reveal ulcers or a gray membrane, in which case stool should be checked for *Clostridium difficile*. Barium x-ray demonstrates a "thumb print" or pseudotumor pattern.

IV fluids and antibiotics are frequently sufficient, although resection of the affected portion of the colon may be necessary in the case of irreversible damage.

Toxic Megacolon

Dilation, usually of the transverse colon, exceeds 6 cm in diameter for the diagnosis of toxic megacolon to apply. In adults, this condition is preceded by inflammatory bowel disease (e.g., ulcerative colitis and Crohn's), whereas in children, Hirschsprung's disease (absence of colonic nerve plexus) is the more common etiology. Toxic megacolon can result in septicemia, generalized peritonitis, or perforation and carries a high mortality rate.

Patients are severely ill, with high fever, abdominal pain, and rebound tenderness.

Leukocytosis is present.

Abdominal x-rays show intraluminal gas along a continuous segment of very dilated bowel.

Patients must be NPO (nothing by mouth) with IV fluid replacement and electrolyte maintenance as needed. Antibiotics and steroids are administered in inflammatory bowel disease. Passage of a rectal tube may alleviate megacolon but may cause a perforation. Surgery may be necessary.

Irritable Bowel Syndrome

Irritable bowel syndrome is a common disorder involving chronic GI complaints, often associated with psychiatric symptoms.

Patients complain of chronic, crampy abdominal pain, bloating, flatulence, and diarrhea or constipation.

Irritable bowel syndrome is a diagnosis of exclusion, and lactose intolerance must be ruled out. Presumptive diagnosis may be made in the context of chronic symptoms without weight change or findings on physical exam.

Dietary bulk supplements, anticholinergics, and antidiarrheals are generally sufficient, and tricyclic antidepressants may be helpful.

Colonic Polyps

Colonic polyps are small tissue masses projecting into the colonic lumen. Polyps may be sessile or pedunculated and mucosal, submucosal, or muscular in origin. They have a variety of etiologic and histologic types. Most neoplastic polyps are adenomas. Other polyps may be inflammatory, hyperplastic, or hamartomatous (juvenile or Peutz-Jeghers).

Adenomatous polyps are found in 50% of 70-year-olds. These premalignant adenomas are probably the origin of most large-bowel adenocarcinomas. Cancer is found in only 1% of adenomas less than 1 cm in diameter, but it is found in 45% of adenomas more than 2 cm in diameter, making size an important predictor of histology. Villous adenomas are more frequently malignant than tubular adenomas. Sessile polyps are more often malignant than pedunculated polyps.

Familial adenomatous polyposis is a rare, autosomal dominant condition involving multiple polyps that eventually develop into colorectal cancer if untreated.

Polyps are generally asymptomatic. Larger lesions can cause intermittent bleeding and changes in bowel habits, such as increased frequency, constipation, or tenesmus.

Polyps may be felt on digital rectal exam, and barium x-ray can also show lesions suggestive of polyps. Diagnosis is confirmed with colonoscopy.

Polypectomy can be performed during colonoscopy or laparotomy. Carcinoma in situ does not require further treatment. Segmental resection of the colon may be needed if pathology shows invasive adenocarcinoma.

Colon Cancer

The colon is the second most common site of visceral cancer in Western countries and is more common in women than men. The vast majority of these cancers are adenocarcinoma. Genetic predisposition is known with familial adenomatous polyposis and with two other disorders: cancer family syndrome and hereditary site-specific colon cancer. All of these are autosomal dominant. Other predisposing conditions include ulcerative colitis, schistosomal colitis, history of radiation exposure, and colonic polyps. Increased incidence is seen in higher socioeconomic classes and is probably related to high-fat, high-calorie, low-fiber, and low-calcium diets.

Colon cancer spreads most frequently to regional lymph nodes. Cancer may also spread by direct extension, as seen with the common circumferential growth pattern of left colon lesions, and it can invade nearby structures. Hematogenous spread commonly leads to metastases in the liver or lungs. "Seeding," or transperitoneal metastasis, may cause local implants or generalized abdominal carcinomatosis. The TNM system and Dukes classification are both used for staging.

The American Cancer Society recommends annual digital rectal exams for individuals 40 years of age or older, annual stool occult blood tests after age 50, and flexible sigmoidoscopy every 3–5 years after age 50.

Adenocarcinoma remains asymptomatic for about 5 years. Right-sided colon lesions typically cause weakness secondary to anemia, dyspepsia, and right-sided discomfort or fullness. Left-sided colon cancer more often causes changes in bowel habits from occlusion of the lumen, with alternating constipation and increased frequency, blood-streaked stool, and stool with decreased diameter ("pencil stools"). Metastatic nodes, called Virchow's nodes or sentinel nodes, may be palpated in the supraclavicular region.

In 70% of patients, carcinoembryonic antigen (CEA) is elevated in the serum, but this finding is not specific to colon cancer. CEA therefore is not considered an appropriate screening tool, but it can be useful to detect recurrences.

Barium enema exam and colonoscopy with biopsy are the principal means of diagnosis. Left-sided colon cancer classically appears as an annular, "apple core" filling defect on contrast exam. Right-sided colon cancer generally looks like an intraluminal mass or a constriction associated with a "napkin ring" appearance.

Surgery, with wide resection of the lesion and its lymphatic drainage, is necessary for cure. Resection is also often helpful for palliation to prevent obstruction and bleeding.

Rectal Cancer

Like colon cancer, rectal cancer is usually adenocarcinoma.

The most frequent presenting symptom is persistent hematochezia (blood-streaked stools), which must be evaluated for cancer even in the presence of hemorrhoids. Tenesmus, altered bowel habit, and sensation of incomplete evacuation are also common complaints.

Distal lesions can be palpated on digital exam. Sigmoidoscopy may be needed to biopsy the lesion.

Surgical resection is performed, often with adjuvant radiation therapy.

Volvulus

Volvulus, the rotation of a bowel segment, may result in obstruction with subsequent gangrene from circulatory block. This is a common cause of bowel obstruction in elderly, bedridden patients and in newborns with disorders of intestinal rotation.

Symptoms of colicky pain, abdominal distention, obstipation (complete lack of stool elimination), and late vomiting vary depending on the location of the volvulus.

X-ray may show a "double bubble" sign with an air pocket on each side of the obstruction. Barium enema will show a dilated colon with a "bird's beak" at the point of the volvulus.

Surgical repair is needed in pediatric patients and in adults with a cecal (right-sided) volvulus. Endoscopic decompression may be possible for sigmoid (left-sided) volvulus. Gangrenous sections must be resected.

Intussusception

Intussusception is the telescoping of one bowel segment into an adjacent segment. Usually the terminal ileum slides into the right colon. Intussusception is the most common cause of bowel obstruction in children under 2 years of age. In 95% of patients the etiology is unknown. Hypertrophied Peyer's patches may provide the leading edge, and there is an association with adenovirus infections. Ischemia of the bowel is a serious complication.

Children present with the sudden onset of abdominal pain that occurs in episodes that last about 1 minute. Reflex vomiting may occur early, but vomiting due to the obstruction does not occur until later. "Currant jelly" stool is common due to blood and mucus. Pallor, sweating, and vomiting are the main symptoms in very small infants.

Leukocytosis with a left shift and hemoconcentration are generally present.

A palpable mass may be felt in the right upper quadrant with no cecum palpable in the right lower quadrant. Obstruction can be seen with barium enema.

Administration of the barium enema itself will reduce the intussusception in the majority of patients and should be repeated if unsuccessful. Surgical reduction is needed for the rest, with resection of any gangrenous portions.

Necrotizing Enterocolitis

Necrotizing enterocolitis and sloughing of the intestinal mucosa often progress to perforation. Premature and low–birth weight newborns and older infants suffering from malnutrition and gastroenteritis are most commonly affected. Etiology is unknown.

Infants have bilious vomiting, abdominal distention, bloody stools, and lethargy.

Thrombocytopenia is typically noted.

X-ray shows small-bowel distention and, later, pneumatosis (air in the bowel wall). Perforation, with free peritoneal air on x-ray, occurs in 20% of cases.

Nasogastric suction, total parenteral nutrition, and IV antibiotics should be started immediately. Resection of the necrotic portion is usually necessary.

Gastrointestinal Infectious Disorders

Botulism

Botulism is a syndrome of neuromuscular deficits produced by the *Clostridium botulinum* toxin. In foodborne botulism the toxin is ingested. Home-canned foods are a frequent culprit. Exposure to high heat for 30 minutes kills the spores, and the toxins are easily destroyed by heat. Infant botulism results from ingestion of spores, which then colonize the GI tract and produce toxin in vivo. Honey may contain these spores and should not be given to infants less than 1 year of age. Wound botulism occurs when spores contaminate the wound site and produce toxin.

Foodborne botulism has an abrupt onset 12–36 hours after ingesting the toxin, and it begins with nausea, vomiting, cramps, and diarrhea. Cranial nerve palsies, particularly of the extraocular muscles; fixed, dilated pupils; and diplopia are characteristic signs. Dysphagia may cause aspiration. The muscles of respiration weaken, leading to respiratory failure. Patients remain afebrile. Wound botulism results in neurologic symptoms without GI involvement, and patients have evidence of an injury or puncture wound. In infant botulism, constipation is usually the first sign, followed by cranial nerve symptoms and neuromuscular paralysis.

The toxin is found in serum, feces, or the suspected food.

Induced vomiting and gastric lavage help eliminate any unabsorbed toxin. Hospitalization is mandatory because supportive respiratory treatment may be needed. An antitoxin is available to halt progression of the disease.

Cholera

The enterotoxin from *Vibrio cholerae* causes cholera, a secretory diarrhea. The organism is spread by fecal contamination of water, seafood, and other products. Endemic cases are found along the Gulf Coast of the United States, as well as in Asia, Africa, and the Middle East. Epidemics, usually caused by fecal contamination of water supplies, can occur in any season and affect children and adults equally.

Huge quantities of "rice-water" stools are passed without pain. Diarrhea is not bloody because the bowel mucosa remains intact. Severe dehydration leads to thirst, oliguria or anuria, cramps, weakness, and loss of skin tone. Circulatory collapse may cause cyanosis, stupor, or renal tubular necrosis.

Metabolic acidosis may be severe due to loss of bicarbonate in the stool.

Stool culture.

Maintaining fluid and electrolyte balance is imperative. Tetracycline or doxycycline reduces duration of symptoms.

Shigellosis

Shigella species bacteria cause dystentery (bloody diarrhea) following ingestion of a very small inoculum. Fecal-oral spread and contaminated foods are responsible, and flies act as mechanical vectors. Epidemics occur with overcrowding and insufficient sanitation, and reinfection is possible.

Young children have an acute onset of symptoms, including fever, nausea, vomiting, diarrhea, abdominal pain, and distention. Within 3 days diarrhea becomes severe and bloody, often with pus or mucus. Dehydration can cause death; otherwise, the acute disease resolves within several days. Adults tend to have a milder illness.

Stool culture. Proctoscopy shows an ulcerated, erythematous mucosal surface.

Fluid replacement is critical. Ciprofloxacin can shorten the course in severe disease.

Hemorrhagic Colitis

Hemorrhagic colitis is an infection of enterohemorrhagic *Escherichia coli* type 157, which produces a toxin that damages GI mucosa and vascular endothelial cells. Absorption of this toxin leads to damage in vessels of other organs, particularly the kidneys. The organism has a bovine reservoir, so sporadic cases and outbreaks are due to consumption of unpasteurized milk or the now infamous undercooked beef. Fecal-oral transmission is also possible.

Acute, severe abdominal cramps and watery diarrhea progress rapidly to bloody diarrhea. Fever tends to be low, except when complications arise. An uncomplicated course lasts about 1 week, but a small number of cases are complicated by hemolytic-uremic syndrome or thrombotic thrombocytopenic purpura.

Stool culture.

Supportive care, especially with fluid replacement. Antibiotics do not help to reduce symptoms or duration. Complications require aggressive management.

Staphylococcal Gastroenteritis

Staphylococcal infection results from eating food containing the toxin produced by staphylococci. Foods left at room temperature, particularly milk, cream products, and some meat and fish, provide a fertile breeding ground for this organism.

Within 8 hours after eating, patients experience the abrupt onset of nausea and vomiting, often with cramps, diarrhea, headache, and fever. Complete recovery occurs within 24 hours of onset.

A history of similar illness in others who ate the same food is common. The clinical syndrome, with Gram's stain of the vomitus showing staphylococci, is diagnostic.

Fluid and electrolyte maintenance.

Salmonella Gastroenteritis

Gastroenteritis is the most common of the syndromes caused by *Salmonella*. Infection results from eating foods produced from infected animals, such as meat, milk, poultry, and eggs; from drinking contaminated water; and from fecal-oral transmission.

Patients may be asymptomatic. Symptoms may develop within 2 days of eating infected food. Nausea and cramps are followed by watery or bloody diarrhea, fever, and sometimes vomiting. Illness lasts 1–4 days.

Stool culture.

Supportive care. Antibiotics are indicated only in patients with an increased risk of mortality, because antibiotics prolong excretion of organisms.

Pseudomembranous Colitis

When antibiotic therapy changes the balance of normal intestinal bacteria, overgrowth of a pathogen can result in pseudomembranous colitis, a form of diarrhea associated with exudative "pseudomembranes" in the colon. The bacterium that most often causes this condition is *Clostridium difficile*. Although therapy with any antibiotic may cause this problem, clindamycin, ampicillin, and the cephalosporins are most frequently involved.

 Onset of symptoms usually occurs during a course of antibiotic therapy but may be delayed by as much as 6 weeks. The illness is often mild, but severe, bloody diarrhea with abdominal cramping, fever, and dehydration may occur.

 Finding *C. difficile* toxin in the stool is diagnostic. Stool culture or sigmoidoscopy with visualization of pseudomembranes may also be used.

 Discontinuing antibiotics, if possible, may be sufficient treatment. Oral metronidazole is the treatment of choice in more severe cases.

Viral Gastroenteritis

Nausea, vomiting, diarrhea, and abdominal cramps in viral gastroenteritis may be due to one of several potential viral agents. The Norwalk virus is a common cause of gastroenteritis outbreaks throughout the year. In winter, rotaviruses may cause severe diarrhea in small children. Enteroviruses, particularly Coxsackie virus A1 and echovirus, and adenoviruses are other sources of disease. These syndromes typically resolve without treatment, although hospitalization and rehydration may be needed for severely affected children.

Pancreatic Disorders

Acute Pancreatitis

Nonbacterial inflammation of the pancreas occurs when the pancreatic enzymes digest the pancreas and surrounding tissues. Acute pancreatitis is most commonly caused by gallstone disease (40%) or alcoholism (40%), but it may also be due to hypercalcemia, hyperlipidemia, drugs, or unidentifiable causes.

 Acute epigastric pain radiating to the back is the classic symptom and may be accompanied by nausea and vomiting. Grey Turner's sign (bluish discoloration in the flank) or Cullen's sign (periumbilic discoloration) occurs in only 1–2%. Severe cases may display left pleural effusion, tachycardia, and hypotension or shock.

Serum amylase and lipase are increased. Note that these are not prognostic.

Labs and presentation establish the diagnosis. X-ray findings frequently include a "sentinel loop" (dilated loop of bowel near pancreas) or the "colon cutoff sign" (gas distending the right colon that abruptly stops near the pancreas).

Treatment includes nasogastric suction, fluid replacement, and narcotic analgesics. The patient must be NPO to reduce pancreatic stimulation. Ranson's criteria (see box) are used to predict severity of prognosis.

Ranson's Criteria

The presence of three or more are associated with increased mortality.

On admission:

1. Age >55 years old
2. Serum glucose >200 mg/dl
3. Serum lactic dehydrogenase >350 IU/liter
4. Serum aspartate transaminase (AST) >250 units
5. White blood cell count >16,000/ml

Within 48 hours:

1. Hematocrit drops >10%
2. BUN rises >5 mg/dl
3. Serum calcium < 8 mg/dl,
4. PaO_2 <60 mm Hg
5. Base deficit >4 mEq/liter
6. Fluid sequestration estimated at >6 liters.

Chronic Pancreatitis

Long-term pancreatic inflammation is usually due to chronic alcoholism.

The most common symptom is chronic or recurrent epigastric pain. The patient may also have signs of pancreatic insufficiency, with malabsorption and diabetes mellitus.

Serum amylase and lipase are elevated during acute attacks, but amylase may be normal if the pancreas is fibrotic. Pancreatic calcification can be seen on x-ray. Endoscopic retrograde cholangiopancreatography (ERCP) can establish the diagnosis and rule out pseudocysts and tumors.

Alcohol intake should be stopped. Narcotics may be given for analgesia, although addiction is a common problem. Pancreatic insufficiency is treated with enzyme supplements. Surgery may be palliative.

Pancreatic Pseudocyst

The term pseudocyst describes a walled-off fluid collection with a high enzyme concentration that arises from the pancreas. It is called a pseudocyst because its walls consist of inflamed membranous material, not epithelial tissue as in a true cyst. As a complication of pancreatitis, pseudocysts are generally sterile, although superinfection can lead to abscess formation. Other complications include rupture and hemorrhage.

Symptoms usually appear about 1 week after an episode of acute pancreatitis and include epigastric mass, pain, and mild fever.

Leukocytosis and persistent increased serum amylase are seen.

The cyst can be visualized on ultrasound or CT scan.

Of pancreatic pseudocysts, 40% resolve spontaneously, so expectant management in the first 4–6 weeks is appropriate unless the cyst is expanding rapidly or causing pain. If needed, surgical management involves drainage or excision.

Cancer of the Exocrine Pancreas

Adenocarcinomas of the pancreas are usually ductal in origin and most often located in the head of the pancreas (80%). Middle-aged men are the typical patients. Symptoms are generally not evident until the tumor has spread locally or metastasized, and 5-year survival is less than 2%.

Most patients experience weight loss and abdominal pain that may radiate to the back. Obstructive jaundice occurs if the tumor is in the head of the pancreas and impinges on the bile duct. A palpable, nontender gallbladder in a jaundiced patient is a classic sign (Courvoisier's law). If the tumor is in the body or tail, splenic vein obstruction may result, causing splenomegaly or gastric and esophageal varices.

Hyperglycemia is evident in 25–50% of patients. Bilirubin and alkaline phosphatase are elevated if bile obstruction occurs.

Ultrasound, CT, or ERCP locates the tumor, and biopsy confirms the diagnosis.

Resection is indicated for localized disease, but patients usually present with advanced disease and treatment is generally palliative. Exocrine pancreas insufficiency and diabetes mellitus are treated medically. No chemotherapy has been shown to be effective.

Cancer of the Endocrine Pancreas

In cancer of the endocrine pancreas, islet-cell tumors may be nonfunctioning, leading primarily to obstructive symptoms, or functioning, with increased secretion of one of the pancreatic hormones. Some are found in syndromes of multiple endocrine neoplasia (MEN) (see Chap. 4). The functioning tumors are discussed below.

- **Insulinoma**, a rare tumor, causes insulin hypersecretion, and symptoms result from **hypoglycemia**. CNS changes begin with headaches, confusion, motor weakness, visual problems, and personality changes; it can progress to seizures and coma. **Whipple's triad** confirms that hypoglycemia is the source of the symptoms. It requires that symptoms occur while fasting, that hypoglycemia is present, and that carbohydrate intake relieves the symptoms. Diagnosis is supported when fasting insulin levels remain high and by a C-peptide suppression test, if necessary. (C-peptide is manufactured with the insulin molecule and is then cleaved. If it is present, the insulin is endogenous; if absent, the insulin is exogenous.) Only 10% of insulinomas are malignant, so surgical cure rates are high.
- In **Zollinger-Ellison syndrome**, gastrin-producing tumors cause excess acid secretion and peptic ulceration. Multiple, small tumors are frequently present, and half of these tumors are malignant. Aggressive **peptic ulcers**, often in atypical sites, may bleed, perforate, or cause obstruction. Serum gastrin is the most reliable diagnostic measure. H_2-receptor antagonists (cimetidine, ranitidine) and omeprazole relieve symptoms, but surgical resection may be needed for cure.
- **VIPoma** is a non-beta islet-cell tumor that produces vasoactive intestinal peptide (VIP), which affects blood flow to the GI tract. Also called "WDHA," VIPoma usually involves *w*atery *d*iarrhea, *h*ypokalemia, and *a*chlorhydria. Diarrhea may be present for years before diagnosis and may be accompanied by dehydration. Weakness, nausea, vomiting, and abdominal cramps are also common. Unexplained secretory diarrhea suggests VIPoma, but diagnostic tests are unreliable. Exploratory laparotomy is the best means of diagnosis, although resection may not be curative.
- **Glucagonoma**, a tumor of the alpha islet cells, is rare and slow-growing; 80% of patients are women, and 80% of tumors are malignant. Weight loss, anemia, and dia-

betes are present. **Necrolytic migratory erythema** is a characteristic exfoliating lesion of the extremities. Elevated glucagon levels and angiography suggest the diagnosis, and resection is indicated.

Liver and Biliary Disorders

Glycogen Storage Diseases

Glycogen storage diseases belong to a group of rare, usually autosomal recessive disorders with varying degrees of severity. Specific defects in carbohydrate metabolism lead to abnormal glycogen accumulation in the liver, muscle, nerves, heart, and other organs. Glycogen stores can be visualized on MRI. Tissue biopsy and enzyme assay confirm the diagnosis. Etiologies include:

- **Pompe's disease**, an alpha-1,4-glucosidase deficiency that is fatal by age 2, with glycogen build-up in many organs.
- **von Gierke's disease**, a glucose-6-phosphatase deficiency that leads to enlarged liver and kidneys, growth retardation, and electrolyte abnormalities.
- **McArdle's disease**, a milder disorder in which muscle phosphorylase is absent. Patients experience cramps and myoglobinuria after exercise. Limiting physical activity and increasing fluid intake help to minimize the symptoms, and diuresis after exertion prevents the myoglobinuria from progressing to renal failure.

Jaundice

Yellowing of the skin and sclera is due to elevated serum bilirubin. Jaundice may be categorized as prehepatic, hepatic, or posthepatic in origin. The most common cause of **prehepatic jaundice** is hemolysis, because hemoglobin breakdown causes increased bilirubin production. Two other prehepatic disorders are Gilbert's disease and the Crigler-Najjar syndrome. **Hepatic jaundice** may be hepatocellular (acute hepatitis, chronic cirrhosis) or cholestatic (primary biliary cirrhosis, toxic drug jaundice, cholestatic jaundice of pregnancy). Biliary obstruction is the most common cause of **posthepatic jaundice**, due to a tumor, gallstones, or biliary stricture.

SIGNS & SYMPTOMS

Yellow skin, scleral icterus, and pruritus are the most common symptoms. Patients may have hepatomegaly and signs of cirrhosis. Patients with choledocholithiasis (stones blocking the bile duct) may also have biliary colic, fever, and chills. Hepatitis may cause tenderness over the liver. With posthepatic obstruction, patients may note light stools and dark urine, due to urinary excretion of bile metabolites.

LABS

Increased bilirubin is in the unconjugated form with prehepatic disease. A mixture of conjugated and unconjugated bilirubin is typical of hepatocellular disease. Conjugated bilirubin is increased in intrahepatic cholestasis and posthepatic disease. Some loss in the urine (bilirubinuria) occurs because conjugated bilirubin is water-soluble. With posthepatic obstruction, serum aspartate transaminase (AST) and lactic dehydrogenase (LDH) will also be elevated. Alkaline phosphatase may be elevated in cases of intrahepatic cholestasis, cholangitis, or extrahepatic obstruction.

Ultrasound is commonly used to diagnose liver and biliary disorders.

DIAGNOSIS

Treat the underlying disorder. The most common are discussed separately below.

TREATMENT

Viral Hepatitis

Any inflammatory processes in the liver is referred to as hepatitis, including viral, alcoholic, or drug-induced hepatitis. The five major hepatatrophic viruses are discussed here. Acute infection may precede chronic hepatitis, which is diagnosed when the disease lasts more than 6 months. Chronic persistent hepatitis is a benign condition, but chronic aggressive or active hepatitis can lead to liver failure, cirrhosis, and cancer. These five viruses are currently the most well-established:

- **Hepatitis A virus** (HAV) is spread by fecal-oral contact and contaminated food, with shellfish a common culprit. Epidemics may be water or foodborne, and sporadic cases are common as well. Fecal shedding ends before onset of symptoms. Infection is acute, often subclinical, and confers lifelong immunity (Fig. 1-1A).

- **Hepatitis B virus** (HBV) causes hepatitis B, sometimes with a concurrent infection of the hepatitis D virus. The Dane particle, which is the infective agent of HBV, is transmitted through contact with infected body fluids. Injection drug use, sexual contact, and vertical transmission in pregnancy are the most common modes of spread. (Transfusions are a less frequent source of infection now that donor blood is routinely screened.) HBV can cause subclinical infection, acute or chronic hepatitis, or cirrhosis, and it is associated with hepatocellular carcinoma.

  The HBV surface antigen (HBsAg) appears first during the incubation and then usually disappears, while antibody against it (anti-HBs) appears later during the patient's recovery and lasts a lifetime. When anti-HBs does not develop, HBsAg persists and the patient becomes a carrier. HBV core antigen (HBcAg) is found in liver cells, but in serum only anti-HBc can be detected, usually as symptoms begin. Anti-HBc immunoglobulin M (IgM) develops first, followed by IgG, which is present throughout the patient's life. The e antigen (HBeAg) reflects viral replication and greater infectivity, whereas high levels of anti-HBe indicate a good prognosis (Fig. 1-1B, C).

- **Hepatitis C virus** (HCV) is the most common source of posttransfusion hepatitis, and it may be responsible for many diagnoses of idiopathic hepatitis. Chronic carriers may be healthy, or they may suffer from chronic hepatitis, cirrhosis, or hepatocellular carcinoma.

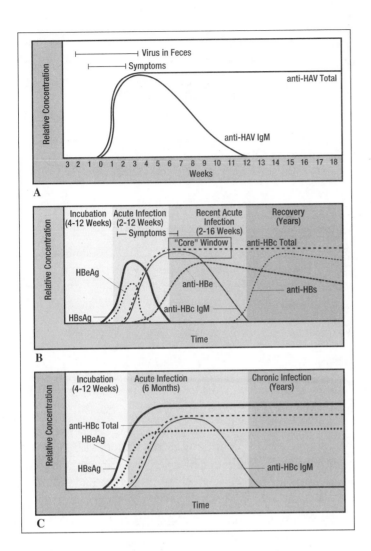

Fig 1-1. Hepatitis serological profiles. A. Hepatitis A serologies. B. Typical hepatitis B serologies. C. Hepatitis B chronic carrier serologies. (Redrawn from J Wallach. *Interpretation of Diagnostic Tests*, Fifth Edition. Boston: Little, Brown, 1992.)

- **Hepatitis D virus** (delta agent) can replicate only when HBV is present, so it occurs only as a coinfection of HBV. Manifestations of this agent are either more severe hepatitis or an exacerbation of chronic disease.
- **Hepatitis E virus** (HEV) is a major cause of waterborne hepatitis in underdeveloped countries. It is spread by fecal-oral contact and is associated with high mortality among pregnant women.

Symptoms of hepatitis range from low-grade fever to fulminant liver failure. A prodrome of malaise, fever, nausea, and vomiting is followed by darkening of the urine (bilirubinuria) and jaundice. Jaundice may persist while other symptoms fade. Full recovery of acute infection generally requires about 4 weeks.

Alanine aminotransferase (ALT) and aspartate transaminase (AST) are elevated, bilirubin is high, and alkaline phosphatase may be mildly increased. White blood cell count (WBCs) is usually normal to low.

In HAV, IgM antibody is present during the illness, and IgG indicates prior infection. For HBV, HBsAg is present prior to onset of symptoms, and anti-HBs follows the illness. During the symptomatic phase, anti-HBc IgM should be tested, as it is the only marker present during the illness itself. New tests are available for HCV, but this is often a diagnosis of exclusion.

Hepatitis usually resolves with only supportive care. Chronic, untreatable infection develops in 5–10% of HBV cases and 50% of HCV cases, and this may lead to cirrhosis or hepatocellular carcinoma.

Immunoglobulin (IG) is recommended for travelers and for contacts of HAV-infected patients. Hepatitis B immunoglobulin (HBIG) is given following needlestick exposure to HBV-infected blood and to newborns of HBV-positive mothers. Vaccination against HBV is very effective and is recommended for newborns and health care providers. It is given as a series of three injections over 6 months.

Cholelithiasis

Cholelithiasis, stones in the gallbladder, is a common disorder and is usually asymptomatic. Incidence increases with age. Other risk factors include female gender, multiparity, and obesity. These can be remembered as "the 4 Fs": "female, fertile, forty, and fat." Native Americans have a particularly high rate of cholelithiasis. Most patients (75%) have cholesterol stones. Other stones contain primarily calcium or bile pigments from hemoglobin breakdown.

Biliary colic results from transient blockage of the cystic duct (Fig. 1-2). This episodic pain in the right upper quadrant may be accompanied by nausea and vomiting. It is frequently precipitated by fatty meals. Only 2% of patients with asymptomatic gallstones develop symptoms each year, most frequently from cholecystitis or gallstone pancreatitis.

Ultrasound. X-ray is not helpful because only a small percentage of gallstones are radiopaque.

Cholecystectomy is performed on symptomatic patients and as prophylaxis for patients with large stones or a calcified gallbladder. Calcification of the gallbladder is associated with carcinoma.

Cholecystitis

Cholecystitis is an inflammation of the gallbladder usually associated with gallstones; however, acalculous cholecystitis may occur in patients on total parenteral nutrition or in

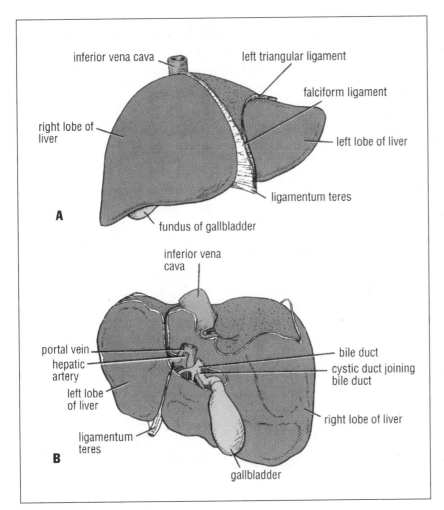

inferior vena cava

left triangular ligament

falciform ligament

right lobe of liver

left lobe of liver

ligamentum teres

A

fundus of gallbladder

inferior vena cava

portal vein

hepatic artery

left lobe of liver

ligamentum teres

B

bile duct

cystic duct joining bile duct

right lobe of liver

gallbladder

Fig. 1-2. A. Anterior view of liver. B. Posterior view of liver. (From R Snell. *Clinical Anatomy for Medical Students*, Fifth Edition. Boston: Little, Brown, 1995.)

ill patients after additional trauma. Symptoms may be acute or chronic, causing scarring of the gallbladder. Some frequent complications include choledocholithiasis (stones blocking the bile duct), cholangitis (inflammation of the bile duct), pancreatitis, ileus, empyema, and perforation. Chronic, mild cholecystitis can lead to acute, severe cholecystitis or gallbladder adenocarcinoma.

SIGNS & SYMPTOMS

Biliary colic starts suddenly and often occurs postprandially. Patients with acute cholecystitis have severe right upper quadrant pain, pain referred to the right scapula, and low fever. One-third have a palpable gallbladder. Pain is steady and abates slowly. Patients tend to curl up and shift position frequently. A positive Murphy's sign of inspiratory arrest during palpation over the gallbladder reflects likely cholecystitis. Milder symptoms of chronic cholecystitis may occur in episodes or almost continuously.

LABS

Leukocytosis and mildly increased serum bilirubin and alkaline phosphatase often occur with acute cases. Increased amylase indicates a stone in the common bile duct and associated pancreatitis.

Ultrasound can show the presence of gallstones but is not as accurate as a HIDA scan. This procedure uses radioisotopes, which are taken up by the liver and excreted in the bile. Nonvisualization of the gallbladder indicates cystic duct obstruction.

Cholecystectomy is the treatment of choice, though percutaneous cholecystostomy, lithotripsy, and stone dissolution are also options.

Cholangitis

Bacterial infection of the bile ducts is symptomatic only when accompanied by biliary obstruction. Frequent causes are choledocholithiasis, biliary strictures, and neoplasm. Bacteria are generally of enteric origin.

Charcot's triad is classic: biliary colic, jaundice, and fever. Bacteremia is common.

Leukocytosis, increased serum bilirubin, and increased alkaline phosphatase are present.

Ultrasound is usually diagnostic but may be supplemented with ERCP or CT scan.

IV antibiotics are administered. Drainage is needed only for severe cases.

Liver Cancer

Liver cancer is an uncommon cancer associated with chronic HBV and HCV infection, as well as with cirrhosis, liver flukes, and aflatoxins (fungus metabolites). Metastatic cancer to the liver is 20 times more frequent than primary liver cancer and most frequently arises from breast, lung, and colon cancers. Complications include intra-abdominal hemorrhage, portal vein obstruction, Budd-Chiari syndrome (thrombosis of the hepatic vein causing ascites and cirrhosis), and liver failure. Benign hepatic adenomas are seen almost exclusively in women taking oral contraceptive pills.

Right upper quadrant pain may be referred to the right shoulder. Other signs include weight loss, jaundice, hepatomegaly, or a bruit over the liver.

Elevated transaminases, bilirubin, and alkaline phosphatase. Patients may have elevated alpha-fetoprotein, HBsAg, or anti-HCV.

Tumors are usually seen on CT, MRI, or ultrasound. Biopsy confirms the diagnosis.

Options include partial hepatectomy, liver transplantation, ethanol injection to induce necrosis, and arterial chemoembolization. Prognosis is poor.

Hepatic Abscess

Most frequently due to enteric bacteria or amebae, hepatic abscesses usually form after spread of infection from biliary or abdominal infections. An underlying malignancy is present in 40% of patients. Complications include formation of multiple abscesses, rupture, septicemia, and liver failure.

Onset may be insidious, but symptoms eventually include spiking fever, chills, right upper-quadrant pain, and tender hepatomegaly. Jaundice is often seen with multiple abscesses.

Ultrasound or CT scan shows abscesses.

Antibiotics are administered. Percutaneous suction catheters are used to drain the abscess. Surgical treatment is only rarely indicated.

Subphrenic Abscess

Subphrenic abscesses, abscesses under the diaphragm and above the transverse colon, result from direct contamination after abdominal surgery, peritonitis, or extension from an adjacent site. Fifty percent occur on the right, 25% on the left, and 25% are in multiple sites.

About 1–2 months after abdominal surgery, patients develop fever and other nonspecific symptoms. Abdominal pain and tenderness may be present, often with paralytic ileus. Cough, dyspnea, and chest or shoulder pain result from diaphragmatic irritation, and decreased breath sounds, rales, rhonchi, and dullness to percussion of the chest may be present.

Leukocytosis and anemia are common.

Chest x-ray shows ipsilateral effusions and an elevated hemidiaphragm. Abdominal films may show gas in the abscess, displaced organs, or a soft-tissue mass. Ultrasound or CT scan generally help in the diagnosis.

Surgical or percutaneous drainage, and antibiotics.

Alcohol-Related Hepatic Disease

Alcoholic liver damage occurs in three progressive stages. Hepatic steatosis, or fatty liver, is the first stage. Fat deposits in the liver cause hepatomegaly and mild enzyme changes, but this pathology is reversible with cessation of alcohol intake. The second stage of disease is alcoholic hepatitis. Biopsies show characteristic changes in tissue, including inflammation and necrosis. The third stage is cirrhosis, discussed in further detail below.

Alcohol-related changes may be clinically silent or may involve fever, abdominal pain, anorexia, nausea and vomiting, or signs of portal hypertension.

Elevated ALT, AST, gamma-glutamyl transpeptidase (GGT), alkaline phosphatase, and bilirubin are commonly seen. In contrast to viral hepatitis, AST levels are generally higher than ALT levels. PT is prolonged due to a reduction in clotting factors, especially II, VII, IX, and X.

Diagnosis is made from clinical signs and labs. If necessary, a biopsy can confirm diagnosis.

Cessation of alcohol intake and supportive care are the keys to treatment.

Alcohol Use

Typically, we associate the effects of alcohol with liver disease and cirrhosis, but a number of other illnesses are caused by alcohol ingestion, including GI, cardiovascular, psychiatric, neurologic, and respiratory problems. Alcohol is also associated with cancers, injury, death, and adverse pregnancy outcomes.

GI problems associated with alcohol include gastritis, peptic ulcer disease, hepatitis, cirrhosis, and pancreatitis. Cardiovascular diseases include ischemic heart disease, cardiomyopathy, and arrhythmias. Nutritional deficiencies and anemia are also seen more often in chronic alcohol users. Aspiration pneumonia is common in alcoholics.

Depression and suicide are often alcohol-related, as are many neurologic disorders, such as delirium, dementia, Wernicke's disease, Korsakoff's disease, and other neuropathies. Cancers associated with alcohol use include oropharyngeal, stomach, hepatocellular, and colon cancer.

Alcohol has been established as the primary cause of injury-related death, including motor vehicle accidents and drowning. Complications resulting from alcohol use during pregnancy include premature labor, low birth weight, and fetal alcohol syndrome (discussed in more detail in Chap. 8).

Cirrhosis

In cirrhosis, insults to liver tissue cause necrosis and fibrosis. The development of regenerative nodules follows, replacing healthy liver cells. Alcohol is the most common cause of cirrhosis in the United States, and 15% of alcoholics develop the condition. Other causes of cirrhosis include viral infection, chronic obstruction of the common bile duct, autoimmune disease, chronic heart disease, and metabolic disorders, though many cases are idiopathic. After diagnosis, 30% of patients die within 1 year. Cirrhosis is the third leading cause of death in 45- to 65-year-olds in the United States.

SIGNS & SYMPTOMS

Patients may be asymptomatic for years or may experience nonspecific symptoms of weakness, weight loss, and malaise. Reduced bile salt excretion can cause fat malabsorption and deficiencies of the fat-soluble vitamins (vitamins A, D, E, K). A dramatic upper GI hemorrhage from esophageal varices may be the presenting symptom. Common physical exam findings of chronic liver disease include hepatomegaly, splenomegaly, jaundice, wasting, ascites, vascular spiders, caput medusae (superficial venous collaterals visible on the abdominal wall), palmar erythema, Dupuytren's palmar contractures, peripheral neuropathy, testicular atrophy, and gynecomastia. Cirrhosis is frequently complicated by portal hypertension, ascites, bleeding varices, hepatic encephalopathy, and hepatoma.

LABS

Decreased serum albumin (due to decreased synthetic activity by the liver), anemia, and increased PT (due to decreased vitamin K absorption and decreased liver synthesis of clotting factors).

Diagnosis can be made from history, clinical presentation, and labs.

Cirrhosis is incurable and irreversible, but the disease generally does not progress if the offending agent is removed. Alcohol intake must stop in the case of alcoholic cirrhosis. Corticosteroids can prevent worsening of cirrhosis due to inflammation. Other causes should be treated whenever possible. Liver transplantation may improve the long-term prognosis.

Portal Hypertension

Elevated pressure in the portal vein is generally due to cirrhosis, other liver disease, or extrahepatic portal vein occlusion. Ascites, secondary hypersplenism, and variceal bleeds occur due to increased pressure in the portal vein. Hepatic encephalopathy occurs because the liver cannot adequately filter the blood. Diagnosis and treatment of portal hypertension depend on the presenting symptoms, and these complications are discussed in detail below. Diuretic drugs may be used to prevent fluid overload, and a portocaval shunt may be needed for serious complications.

Esophageal Varices

Esophageal varices are tortuous, collateral veins, usually esophageal or gastric, that expand to circumvent congested hepatic blood flow. They may rupture, causing upper GI bleeding. The 50% death rate from bleeding varices reflects severe hemorrhage in the presence of existing severe liver disease.

Varices are asymptomatic until rupture leads to hemorrhage with hematemesis or melena (black tarry stool).

The diagnosis is suggested by an upper GI bleed in the context of cirrhosis or portal hypertension, and it is confirmed by esophagoscopy.

For bleeding varices, controlling bleeding and replacing fluid and blood loss are crucial. The most common measures to control bleeding include vasopressin, balloon tamponade, endoscopic sclerotherapy, transjugular intrahepatic portosystemic shunt (TIPS), and invasive surgical treatment, such as emergency portosystemic shunt placement. Several of these procedures may also be performed as prophylactic or therapeutic treatment in nonbleeding patients. Despite intervention, prognosis is poor.

Hepatic Encephalopathy

Hepatic encephalopathy is a reversible metabolic neuropathy seen in patients with chronic liver disease and with portocaval shunts. Decreased detoxification by the liver and shunting of blood around the liver lead to exposure of the brain to toxins absorbed from the gut. Possible agents responsible for this effect are ammonia, amino acid neurotransmitters, and other neurotoxins. Altered mental status is exacerbated by increased protein absorption, whether dietary or from an upper GI bleed, by azotemia from dehydration, and by some medications.

Altered consciousness, ranging from lethargy to coma, and abnormal neuromuscular activity, such as asterixis (a wrist-flapping tremor).

Arterial ammonia and cerebrospinal fluid (CSF) glutamine are elevated. Electroencephalogram (EEG) is abnormal.

Diagnosis is made from clinical presentation and above labs.

Eliminate or control the precipitating factor. Reduce dietary protein and administer lactulose, neomycin, or metronidazole to decrease intestinal absorption of ammonia.

Ascites

Ascites, fluid collection in the peritoneal cavity, is most frequently a complication of hepatic disease. It results from a combination of sodium and water retention by the kidneys, low plasma osmotic pressure due to hypoalbuminemia, and elevated hydrostatic pressure in hepatic sinusoids or portal veins.

Abdominal fluid collection can be demonstrated by percussion or the presence of a fluid wave or shifting fluid.

Paracentesis shows the same concentration of albumin in the ascitic fluid as in the serum. An increased concentration of albumin in the ascitic fluid suggests malignant ascites. LDH levels exceeding 60% of serum levels indicate malignant or infected ascites. An increased ascitic white count suggests infection.

Sodium restriction, diuretics, and therapeutic paracentesis all help to control ascites. A portocaval shunt or peritoneal-jugular (LeVeen) shunt may be useful.

Acute Disorders

Upper Gastrointestinal Bleeding

Bleeding from the upper GI tract is most often due to peptic ulcer disease, gastritis, esophageal varices, and Mallory-Weiss tears (gastroesophageal tears due to wretching). Although signs of portal hypertension seen during the exam may suggest bleeding varices, 50% of cirrhotic patients with upper GI bleeds actually have a peptic ulcer.

Hematemesis usually indicates a rapid bleed. A "coffee ground" appearance to the vomitus means that the blood has been in the stomach long enough to be partially digested. Melena (black tarry stool) usually reflects an upper GI source, while hematochezia (bright red blood in the feces) is usually due to a lower source but may also occur with a rapid upper GI bleed.

A guaiac test detects occult blood in the stool or vomit. Bloody aspirate from a nasogastric tube confirms an upper GI source. Upper endoscopy shows the source of bleeding in a majority of patients, but angiography or an upper GI series may be needed to diagnose the rest.

If the patient is not stable, fluid replacement and ice water lavage to reduce bleeding are important initial steps. Most often, patients with a Mallory-Weiss tear will stop bleeding spontaneously, and only monitoring and supportive care are needed. Treatment of specific lesions is discussed under the topics of peptic ulcer disease, esophageal varices, and gastritis.

Lower Gastrointestinal Bleeding

Lower GI bleeding is defined as bleeding from a site distal to the ligament of Treitz. Chronic hematochezia (bright red blood in the feces) can originate from carcinoma, polyps, hemorrhoids, or fissures. Etiologies of heavy bleeding include diverticular disease, angiodysplasia (an abnormal mass of blood vessels in the intestinal wall), ulcerative colitis, or infectious colitis.

Passage of bright red blood suggests a lower GI bleed but can occasionally originate from a briskly bleeding upper GI source. Melena indicates a proximal source of blood.

Rectal examination with anoscopy or sigmoidoscopy can demonstrate most lesions. Colonoscopy, x-ray, radionuclide scan, or angiography may be helpful. Bloody aspirate from a nasogastric tube indicates an upper GI source.

Transfusion is needed less frequently than with upper GI bleeds. Some lesions, such as angiodysplasia, are treated colonoscopically. Intra-arterial vasopressin may be useful with other lesions, particularly diverticular hemorrhage. Surgery is needed if the above therapies are ineffective and usually consists of segmental colonic resection.

Intestinal Perforation

Varied lesions can result in intestinal perforation, including ulcers, obstruction, inflammatory bowel disease, appendicitis, and malignancies. Symptoms include abdominal pain and rigidity with guarding and rebound tenderness. X-ray may show free air under the diaphragm. Definitive diagnosis is surgical, and the perforation must also be corrected surgically. Antibiotics must be given to prevent infection.

Acute Abdomen

Acute abdomen refers to any acute, nontraumatic disorder with primarily abdominal manifestations. Urgent surgery is often indicated. Disorders may involve the GI tract, liver, spleen, biliary tree, pancreas, urinary tract, vasculature, peritoneum, or uterus and ovaries. Visceral pain (usually due to distention, inflammation, or ischemia) is generally diffuse, dull, and poorly localized. Parietal pain from direct irritation of the peritoneum is easier to localize. Other features used in diagnosis are onset, progression, and character of the pain.

Some common symptoms associated with abdominal pain are fever, nausea and vomiting, constipation, and diarrhea. "Guarding" refers to the involuntary spasm of abdominal muscles, causing board-like rigidity on exam, due to peritoneal inflammation. Jaundice, hematochezia, hematemesis, and hematuria indicate specific disorders. Costovertebral angle tenderness is seen with pyelonephritis.

A full lab work-up may include hemoglobin and hematocrit to monitor bleeding; WBC and differential to detect infection; beta–human chorionic gonadotropin (β-HCG) to rule out pregnancy; electrolytes, blood urea nitrogen (BUN), and creatinine to assess kidney function; amylase to detect pancreatic involvement; liver function tests (LFTs) and clotting studies to show liver abnormalities; and stool studies for occult blood or for organisms.

X-ray is often useful to diagnose the cause of an acute abdomen. For example, free air under the hemidiaphragm is often seen with perforated ulcers. Contrast x-rays may be used later to evaluate for specific diagnoses. Angiography is particularly useful to evaluate a hemorrhage. Other commonly used exams include ultrasound, CT, endoscopy, paracentesis, culdocentesis, or laparoscopy.

Treat the underlying disorder. (Common etiologies are discussed in detail throughout this chapter.)

Table 1-3. Common causes of obstructions

	Duodenum	Jejunoileum	Large bowel
Neonate	Atresia Volvulus Congenital bands	Meconium ileus Volvulus Atresia Intussusception	Hirschsprung's Atresia
Adult	Duodenal or pancreatic cancer	Incarcerated hernias Adhesions	Tumors Diverticulitis Volvulus

Intestinal Obstruction

The three most common causes of mechanical obstruction of the bowel are adhesions, hernias, and tumors (Table 1-3). Compromise of the blood flow can lead to ischemia and infarction.

Abdominal cramps, distention, and obstipation are typical. Vomiting is common with small-bowel obstruction but occurs late and is often feculent with large-bowel obstruction. More severe pain, a tender abdomen, and increased distention accompany a strangulating obstruction. Scars, hernias, or a mass may be present on physical exam. High-pitched, hyperactive ("tinkling") bowel sounds are typical.

Abdominal x-ray shows proximal distention in large-bowel obstruction and dilated loops of bowel with air-fluid levels in small-bowel obstruction.

Nasogastric suction may relieve small-bowel obstruction secondary to adhesions. Otherwise, a laparotomy is necessary, with surgical treatment of the source of obstruction. Rehydration of a vomiting patient is crucial.

Ileus

Ileus, a paralytic obstruction of the bowel, occurs due to loss of peristalsis. Infection is a common etiology, along with ischemia, vascular injury, and metabolic disorders. Postoperative ileus, resulting from anesthesia and intestinal manipulation, resolves within a few days.

Cramps, distention, vomiting, and obstipation with hypoactive or absent bowel sounds.

X-ray shows gaseous distention of affected segments.

Options include colonoscopic decompression or cecostomy. Postoperative patients should be kept NPO until ileus resolves.

TREATMENT

Congenital Disorders

Pyloric Stenosis

Pyloric stenosis, muscular hypertrophy of the pyloric valve, causes obstruction, most often in boys. This hypertrophy begins at birth; signs of obstruction begin to appear at age 2–4 weeks. Projectile vomiting and visible peristaltic waves suggest this diagnosis, which is supported by palpation of an olive-sized mass in the right epigastrium. Barium swallow x-ray confirms the diagnosis, showing the "string sign" of a narrowed lumen. Surgery is curative.

Diaphragmatic Hernia

Diaphragmatic hernia, protrusion of parts of the GI tract through the diaphragm and into the thorax, generally occurs on the left side and may result in a hypoplastic left lung. Respiratory distress, a sunken abdomen, and bowel sounds over the left hemithorax indicate this disorder. X-ray is confirmatory. Large hernias are often fatal because of poor lung development. Small defects can be corrected surgically, though pulmonary effects persist.

Meconium Ileus

Meconium ileus is an early sign of cystic fibrosis. Infants with this disorder have abnormally thick meconium containing undigested protein. Loops of intestine can often be palpated, and in utero volvulus may occur and infarct. Infarcted bowel segments often reabsorb, resulting in atresia or cyst formation. A positive sweat test confirms the diagnosis of cystic fibrosis.

Hirschsprung's Disease

Also called congenital megacolon, Hirschsprung's disease is caused by the absence of autonomic nerve innervation of the bowel wall. Continuous small muscle spasm causes partial obstruction, and the proximal bowel segment becomes massively dilated. Toxic enterocolitis is a complication of untreated disease. Distention, obstipation, and late vomiting are key features, and barium enema x-ray shows a dilated proximal segment and a narrowed distal segment. Rectal biopsy, demonstrating the absence of nerve ganglia, is confirmatory. A colostomy is necessary for immediate management. Later, the aganglionic segment should be resected.

Cardiovascular Disorders

Hypertension

Essential (Idiopathic) Hypertension

Hypertension is defined as systolic blood pressure (BP) greater than 140 mm Hg or diastolic blood pressure greater than 90 mm Hg. It affects about 20% of the U.S. population. Of all cases of hypertension, 90–95% are essential hypertension—that is, without an identifiable cause. Prevalence increases with age and is greater in blacks. Sequelae of uncontrolled hypertension include strokes, heart attacks, renal disease, and aortic dissection.

SIGNS & SYMPTOMS

Most patients are asymptomatic. Others complain of headaches, visual disturbances, and nausea or vomiting if BP elevation is severe. On fundoscopic exam, arteriovenous "nicking" (discontinuity in the appearance of a retinal vein due to thickened arterial walls) and "cotton wool spots" (infarction of the nerve fiber layer of the retina) may be seen. A loud systolic click at S2 may be audible, with evidence of left ventricular enlargement on exam or electrocardiogram (ECG).

DIAGNOSIS

Diagnosis requires measurements of elevated BP on three separate visits. The patient should sit quietly for about 10 minutes before the measurement for greatest accuracy. Medication should not be started after only one reading of high BP because the elevated measure may indicate only "white coat" hypertension, brought on by the physician visit.

TREATMENT

Weight loss, reduction of salt and alcohol intake, smoking cessation, and stress reduction may reduce BP substantially. Classes of antihypertensive medications include diuretics, adrenergic blockers, calcium channel blockers, and angiotensin-converting enzyme (ACE) inhibitors. Diuretics or beta-blockers are ordinarily used for initial therapy; however, ACE inhibitors may be beneficial in diabetics to prevent renal disease, and calcium channel blockers are useful for patients with poor lipid profiles. Table 2-1 lists common contraindications for antihypertensives. It is important to determine medication compliance before adding or changing medications in uncontrolled hypertension, since about half of patients are noncompliant after 1 year.

Table 2-1. Contraindications of hypertensive drugs

Condition	Contraindicated drugs	Reason
Asthma/COPD	Beta-blockers	May cause bronchoconstriction
Diabetes mellitus	Thiazide diuretics	Promotes impaired glucose tolerance
	Beta-blockers	May mask signs and symptoms of hypoglycemia
Cardiac failure	Beta-blockers	Reducing contractility of an already compromised
	Calcium channel blockers	heart can cause decompensation.
Pregnancy	Thiazide diuretics	Increased blood volume is normal in pregnancy and should not be reduced.
	ACE inhibitors	Fetal complications

COPD = chronic obstructive pulmonary disease.
ACE = angiotension-converting enzyme.

Hypertensive emergencies occur when extreme elevation of blood pressure leads to conditions such as unstable angina, encephalopathy, or myocardial infarction. Immediate blood pressure reduction with intravenous antihypertensives, such as diazoxide or sodium nitroprusside, is required. Sublingual nifedipine may also reduce blood pressure quickly.

Secondary Hypertension

Secondary hypertension is elevated blood pressure with an identifiable underlying cause. It constitutes only 5–10% of all cases of hypertension. The six major causes are listed below. Most of these disorders are addressed in other chapters; therefore, this list contains only a brief summary of each disorder.

- **Estrogen** in birth control pills causes hypertension in about 5% of women taking oral contraceptives. Treatment involves discontinuation of estrogen or switching to a progestin-only pill.
- Several **renal diseases** are associated with hypertension, probably due to dysfunction in the renin-angiotensin-aldosterone system. Depending on the level of residual kidney function, dialysis and antihypertensives may be necessary.
- **Renovascular hypertension**, or renal artery stenosis, is caused by a thickening of the renal artery wall. In young women, the condition is due to **fibromuscular hyperplasia** (an abnormal thickening of the muscular portion of the artery wall). In older patients, it is often caused by atherosclerotic changes. A renal artery bruit may be heard on exam. Treatment involves angioplasty or surgery.
- **Hyperaldosteronism** and **Cushing's syndrome** often lead to hypertension and are usually due to adrenal adenomas. They should be suspected in patients who are hypokalemic prior to the initiation of antihypertensive treatment. Diagnosis is confirmed with computerized tomography (CT) or magnetic resonance imaging (MRI). Treatment involves surgical excision of the adenoma.
- **Pheochromocytoma** is an adrenal tumor that secretes epinephrine and norepinephrine. It is characterized by rapid, wide swings in BP and by orthostatic hypotension. Diagnosis is via the detection of high levels of urinary catecholamine metabolites. CT or MRI scan may help localize the tumor. Treatment involves surgical excision.
- **Coarctation of the aorta** is a congenital narrowing of the aortic arch just past the origin of the left subclavian artery. Hypertension develops in childhood. It is present in the arms but absent in the legs, so BP measurements of all four extremities are useful for diagnosis. Femoral pulses are weak and delayed when compared to the carotid or radial pulse. The ECG may show left ventricular hypertrophy. Treatment is through surgical correction.

Congenital Heart Disease

Congenital heart defects occur in about 1% of all children (Fig. 2-1). They may result in **left-to-right shunts**, in which blood that has been through the lungs is shunted back to the venous side of the heart and goes through the lungs again, or **right-to-left shunts**, in

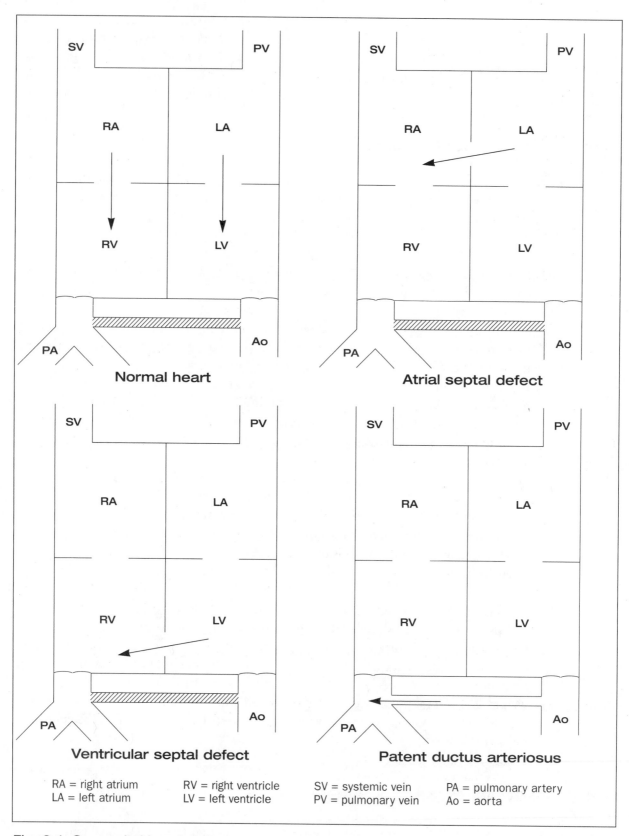

Fig. 2-1. Congenital heart defects.

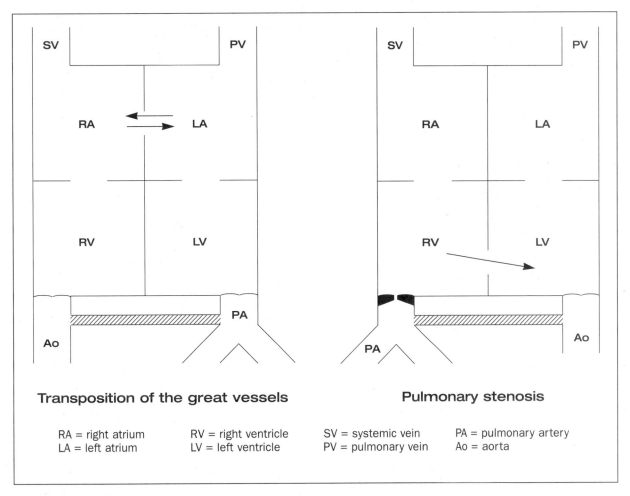

Transposition of the great vessels   Pulmonary stenosis

RA = right atrium   RV = right ventricle   SV = systemic vein   PA = pulmonary artery
LA = left atrium   LV = left ventricle   PV = pulmonary vein   Ao = aorta

Fig. 2-1. (continued)

which blood that has not been oxygenated in the lungs goes directly into the arterial circulation. Intrauterine risk factors for congenital heart disease include alcohol and drug use, exogenous hormones (e.g., birth control pills), lithium, and congenital infection.

Atrial Septal Defect

Atrial septal defect (ASD) describes an opening between the left atrium and right atrium, usually due to a patent foramen ovale. This condition usually results in a left-to-right shunt, so that blood volume is increased on the right side.

SIGNS & SYMPTOMS

A systolic ejection murmur is usually heard at the pulmonic area (second intercostal space to the left of the sternum). This results from increased blood velocity in the pulmonary artery. The hallmark heart sound is a widely split, fixed S2, due to increased right-sided blood volume delaying closure of the pulmonic valve.

ECG may show right ventricular conduction abnormalities. Echocardiography is usually diagnostic.

Very small defects may not need treatment. Larger ones require surgical correction.

Ventricular Septal Defect

Ventricular septal defect (VSD) describes an opening between the left and the right ventricles, usually due to a defect in the interventricular septum. VSD is the most common type of congenital cardiac defect. It results in a left-to-right shunt due to the greater power of the left ventricle.

The hallmark heart sound is a pansystolic murmur, heard best along the left sternal border. A thrill (vibration felt with a hand on the patient's chest) is commonly associated with the murmur.

ECG may show left and/or right ventricular hypertrophy. Echocardiography is diagnostic.

Small ventricular septal defects may need no treatment, but larger defects require surgical repair. About 25% of patients will develop **Eisenmenger's syndrome**, a condition in which the direction of the shunt becomes reversed (left-to-right shunt becomes right-to-left) due to increased pulmonary vascular resistance. This situation results in cyanosis and, eventually, heart failure.

Patent Ductus Arteriosus

Patent ductus arteriosus (PDA) occurs when the ductus arteriosus, a bypass that shunts blood from the pulmonary artery to the aorta during fetal life, does not close properly. This state results in a left-to-right shunt due to the greater systemic BP.

The hallmark heart sound is a continuous "machinery" murmur throughout systole and diastole. A thrill may also be felt, and a widened pulse pressure may be noted on blood pressure measurement.

ECG shows left ventricular hypertrophy. Echocardiography is diagnostic. Cardiac catheterization may also be used to establish the presence and severity of a shunt.

Indomethacin injection may produce closure in the first few days of life. Small PDAs may not require correction. If correction is necessary in later life, surgical ligation of the ductus may be performed.

Transposition of the Great Vessels

In transposition of the great vessels, the aorta arises from the right ventricle and the pulmonary trunk arises from the left ventricle, resulting in a "transposition" of normal anatomy. There is usually an ASD allowing oxygenated and deoxygenated blood to mix. Without an ASD, this defect is incompatible with life.

Newborns with transposition show extreme cyanosis immediately after birth, but most newborns are otherwise healthy.

Chest x-ray reveals narrowing of the base of the heart, and the normal pulmonary artery markings may be absent. Diagnosis is confirmed with echocardiography and catheterization.

Immediate palliative treatment includes balloon septostomy or a prostaglandin injection, allowing the ASD to remain open. Surgical correction is performed later in infancy.

Tetralogy of Fallot

Tetralogy of Fallot is a classic syndrome that consists of four abnormalities: VSD, right ventricular hypertrophy, pulmonary stenosis, and an overriding aorta. Because of the pulmonary stenosis, there is a right-to-left shunt, with passage of deoxygenated blood from the right ventricle to the left ventricle and into the systemic circulation.

Depending on the severity of the pulmonary blood flow restriction, infants may develop cyanosis and a right ventricular ejection murmur shortly after birth. Associated symptoms include anxiety, "air hunger," and changes in level of consciousness, especially after activity.

Chest x-ray shows a small heart and concave pulmonary artery segment. ECG shows right ventricular hypertrophy and right axis deviation. Diagnosis is confirmed with echocardiography and catheterization.

Prostaglandin injections may be given initially to maintain a PDA and preserve the flow of oxygenated blood into the systemic circulation. Surgical correction is the definitive treatment.

Pulmonary Stenosis

Pulmonary stenosis results when the pulmonary valve cusps are fused together or the pulmonary trunk is very small and obstructive to blood flow. There may be an associated ASD or VSD, which results in a right-to-left shunt.

The hallmark heart sound is a high-pitched systolic murmur with a soft or absent S2. Since the pulmonic valve is nonfunctional, the pulmonic component of S2 is weak. A parasternal lift and prominent thrill may also be noted.

ECG shows right ventricular hypertrophy. Echocardiography is diagnostic.

If mild, no treatment may be needed. Severe stenosis, however, can cause heart failure or sudden death. Treatment consists of balloon valvuloplasty to enlarge the pulmonic valve.

Endocardial Cushion Defect

The endocardial cushions are embryonic structures necessary for normal development of the atrioventricular valves, atrial septum, and ventricular septum. Malformation of these cushions may result in complex combinations of valvular and septal defects. One frequent manifestation is a common atrioventricular (AV) canal, a defect producing a two-chambered heart in which the atria are connected by an ASD, the ventricles are connected by a VSD, and only one AV valve exists. Another frequent manifestation is an ostium primum defect, in which an ASD is associated with minor AV valve abnormalities.

Signs and symptoms depend on the exact defects present but are generally those of ASD and VSD (described above). Mitral and tricuspid valve murmurs are also common.

ECG may show distinctive axis deviations, depending on the defect present. Echocardiography and cardiac catheterization are diagnostic, revealing the valvular and septal abnormalities.

The need for treatment depends on the severity of the defect. Surgical treatment may be required to prevent congestive heart failure in later life. Patients who do not receive appropriate treatment may later develop Eisenmenger's syndrome, in which severely increased pulmonary resistance results in a directional change of shunted blood.

Coarctation of the Aorta

Coarctation of the aorta is a localized narrowing of the aortic arch immediately distal to the origin of the left subclavian artery. A bicuspid aortic valve is present in 25% of cases.

Hypertension is present in the arms but not in the legs. Femoral pulses are weak and delayed when compared to upper-extremity pulses. Patients may have leg claudication on exertion. On exam, a midsystolic or continuous murmur is heard best in the back. A diastolic murmur caused by aortic insufficiency (due to bicuspid valves) may be present.

ECG reveals left ventricular hypertrophy. X-ray may show "scalloping" of ribs due to enlarged intercostal arteries. These vessels provide collateral circulation from the internal thoracic artery. MRI and cardiac catheterization are used for definitive diagnosis.

All patients under age 20 should undergo resection of the stenosed portion of the aorta. Patients under 40 should have surgery if other cardiac risk factors are great (e.g., uncontrolled hypertension). Patients over 50 generally do not undergo surgery because the risks involved are high.

Inflammatory Conditions

Rheumatic Fever

Rheumatic fever is a complication that occurs 1–4 weeks following an infection with group A *Streptococcus* (*S. pyogenes*). Current theories suggest that streptococcal infections can induce the generation of auto-antibodies that attack the heart valves and joints. In Western countries, the incidence of rheumatic fever is extremely low due to sanitation and antibiotic treatment of streptococcal infections, but it remains a major public health problem in developing countries. Attack rates are about 3% in patients with untreated exudative streptococcal pharyngitis.

A migratory arthritis, with hot, painful, swollen joints, is the most common manifestation. Endocarditis, which can result in permanent mitral or aortic regurgitation or stenosis, and pericarditis may also be present. Other manifestations include subcutaneous nodules on extensor surfaces, chorea, and erythema marginatum, a transient, painless rash.

Laboratory evaluation reveals an increased sedimentation rate and an elevated white blood cell (WBC) count. Diagnosis relies on the presence of clinical manifestations in the setting of a recent streptococcal infection, which is reflected by elevated antistreptolysin O titers.

Aspirin is the treatment of choice, although severe carditis may require corticosteroids. If severe, cardiac damage may result in long-term scarring and subsequent heart failure. Patients should be given antibiotic prophylaxis before receiving dental work or surgery to prevent bacterial endocarditis.

Currently, prevention guidelines advocate throat cultures in all patients with pharyngitis. If the culture is positive for group A streptococci, patients should receive a 10-day course of penicillin. Erythromycin can substitute for penicillin in penicillin-allergic patients. This treatment prevents rheumatic fever even if started several days after the onset of pharyngitis.

Bacterial Endocarditis

Bacterial infection of the heart lining or valves can result in temporary or permanent damage. This condition is seen most often in patients with preexisting heart abnormalities (e.g., congenital defects or damage from rheumatic disease), in intravenous (IV) drug users, or in patients with prosthetic heart valves, although patients without these risk factors may also be affected.

Acute bacterial endocarditis (ABE) is usually caused by *Staphylococcus aureus*, *Streptococcus* (group A or *Streptococcus pneumoniae*), and *Neisseria gonorrhoeae*. Subacute bacterial endocarditis (SBE) is usually caused by streptococcal species, including viridans *Streptococcus*, and often occurs on abnormal or artificial valves following bacteremia.

Both ABE and SBE are characterized by fevers, chills, night sweats, fatigue, weight loss, and arthralgias, although the course of SBE is much more indolent than that of ABE. Physical exam is significant for new heart murmurs, petechiae over the upper half of the body, and splinter hemorrhages under the fingernails. Other manifestations include Osler's nodes (painful, red nodules on the tips of fingers and toes) and Roth's spots (hemorrhagic retinal lesions). These physical signs are due to small septic emboli from the infected vegetation, which can also cause infarcts or abscesses in the brain, kidney, and other organs.

Risk factors, such as artificial valves or IV drug use, combined with the above presentation suggest the diagnosis. Blood cultures should be drawn to check for bacteremia, although negative cultures do not rule out the diagnosis. Echocardiography may show vegetations on the valvular leaflets.

Rapid antibiotic treatment is essential, since fatality rates can be high, depending on the organism. Antibiotics are necessary for several weeks following the infection, regardless of clinical resolution of symptoms. If valves are permanently damaged, artificial valves may need to be placed surgically.

Major attention must be paid to patients with abnormal or prosthetic valves who undergo dental or surgical procedures, since these often cause transient bacteremia. Prophylactic antibiotics should be given before these procedures.

Noninfective Endocarditis

In noninfective endocarditis, fibrin and thrombi can form vegetations on the heart valves even in the absence of an infectious cause. This type of endocarditis often results from trauma, deposition of immune complexes, and hypercoagulability. One frequent type of noninfectious endocarditis is Libman-Sacks disease, which strikes up to 40% of patients with systemic lupus erythematosus (SLE). Libman-Sacks disease is characterized by platelet and fibrin vegetations on the valvular leaflets. Sequelae of noninfective endocarditis include emboli and vascular obstruction.

Patients are often asymptomatic but may have audible regurgitant murmurs on exam. Arterial emboli may result in stroke or other tissue infarction.

Blood cultures to rule out bacterial endocarditis will be negative. Echocardiography may reveal vegetations on the valves. The presence of an associated disease, such as SLE, also suggests the diagnosis.

Treatment involves anticoagulation with heparin and coumadin. Infectious endocarditis must be ruled out, since inadvertent anticoagulation of infected patients can lead to severe hemorrhage and death.

Cardiovascular Treatment Issues

Dietary Measures

Diet plays a large role in the development of heart disease. Initial treatment for most acquired heart diseases involves dietary restrictions. In general, salt intake should be maintained between 4.5 and 6.0 g per day, serum cholesterol less than 300 mg per day, and fat intake less than 30% of total caloric intake. Since most dietary modifications require the development of new, lifelong habits, however, the success of dietary treatment measures is quite variable and depends primarily on patient motivation.

Medication

Only about half of patients who take antihypertensive medications are compliant after 1 year, and rates are similar for other cardiac medications. Lack of compliance should be considered when there is insufficient improvement in the patient's condition. If necessary, compliance can be checked with pill counts and blood tests. Other issues that may affect compliance are the cost of the drug, the dosing schedule (the more often it needs to be taken, the lower the compliance), and possible side effects.

Special Concerns of the Elderly

Many patients with chronic cardiac conditions are elderly and require special attention. Falling is a major concern in the elderly, so drugs with side effects such as orthostatic hypotension and sedation should be monitored. The orthostatic hypotension associated

Table 2-2. Strategies for medical visits with the elderly

1. Review all medications. Ask the patient to bring all pill bottles to each medical visit.
2. Question patients regarding their use of over-the-counter drugs. More than 75% of older patients are frequent users, and they may be unaware of potential interactions of their prescription medications.
3. Assess the benefits and side effects of each medication and reduce their total number or dosage if possible.
4. If possible, select medications that are not centrally acting, that do not cause postural hypotension, and that have shorter durations of action.
5. Ensure that the patient's symptoms are not caused by other drugs.
6. Initiate medications at dosages lower than the usual adult dosage, since metabolism and clearance rates are generally lower in the elderly. Serum albumin levels are also decreased, so albumin-bound drugs may reach toxic concentrations at lower doses.

Table 2-3. Common drugs and their drug reactions in the elderly

Drug type	Side effect
Blood pressure drugs	Postural hypotension
Digitalis	Toxicity, depression, confusion, anorexia (can occur even at therapeutic levels)
Anticoagulants	Increased risk of bleeding after minor falls
Diuretics	Dehydration (do not routinely give for ankle edema; use compression stockings)

with antihypertensives frequently precipitates falls. The patient's state of hydration and visual acuity are also important considerations. Since many elderly patients have more than one chronic condition, polypharmacy may become a major concern and should be monitored carefully to reduce side effects. Table 2-2 discusses strategies for medical visits with elderly patients. A list of common drug reactions in the elderly is presented in Table 2-3.

Common Symptoms of Heart Disease

Palpitations are the perception of the heartbeat by the patient. Palpitations can be associated with cardiac and noncardiac conditions, including anxiety, anemia, and thyrotoxicosis. They may also be a symptom of cardiac valve disorders or arrhythmias.

Dyspnea is a sensation of difficulty breathing. Dyspnea associated with cardiac conditions usually occurs on exertion and indicates the presence of systolic dysfunction or valvular disease. Orthopnea (dyspnea while lying down) arises because of increased venous return to the heart. Patients often sleep on a number of pillows because elevation of the head can relieve the orthopnea. Paroxysmal nocturnal dyspnea refers to a sudden episode of difficulty breathing that awakens the patient from sleep and is relieved by sitting or standing.

(continued)

Cyanosis is a bluish-gray discoloration of the skin due to a lack of oxygen. Poorly oxygenated blood may result from anemia or hypoventilation. Cyanosis in newborns may indicate a congenital defect. Cyanosis of the fingers and hands may be indicative of Raynaud's phenomenon, idiopathic vasoconstriction, or complex rheumatic diseases.

Edema is an excessive extravascular fluid accumulation. In patients with cardiac disease, dependent edema is generally attributable to heart failure. Signs include dependent swelling of legs, ascites, and pulmonary edema.

Syncope (fainting) refers to a transient loss of consciousness. Generally, patients complain of lightheadedness, nausea, and sweating. Cardiovascular causes include arrhythmias, flow obstruction, and arteriovenous (AV) blocks. The most common etiology of syncope is vasovagal faints, due to increased vagal tone. Other common causes are orthostatic hypotension and hyperventilation. It is important to differentiate syncope from possible seizure disorders.

Fatigue is a sensation of tiredness, not unlike what you're experiencing now as you prepare for the Boards. It is an extremely common presenting symptom, with many possible etiologies. A good history often reveals a likely cause for fatigue, such as inadequate rest, poor nutrition, or excessive stress. However, it is important to also consider endocrine disorders, anemia, rheumatic diseases, and depression. Cardiac causes of fatigue occur with overwork of the heart and may result in inadequate cardiac perfusion or in heart failure.

Chest pain can be caused by cardiac disease, pleuritic pain, esophageal/gastrointestinal pain, or chest wall pain. Cardiac pain, such as that stemming from angina, heart attack, or pericardial disease, is described in more detail later in this chapter. Pleuritic pain is aggravated by deep breathing. Esophageal and gastric pain usually result from esophageal reflux, although chest pain may be seen in the context of gastritis, peptic ulcer disease, and pancreatitis. Chest wall pain refers to musculoskeletal discomfort and is usually benign.

General Clinical Conditions

Premature (Ectopic) Beats

Premature beats are caused by the generation of an impulse from outside the sinoatrial node. Classifications include supraventricular ectopics, which denote a beat arising from the atria, and ventricular ectopics, which denote a beat of ventricular origin. Common causes of ectopic beats include caffeine and nicotine, but ectopic beats are often idiopathic. Ectopic beats, however, may signify the presence of a more serious cardiac arrhythmia or other disorder.

Sinus Bradycardia

Sinus bradycardia is defined as sinus rhythm with a heart rate of less than 50 beats per minute (bpm). In healthy individuals and well-conditioned athletes, bradycardia is a normal finding; however, bradycardia in

(continued)

elderly or cardiac patients may be associated with syncope, and may exacerbate ectopic arrhythmias. Some individuals may require a pacemaker.

Diastolic Dysfunction

Difficulty in the filling of the ventricles in diastolic dysfunction usually occurs from fibrosis or scarring, resulting from extensive hypertrophy or from previous ischemic attacks. This results in backup of blood flow and vascular congestion. Diastolic dysfunction can occur in isolation, without significant changes in systolic performance.

Systolic Dysfunction

Difficulty in the ejection of blood from the ventricles in systolic dysfunction can be due to decreased contractile function, abnormalities of the ventricular wall, or obstructed outflow. It generally results from valvular abnormalities or ventricular ischemia, usually caused by chronic coronary artery disease (CAD) and myocardial infarctions (MIs). The resulting decrease in cardiac output may lead to congestive heart failure.

Hypovolemia

Hypovolemia refers to a condition of decreased intravascular fluid volume or blood supply. Direct blood losses (e.g., hemorrhage) or other fluid losses (e.g., excessive vomiting or diarrhea) may cause the decrease in volume. Inadequate fluid intake, especially in the elderly or homeless, is another frequent etiology. Iatrogenic causes, such as diuretic use, are also common. Physical manifestations of hypovolemia include loss of skin turgor, postural hypotension, and tachycardia. Treatment consists of rehydration. IV fluids are necessary if the patient cannot tolerate oral intake or if dehydration is severe. The hematocrit should be followed closely. It may initially be normal or even high due to hemoconcentration, but may drop rapidly with rehydration.

Cardiac Arrest

In cardiac arrest, complete cessation of spontaneous cardiac contractions results in the loss of systemic circulation. Cardiac arrest presents with loss of consciousness, pulselessness, and cyanosis. Common causes are ventricular fibrillation, shock, and respiratory depression.

Arterial Diseases

Aortic Aneurysm

An aortic aneurysm is an abnormal, localized dilatation of the aorta. Most aortic aneurysms occur in the abdomen and are usually caused by atherosclerosis, which gradually weakens the vascular wall. Hypertension, smoking, a family history of abdominal aneurysms, trauma, and vasculitis may also be contributing factors. Marfan's syndrome and syphilis are primary causes of thoracic aortic aneurysms but may cause abdominal aneurysms as well.

Patients with abdominal aneurysms are often asymptomatic but may complain of a deep, boring pain in the lower back. On exam, a pulsating, tender mass in the abdomen may be palpated. Thoracic aneurysms may be associated with hemoptysis, dysphagia, hoarseness, and cough, due to compression of adjacent structures.

Abdominal x-ray may reveal aortic calcifications. Ultrasound can help localize and assess the size of the aneurysm. Aortography, CT, and MRI may provide additional information. Thoracic aneurysms can also be assessed with transesophageal ultrasound.

Treatment depends on the size of the aneurysm. For abdominal aneurysms, surgical repair is generally recommended for aneurysms larger than 4 cm in diameter; aneurysms smaller than 4 cm are not at high risk for rupture. Thoracic aneurysms should be resected if greater than 7 cm; however, aneurysms in Marfan's syndrome should be removed at smaller sizes because of their tendency to rupture. Surgery consists of resection of the aneurysmal portion and replacement with a synthetic graft.

Dissecting Aortic Aneurysm

Dissection of an aortic aneurysm is a disease characterized by a splitting of the aortic wall between the medial and adventitial layers. Hypertension producing degenerative changes of the aortic wall causes most dissections, but congenital tissue disorders may also contribute.

Patients complain of the sudden onset of a tearing or "ripping" in their chest. Physical exam reveals weak or absent pulses and the murmur of aortic insufficiency, due to disruption of the valve.

Differentiation between a dissecting aneurysm and an MI is crucial, since treatments differ. Increased WBC count is a common but nonspecific finding of dissecting aneurysm. Anemia may also be noted if significant bleeding occurs into the space created by the separation of tissue layers. While the ECG is abnormal in an MI, it is generally normal in dissecting aneurysms. Chest x-ray shows a widening of the aorta. As with all aneurysms, ultrasound, CT, and aortography can provide a definitive diagnosis.

Mortality from dissecting aneurysms is extremely high, so patients should be monitored in the intensive care unit and given medications that reduce cardiac contractility. Surgery is indicated in almost all cases.

Peripheral Arterial Vascular Disease

Peripheral arterial vascular disease refers to arterial occlusion in the extremities, usually as a result of atherosclerosis. The resulting ischemia may be acute or chronic. Chronic ischemia of the lower extremities may result in **intermittent claudication**, in which an exercising muscle receives insufficient oxygenated blood. This condition may progress to complete occlusion of the vessel over time. Acute occlusion may also occur, usually as a result of embolization of an atherosclerotic plaque. Diabetics have an increased risk of developing arterial vascular disease due to changes in their microvascular circulation.

The classic pentad of peripheral ischemia consists of "the 5 Ps": **p**ain, **p**allor, **p**ulselessness, **p**aresthesias, and (in late stages) **p**aralysis. Associated findings are ulcerations and dry skin with poor hair and nail growth. The patient may complain of exercise-associated muscle pain and weakness.

The above signs and symptoms, especially in the context of systemic atherosclerosis (e.g., a history of MI), should suggest the diagnosis. X-rays are generally not helpful. Doppler ultrasound is fairly accurate in assessing the extent of occlusion.

Patients with intermittent claudication should begin a regimen of daily walking to increase collateral circulation. Patients at risk for developing progressive ischemia (such as diabetics) should be taught to perform daily foot inspection and care to detect and prevent ulceration. Primary disorders, such as diabetes, should be well controlled. Clots that develop may be treated with angioplasty or bypass grafting. Significant or prolonged ischemia may require amputation.

Functional Arterial Vascular Disorders

The set of functional arterial vascular disorders describes conditions resulting from excessive vascular constriction or spasm. Raynaud's phenomenon and acrocyanosis are the most frequently seen functional arterial vascular disorders.

Raynaud's phenomenon consists of pallor and cyanosis of the fingers and toes, often followed by reddening due to compensatory hyperemia. It is caused by vasospasm of the digital arteries. Most cases of Raynaud's phenomenon are idiopathic, occurring predominantly in young women. It is also seen in SLE and other connective tissue disorders. Mild cases may need no medical treatment, but the extremities should be kept warm if possible. More severe cases may be treated with vasodilators.

Acrocyanosis involves pallor and cyanosis of the hands and feet secondary to vasospasm of the microcirculation. Aside from keeping the extremities warm, no treatment exists. Vasodilators are ineffective.

Mitral Valve Disorders

Mitral Stenosis

Mitral stenosis describes narrowing and calcification of the mitral valve, resulting in obstructed blood flow from the left atrium to the left ventricle. The continued resistance to flow results in left atrial enlargement, and the backup of this flow results in pulmonary hypertension and right ventricular hypertrophy. Rheumatic fever causes almost all cases of mitral stenosis.

Symptoms usually occur 10–20 years after the stenosis has developed. Progressive dyspnea and fatigue are common, although patients with severe mitral stenosis can be completely asymptomatic. Auscultation reveals an "opening snap" after S2, followed by a low-pitched, diastolic rumble. Patients may exhibit a reddish-purple rash across the cheekbones (mitral facies).

The clinical presentation is suggestive of mitral stenosis. Depending on the advancement of disease, ECG may show left atrial enlargement and right ventricular hypertrophy. Chest x-ray may also show left atrial enlargement, as well as calcification of the mitral valve. Echocardiography confirms the diagnosis.

Beta-blockers and calcium channel blockers decrease heart rate and reduce preload. Symptoms of right heart failure should be treated with diuretics. Significant atrial enlargement may precipitate atrial fibrillation, which may require anticoagulation. Surgical valvuloplasty or valve replacement provides long-term relief.

Mitral Regurgitation

Mitral regurgitation occurs when the mitral valve becomes incompetent, resulting in systolic backflow of blood from the left ventricle into the left atrium. It usually results from mitral valve prolapse, in which part of the mitral valve is "floppy" and falls back into the atrium. Other causes include rheumatic fever and dysfunction of the papillary muscle or chordae tendineae.

Patients may complain of palpitations or dyspnea on exertion; however, many remain asymptomatic. On auscultation, a harsh, blowing, holosystolic murmur is heard at the apex. S2 may be widely split, but it will widen normally on inspiration. Mitral valve prolapse is associated with a midsystolic click.

Chest x-ray shows left atrial enlargement and left ventricular hypertrophy. Echocardiography provides the definitive diagnosis.

Beta-blockers provide symptomatic relief, but valve replacement is indicated. Because mitral valve abnormalities are associated with endocarditis, prophylactic antibiotics are indicated for procedures that might produce bacteremia (e.g., surgery, dental visits).

Aortic Valve Disorders

Aortic Stenosis

Aortic stenosis describes narrowing of the aortic outflow tract, resulting in obstructed blood flow from the left ventricle to the aorta and systemic circulation. Aortic stenosis almost always results from congenital bicuspid aortic valves, present in 1% of the population, which undergo progressive fibrosis and calcification. Other causes include sclerosis and calcification in the elderly and rheumatic heart disease.

The classic triad of symptoms is angina, dyspnea on exertion, and syncope. The patient's pulse is often weak and prolonged, and a crescendo-decrescendo systolic ejection murmur is frequently heard at the left sternal border, radiating to the carotid arteries.

ECG indicates left ventricular hypertrophy and may show T-wave inversion. Chest x-ray may reveal a calcified aortic valve and a dilated ascending aorta. Echocardiography or cardiac catheterization provides the definitive diagnosis.

Beta-blockers can help slow heart rate and improve coronary flow. If symptoms are severe, valvuloplasty or valve replacement is indicated. Stenosis often recurs after valvuloplasty.

Aortic Regurgitation

Aortic regurgitation occurs when the aortic valve becomes incompetent, resulting in diastolic backflow of blood from the aorta into the left ventricle. In children, the most common cause is a congenital ventricular septal defect with associated aortic valve prolapse. In adults, the most common cause of mild aortic regurgitation is a bicuspid aortic valve. Rheumatic heart disease, tertiary syphilis, and idiopathic degeneration are the most common causes of severe aortic regurgitation.

Dyspnea on exertion, angina, and orthopnea may be present, although most patients remain asymptomatic for many years. On physical exam, a "water hammer" pulse may be noted, characterized by a rapid upstroke and downstroke. This pulse may be heard as a "pistol shot" over the femoral arteries. A widened pulse pressure (difference between the systolic and the diastolic BPs) may also be present. A pulsatile whitening of the fingernails may be elicited under slight pressure (Quincke's sign).

On cardiac exam, a pandiastolic decrescendo murmur may be heard best at the second intercostal space. An additional diastolic rumble (Austin-Flint murmur) may be noted as the blood flowing through the incompetent aortic valve strikes the mitral valve.

Chest x-ray usually reveals an enlarged heart with a dilated aorta. ECG tracings are usually consistent with left ventricular hypertrophy. Echocardiography and catheterization are diagnostic.

Medical management consists of afterload reduction with ACE inhibitors, calcium channel blockers, or nitrates. Digitalis can increase stroke volume and cardiac output. Valve replacement surgery is the therapy of choice if the patient begins to develop heart failure.

Vasculitis

Vasculitis refers to inflammation of the blood vessels. In addition to the etiologies listed below, vasculitis may occur as part of connective tissue syndromes, such as systemic lupus erythematosus, which are described in more detail in Chap. 14.

Polyarteritis Nodosa

Polyarteritis nodosa is the inflammation of medium-sized muscular arteries, followed by ischemia in the tissues supplied by these arteries. The condition is idiopathic but may be related to hypersensitivity reactions to drugs and viruses. Men are afflicted three times more often than women. While it usually occurs between the ages of 40 and 50, polyarteritis nodosa can strike at any age. Affected organs include the kidneys, liver, heart, and gastrointestinal (GI) tract.

SIGNS & SYMPTOMS

Common symptoms include fever, abdominal pain, neuropathy, weight loss, and asthma. On exam, hypertension and edema may be noted.

LABS

Elevated WBC count, proteinuria, and hematuria are common.

DIAGNOSIS

Because there are no laboratory tests specific to polyarteritis, diagnosis must be confirmed with either biopsy of necrosed areas or angiography revealing aneurysms of medium-sized vessels.

TREATMENT

Possible causative medications should be discontinued. Long-term therapy with corticosteroids and other immunosuppressive agents may be necessary.

Giant Cell Arteritis

Also known as temporal arteritis, giant cell arteritis is characterized by chronic inflammation of the large blood vessels, primarily the carotid and cranial arteries. Giant cell arteritis becomes frequent (1 per 1,000) after age 50, and women are more likely to develop it than men. Severe sequelae such as blindness occur in up to 20% of patients.

SIGNS & SYMPTOMS

Symptoms include severe temporal or occipital headaches and visual disturbances, such as amaurosis fugax (transient blindness in one eye), blurring, and diplopia. Systemic complaints, including arthritis, fever, and weight loss, may also be present. On physical exam, the temporal artery may be swollen, tender, and nodular. There may be an associated bruit.

Diagnosis is made by clinical presentation and is confirmed with temporal artery biopsy. Angiography may assist in the diagnosis.

Because of the risk of blindness, treatment should be initiated immediately if the diagnosis is suspected. Treatment consists of high-dose corticosteroids or other immunosuppressive agents for several weeks to months.

Venous Diseases

Varicose Veins

Varicose veins are superficial veins that have developed incompetent valves, resulting in elongation and reversed blood flow.

Varicose veins may be asymptomatic or may cause aching pain, fatigue, or warmth. Symptoms resolve with leg elevation. Varicose veins may not always be visible, but they may be palpated. Symptoms do not necessarily correspond to the size of the varicosities. Complications include pigmentation (due to blood stasis), eczema, edema, and ulceration.

Diagnosis can be made by visual inspection and clinical presentation. The Trendelenburg test is performed by raising the affected leg above the level of the heart and quickly lowering it. Immediate distention of the leg veins indicates valvular incompetency.

Nonsurgical management includes compression hosiery and leg elevation. Surgical removal of the saphenous veins is discouraged, since they may be required for later bypass graft surgery. Injection sclerotherapy may be performed for both cosmetic and therapeutic reasons.

Arteriovenous Fistula

An arteriovenous (AV) fistula is an abnormal communication between an artery and a vein. This may be congenital or acquired (e.g., in the case of trauma). Superficial AV fistulas may be palpated as warm, pulsating masses, accompanied by a thrill. Signs and symptoms may include ischemia, edema, pigmentation, and varicosities. Embolic complications may arise. Surgery is the treatment of choice.

Deep Venous Thrombosis and Thrombophlebitis

Deep venous thrombosis (DVT) refers to the development of a blood clot in a vein. Thrombophlebitis refers to a secondary inflammation of the clot, resulting in pain, tenderness, and warmth. These symptoms most often occur in the lower extremities. The risk factors that predispose to the development of venous thrombi are referred to as Virchow's triad: injury to the endothelium of the vessel (e.g., trauma), hypercoagulable states (e.g., malignancy, estrogen use), and stasis (e.g., postoperative states).

Budd-Chiari syndrome refers to obstruction of the hepatic vein, usually by thrombosis, as a consequence of the risk factors described above. Patients may experience abdominal pain, ascites, and jaundice over a period of weeks to months. Treatment involves anticoagulation and surgical decompression.

Patients may be asymptomatic or may complain of pain, tenderness, swelling, and warmth of the affected areas. They may also note pain and soreness when walking, which is relieved on leg elevation. A positive Homan's sign (pain on simultaneous foot dorsiflexion and leg elevation) may be present, but this is an unreliable sign of DVT.

The presence of a risk factor combined with the above symptoms suggests the diagnosis. Venography, ultrasound, and plethysmography can confirm the diagnosis but may not be necessary if the clinical evidence is strong.

Superficial thrombophlebitis may require only nonsteroidal anti-inflammatory drugs (NSAIDs) and warm compresses over the involved area. Deep venous thrombi usually require antithrombotic therapy involving acute IV heparin for 1–2 weeks, bringing the partial thromboplastin time (PTT) to twice its normal value, followed by chronic warfarin therapy for several months, maintaining the prothrombin time (PT) at approximately twice its normal value. Thrombolytic therapy, such as streptokinase, is effective only within the first few hours of acute thrombus formation. DVTs should be aggressively treated to prevent the severe complication of pulmonary embolism.

Thromboembolic Disease

In thromboembolic disease, vessels are blocked by clots that have broken loose from a distant source (emboli) or by clots that have formed locally (thrombi). Thromboembolic disease, including stroke, pulmonary embolism, and MI, is one of the leading causes of death in the United States. As in DVTs, Virchow's triad identifies the three factors that can contribute to thromboembolic disease: stasis, hypercoagulable states, and endothelial injury.

Symptoms depend on the location of the clot. MIs cause chest pain and are discussed in detail later in this chapter. Stroke is associated with headache, neurological deficits, and changes in consciousness, and is discussed in more detail in Chap. 15. Pulmonary embolism causes shortness of breath and chest pain and is discussed in Chap. 3.

Clinical manifestations of vascular occlusion in a patient with risk factors for thromboembolic disease (Table 2-4) suggest the diagnosis. Ultrasound, radioactive isotope scanning, and plethysmography aid in localization of the clot.

Table 2-4. Risk factors for thromboembolic disease

Heart disease (especially arrhythmias)
Malignancy
Trauma (including surgery)
Pregnancy or immediate postpartum
Exogenous estrogens
Immobility (leading to blood stasis)
Increasing age
History of previous thromboembolisms

Thrombolytic therapy, such as streptokinase or tissue plasminogen activator (tPA), may be helpful during or immediately after clot formation. Heparin and coumadin may be used to inhibit coagulation.

Prevention strategies for high-risk patients include pneumatic compression stockings, aspirin, and subcutaneous heparin administration. Filters placed in large veins, such as the inferior vena cava, can catch emboli before they reach the lungs.

Arrhythmias

A normal ECG is shown (Fig. 2-2) for reference.

Atrial Flutter

Atrial flutter is caused by the firing of an ectopic focus in the atria, resulting in a rapid atrial firing rate (250–400 bpm). Most impulses are blocked at the AV node, so that the ventricular rate is a fraction of the atrial rate. Atrial flutter is usually associated with preexisting heart disease, including CAD, valvular disease, and pericardial disease.

Patients are usually asymptomatic but may experience palpitations, syncope, and lightheadedness at higher heart rates.

ECG tracing shows a characteristic "saw-tooth" appearance, made up of identical P waves generated by the ectopic atrial focus (Fig. 2-3).

Treatment involves slowing of the ventricular firing rate, if necessary, with digoxin and converting to sinus rhythm with chemical or electrical cardioversion.

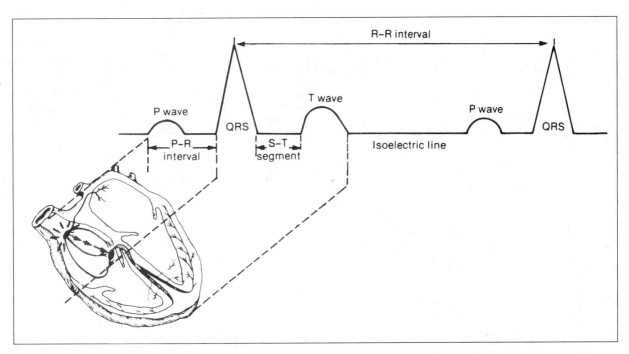

Fig. 2-2. A normal electrocardiogram. The P wave corresponds to atrial depolarization, and the QRS corresponds to ventricular depolarization. (From N Caroline. *Emergency Care in the Streets,* Fifth Edition. Boston: Little, Brown, 1995.)

Atrial Fibrillation

Atrial fibrillation occurs when atrial firing is rapid and disorderly. The irregular impulses reach the AV node and result in sporadic ventricular contraction. Because the atria do not contract efficiently, blood stasis occurs, promoting the formation of an atrial thrombus. This is a major concern, since the thrombus can be a source for pulmonary emboli, strokes, or other systemic emboli.

Patients are usually symptomatic and experience palpitations and chest discomfort. Shortness of breath, lightheadedness, and weakness are also common. The classic physical finding is an irregularly irregular pulse.

ECG tracing reveals an irregular baseline appearance with absent P waves (Fig. 2-4).

Treatment must address the restoration of sinus rhythm, the prevention of emboli, and the underlying cardiac disorder. Control of the ventricular rate is achieved with digoxin followed by cardioversion (either electrical or chemical). If there is evidence of thrombus formation, anticoagulation is required prior to cardioversion.

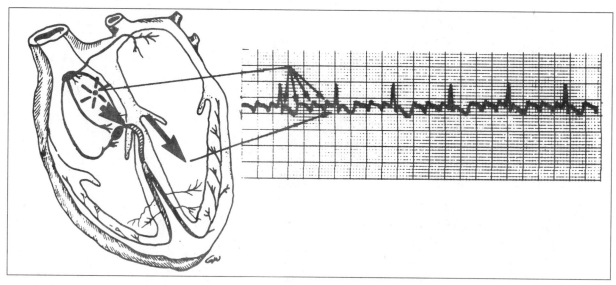

Fig. 2-3. Atrial flutter. (From N Caroline. *Emergency Care in the Streets*, Fifth Edition. Boston: Little, Brown, 1995.)

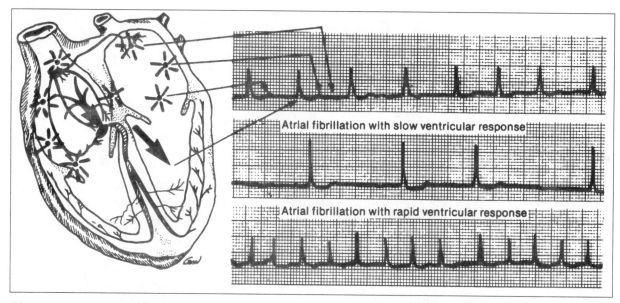

Fig. 2-4. Atrial fibrillation. (From N Caroline. *Emergency Care in the Streets*, Fifth Edition. Boston: Little, Brown, 1995.)

Premature Ventricular Contraction

Premature ventricular contractions (PVCs) are ectopic beats arising from ventricular foci. PVCs are quite common and may be benign in the absence of preexisting heart disease. PVCs on exertion or in the context of heart disease are more significant and may indicate a poor prognosis. Noncardiac causes of PVCs include hyperthyroidism, electrolyte abnormalities, stress, and (our favorite) caffeine. Arrhythmias in which every second or third beat is premature are known as bigeminy and trigeminy, respectively.

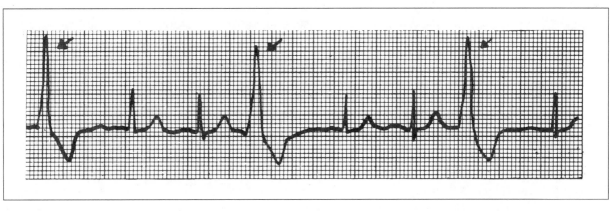

Fig. 2-5. Premature ventricular contractions. (From N Caroline. *Emergency Care in the Streets*, Fifth Edition. Boston: Little, Brown, 1995.)

Patients may be asymptomatic or may experience palpitations or syncope. On exam, extra or skipped beats may be noted.

SIGNS & SYMPTOMS

ECG shows extra QRS complexes that are not preceded by a P wave and are wider than normal QRS complexes (Fig. 2-5).

DIAGNOSIS

No treatment is needed if the patient is asymptomatic and has no cardiac disease. Patients who are symptomatic or have cardiac disease should be treated with beta-blockers or antiarrhythmics.

TREATMENT

Paroxysmal (Supraventricular) Tachycardia

Supraventricular tachycardia (SVT) refers to a rapid arrhythmia arising from the atria. It occurs most often in young patients with normal hearts. This type of arrhythmia is caused by a re-entry rhythm, in which a contractile impulse is repeatedly sent back to the atria through a signaling loop. In AV nodal re-entry, the most common cause, SVT arises from re-entry of a contractile impulse through the AV node. In Wolff-Parkinson-White (WPW) syndrome, a congenital disorder, conduction occurs through an accessory muscle bundle. While AV nodal re-entry is a fairly benign condition, WPW syndrome can precipitate ventricular fibrillation in a patient with atrial fibrillation.

Attacks are characterized by sudden onset and resolution, but they may last for several hours. Heart rate varies from 150 to 250 bpm. Patients may be asymptomatic or may experience mild chest pain, shortness of breath, and the sensation of a racing heart beat.

ECG shows tachycardia and a characteristic pattern of P waves hidden in T waves.

Carotid sinus massage or the Valsalva maneuver may stop the paroxysmal (supraventricular) tachycardia. Drugs such as calcium channel blockers, digoxin, or beta-blockers may help as well. WPW accessory pathways can be surgically ablated.

Ventricular Tachycardia

Defined as three or more consecutive premature ventricular contractions (PVCs), ventricular tachycardia is often associated with MI or other underlying cardiac diseases, although very brief episodes may be benign. The condition is called *torsades de pointes* when it is drug-induced.

As with PVCs, patients may be asymptomatic or experience skipped or extra beats, which also may be noted on physical exam.

ECG shows a series of PVCs, often accompanied by the independent presence of P waves (Fig. 2-6).

Drug treatment includes lidocaine and other antiarrhythmics. Persistent ventricular tachycardia in an unstable patient requires DC cardioversion.

Ventricular Fibrillation

Ventricular fibrillation describes a lack of ordered ventricular contraction, resulting in the absence of cardiac output; it is rapidly fatal. This condition is usually seen after a severe, acute MI, but it can also be seen in patients with "sudden death syndrome."

The lack of cardiac output causes the patient to faint. No pulses are appreciated on exam.

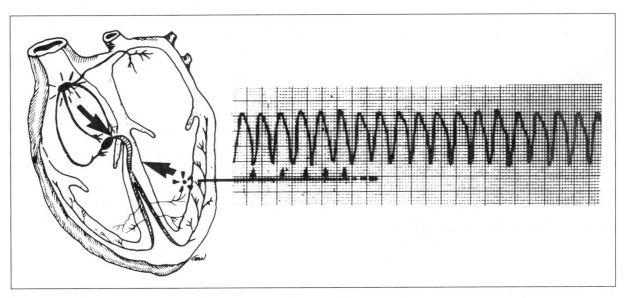

Fig. 2-6. Ventricular tachycardia. (From N Caroline. *Emergency Care in the Streets*, Fifth Edition. Boston: Little, Brown, 1995.)

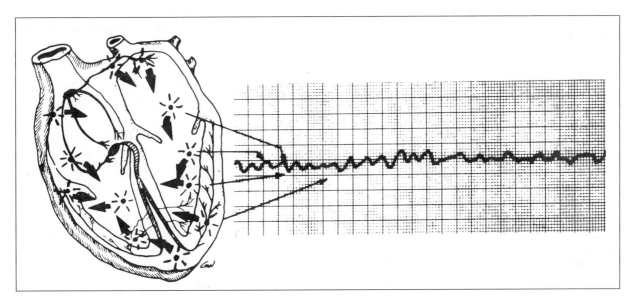

Fig. 2-7. Ventricular fibrillation. (From N Caroline. *Emergency Care in the Streets*, Fifth Edition. Boston: Little, Brown, 1995.)

DIAGNOSIS

Definitive diagnosis requires ECG, which reveals a totally erratic tracing with no identifiable P or QRS waves (Fig. 2-7).

TREATMENT

Call a code and begin cardiopulmonary resuscitation (CPR). Electrical defibrillation is usually necessary. Chemical cardioversion with IV lidocaine may be administered simultaneously.

Heart Failure

Congestive Heart Failure

The term *heart failure* describes a clinical syndrome that may result from many different conditions. Their common factor is the inability of the heart to meet the body's circulatory needs. Conditions that may result in heart failure include valvular heart disease, coronary artery disease, and myocardial heart disease. States that require increased cardiac output, such as anemia, thyrotoxicosis, and pregnancy, can also result in heart failure.

In **left-sided heart failure**, the left side of the heart is physiologically unable to keep up, resulting in left ventricular hypertrophy. Backup of blood into the lungs and subsequent pulmonary hypertension later develop. Conditions that precipitate left-sided failure include congenital defects, CAD, hypertension, and aortic valve disease.

In **right-sided heart failure**, right-sided compromise results in right ventricular hypertrophy and backup of blood into the venous system. The most common cause of right heart failure is left heart failure. Other causes include pulmonary hypertension (caused by factors other than left heart failure), valvular disorders, pulmonary emboli, and atrial septal defects.

Clinical manifestations of left-sided failure include fatigue, dyspnea on exertion, paroxysmal nocturnal dyspnea, orthopnea, and cough. Right-sided failure results in fatigue, neck vein distention, liver enlargement, and peripheral edema. Late-stage symptoms can include ascites, pleural effusions, and severe pitting edema of the lower extremities. The development of acute pulmonary edema is a medical emergency and is addressed in more detail in Chap. 3.

Pooling of blood in the atria during systole can result in an S3, an early diastolic sound that occurs due to rapid filling of the ventricles. An S4, a late diastolic sound caused by a noncompliant ventricle, may be heard due to abnormal relaxation of the hypertrophied ventricle. Both S3 and S4 can be heard in normal patients as well as in other medical conditions and are not specific to heart failure; however, an S3 is the most reliable predictor of heart failure.

Diagnosis may be evident from physical findings as well as from the presence of a precipitating medical condition. Chest x-ray shows increased vascular congestion and cardiac enlargement. Kerley B lines may be present and reflect thickening of the interlobular septa of the lungs from persistent edema. There are no specific ECG findings, but abnormal tracings may indicate the underlying disorder if it is cardiac.

Treatment of the underlying disorder may be possible for valvular disorders or noncardiac disorders such as thyrotoxicosis. Intravascular volume can be decreased with salt restriction and diuretics. Digoxin is given to increase myocardial force. Vasodilators, such as nitrates and ACE inhibitors, are used to reduce preload and afterload.

Cor Pulmonale

Cor pulmonale refers to enlargement of the right ventricle due to pulmonary hypertension, which arises from a reduction of the lung vascular bed or from pulmonary arterial vasoconstriction. The most common underlying pulmonary disorder is reduction of the lung vascular bed. Chronic obstructive pulmonary disease (COPD) is the most common cause of cor pulmonale.

Dyspnea on exertion is the most common symptom. Syncope on exertion, anginal symptoms, and murmurs due to right-sided valvular incompetence may also be present. Signs and symptoms of right-sided heart failure, such as an S3 and S4, distended neck veins, hepatic engorgement, and edema, may be noted in later stages.

The above signs and symptoms in the context of a likely history (e.g., smoking) should suggest the diagnosis. ECG tracings are consistent with right ventricular hypertrophy. Chest x-ray may show signs of right heart enlargement as well as pulmonary vascular congestion.

Treatment includes the use of diuretics and oxygen therapy. Signs of heart failure should be treated as discussed above. Patients are at increased risk of thromboembolism due to polycythemia caused by chronic hypoxia.

Ischemic Disease

Atherosclerosis and Coronary Artery Disease

Atherosclerosis (AS) describes the narrowing of arteries by plaques, which are made up of lipid, smooth muscle, and calcifications. Atherosclerosis is the leading cause of coronary artery disease (CAD) in the United States, and CAD is currently the leading cause of death; however, incidence of CAD has been declining since the 1960s, presumably because of better hypertension diagnosis and control. Risk factors for AS/CAD include male gender, family history of CAD, hypertension, smoking, high cholesterol and lipid intake, diabetes, obesity, sedentary life-style, and stress.

AS can manifest in a number of ways, all involving the presence of ischemia. These manifestations include angina, intermittent claudication, MI, stroke, and mesenteric ischemia. On exam, patients may have high BP, hypertensive retinal changes, tendon xanthomas (yellowish, nodular fatty depositions on tendons), xanthelasma (yellow fatty depositions on eyelids), and S3 or S4 heart sounds.

An exercise stress test (ECG performed while patient is on a treadmill) showing ST changes or a thallium perfusion test showing decreased circulation both indicate CAD. Angiography is the gold standard for both CAD and AS. However, this test is invasive and may only be indicated if surgical intervention is an option.

Reduce precipitating risk factors, including smoking, hypertension, and hyperlipidemia. Angioplasty and bypass surgery may be indicated if the condition is severe.

Angina Pectoris

Angina pectoris refers to chest discomfort on exertion that arises from temporary myocardial ischemia. The most common cause of angina is CAD, although chronic valvular disorders may be involved.

The classic presentation involves substernal pain or pressure that may radiate to the left shoulder, arm, back, or jaw. It is ordinarily triggered by physical activity or stress and lasts a few minutes, with resolution of symptoms by rest or the use of nitroglycerin.

The preceding symptoms indicate the diagnosis. Exercise stress testing and persantine-thallium radionuclide scanning can reveal ischemia during exertion, while coronary angiography can demonstrate obstruction or narrowing of coronary vessels.

Nitroglycerin, administered sublingually, is the immediate treatment of choice for an anginal attack. Long-acting nitrates, beta-blockers, and calcium channel blockers are the preferred forms of chronic therapy. Antiplatelet drugs, such as aspirin, reduce the incidence of more severe coronary events such as unstable angina and MI. Severe angina may require angioplasty or coronary artery bypass grafting for more long-term relief.

Coronary Insufficiency

Coronary insufficiency, also known as unstable angina, describes a change in the status of previously established angina. About one-third of unstable angina patients are likely to develop an MI or sudden death within 3 months; therefore, unstable angina is an emergent medical condition that may require intensive care.

Patients experience anginal attacks of severe chest pain and pressure that are longer or more severe than their previous attacks of angina, and which may occur at rest. Radiation of pain may occur, as in angina pectoris.

Patients with unstable angina should not undergo stress testing. Echocardiography and angiography may be helpful in assessing the specific location of coronary occlusion.

Heparin and aspirin therapy should be instituted on admission. Oxygen, nitrates, beta-blockers, and calcium channel blockers may be useful. Patients with unstable angina may require angioplasty or coronary artery bypass grafting for long-term relief.

Myocardial Infarction

Commonly known as a heart attack, myocardial infarction refers to ischemia and necrosis of the myocardium due to insufficient blood supply. As with angina pectoris and unstable angina, the most common etiology is atherosclerosis. MI is usually caused by the acute development of a thrombus in the coronary arteries.

The majority of patients experience ischemic symptoms in the weeks before the MI, including angina, dyspnea, and fatigue. The onset of the MI is characterized by severe, substernal pressure or pain, with radiation to the left arm, back, or jaw. However, up to 20% of MIs may be "silent," with little or no discomfort. Symptoms of left-sided heart failure, such as pulmonary edema, may develop.

On physical exam, the patient is usually pale and diaphoretic and may be cyanotic, with cool skin and a weak pulse. Heart sounds may be distant, and an S4 is almost always present. A blowing systolic murmur may be heard, indicating papillary muscle necrosis.

ECG changes provide the definitive diagnosis. Transmural infarcts (involving the entire thickness of the myocardium) are associated with abnormal Q waves, while nontransmural infarcts may cause abnormal ST segments and T waves. On laboratory evaluation, creatinine phosphokinase of myocardial origin (CPK-MB) levels begin rising 2–12 hours after the MI, peak after 12–40 hours, and decrease after 24–72 hours. Normal CPK-MB values rule out the diagnosis of acute MI. Serum lactic dehydrogenase (LDH) levels also rise, peaking 3–6 days after the MI, and are used for later diagnosis.

IV morphine will reduce the patient's pain, but morphine must be used judiciously to avoid depressing respiration and myocardial contractility. Adequate arterial PO_2 can be assured with oxygen therapy. Aspirin chewed immediately will help prevent cardiac thrombus formation, and thrombolytic therapy (e.g., tPA and streptokinase) given within 6 hours of the MI can reduce mortality 30–50%. Cardiac work can be reduced with vasodilators such as nitroglycerin, which reduces afterload, and with beta-blockers, which reduce heart rate as well as total cardiac work. Subsequent to a myocardial infarction, chronic aspirin therapy and beta-blockers each reduce mortality by approximately 25%. Antiarrhythmics are not useful.

Primary prevention of MIs involves managing risk factors: quitting smoking, losing weight, avoiding a sedentary life-style, reducing cholesterol intake, and controlling hypertension.

Cardiomyopathies

Cardiomyopathies involve structural or functional abnormalities of the ventricular myocardium.

Congestive Cardiomyopathy

Congestive cardiomyopathy involves left and/or right ventricular dysfunction with subsequent ventricular dilation and heart failure.

Both acute and chronic forms can result from infection, including Coxsackie virus B and *Trypanosoma cruzi* (Chagas' disease). Congestive cardiomyopathy of acute onset is referred to as myocarditis. Chronic congestive cardiomyopathy is far more common, and chronic alcohol abuse is its most common cause. Congestive cardiomyopathy has a bad prognosis, with 70% of patients dying within 5 years.

Patients with chronic dilated congestive cardiomyopathy show signs of both left-sided and right-sided heart failure, including chronic dyspnea, fatigue, neck vein distention, inspiratory rales, and an S3 gallop. Ventricular dilation may cause a murmur of mitral regurgitation.

The clinical presentation suggests congestive heart failure. ECG shows sinus tachycardia. The chest x-ray shows cardiomegaly and pleural effusion. Echocardiography demonstrates ventricular dilation and rules out valvular disorders. Catheterization and MRI can also help if the diagnosis is still not certain.

Underlying disorders, such as chronic alcohol abuse, should be treated. ACE inhibitors, nitrates, low-dose beta-blockers, and diuretics are all useful. Digitalis may increase cardiac contraction. Because of the risk of mural thrombus formation, prophylactic anticoagulants are indicated.

Hypertrophic Cardiomyopathy

Hypertrophic cardiomyopathy refers to a congenital or acquired ventricular hypertrophy that develops under normal afterload. The stiff, noncompliant ventricle cannot readily be filled and may block the outflow of blood. The heart may show endocardial infiltration and thickening. Causes of hypertrophic cardiomyopathy include hemochromatosis and sarcoidosis.

Patients may complain of chest pain, syncope, palpitations, and dyspnea on exertion. Signs of increased venous pressure are evident and include jugular venous distention, ascites, edema, pleural effusion, and rales. An S4 is almost always apparent on exam.

ECG changes demonstrate left ventricular hypertrophy. Echocardiography is diagnostic. Cardiomegaly is not observed on x-ray.

Patients with hypertrophic cardiomyopathies have a poor prognosis, with a 20% mortality after 5 years. Beta-blockers and verapamil can both increase cardiac compliance, improving diastolic ventricular function. Valve replacement or removal of septal muscle is reserved for only the most severe cases.

Pericardial Diseases

Acute Pericarditis

Acute pericarditis can follow MIs or upper respiratory tract viral infections. It can also occur in the setting of collagen vascular diseases such as SLE; tubercular, streptococcal, and staphylococcal infections; drug use, including isoniazid (INH) and hydralazine; pericardial metastasis, especially from the breast or the lung; and uremia.

Inspiratory chest pain is the most common symptom. Position changes may relieve pain. A friction rub, a scratchy, leathery sound present throughout diastole and systole, is the characteristic sign of acute pericarditis. Pulsus paradoxus, an exaggerated drop in systemic blood pressure with inspiration, is also present.

The friction rub demonstrated on exam confirms the diagnosis. Echocardiography shows pericardial effusion. ECG findings are nonspecific.

Treatment of a known underlying disorder can be curative. NSAIDs decrease pericardial inflammation and associated chest pain. Steroids are used with intractable cases.

Chronic Constrictive Pericarditis

Chronic constrictive pericarditis arises as a reactive, diffuse thickening of the pericardium following pericardial inflammation. Pericardial changes result in decreased cardiac compliance, which causes decreased cardiac output. Any cause of acute pericarditis can lead to chronic constrictive pericarditis.

Patients usually present with a history of dyspnea on exertion and orthopnea. They may have signs of right-sided failure, such as jugular venous distention, ascites, and edema. Kussmaul's sign (increasing neck vein distention with inspiration) and pulsus paradoxus are present. Distant heart sounds are heard on exam.

Chest x-ray shows pericardial calcifications in 50% of patients. Echocardiography is not useful in the diagnosis. Cardiac catheterization is most diagnostic, showing equal diastolic pressures in all four chambers.

Surgical removal of the pericardium is curative.

Pericardial Effusion

Pericardial effusion involves an accumulation of fluid in the pericardial space. In acute pericarditis the fluid is exudative, but in neoplasms or fibrosis the fluid is transudative. If filling occurs rapidly, the fluid compresses the heart and causes tamponade.

Patients with pericardial effusion may be asymptomatic, especially if fluid accumulates slowly; however, if ventricular filling is limited, patients may present with symptoms of congestive heart failure. On exam, heart sounds are distant and a friction rub may be audible.

Chest x-ray shows symmetrical enlargement of the cardiac silhouette. Echocardiography demonstrates the pericardial fluid and is diagnostic. Fluid removed from the pericardial sac by pericardiocentesis can be evaluated for infectious causes, (e.g., TB), collagen vascular diseases, and cancer.

Treatment of a pericardial effusion is identical to treatment of acute pericarditis. Fluid can be aspirated for symptom relief.

Cardiac Tamponade

Cardiac tamponade occurs when pericardial fluid compresses the heart and drastically reduces cardiac output. This is a life-threatening condition.

Patients present with dyspnea, fatigue, and orthopnea. Pulsus paradoxus, neck vein distention, and a narrowed pulse pressure may be noted. Kussmaul's sign is absent.

Chest x-ray shows an enlarged heart, and echocardiography demonstrates the pericardial effusion. Catheterization, showing equal left and right atrial pressures, is rarely necessary to confirm the diagnosis.

Removal of fluid by emergency pericardiocentesis restores cardiac output.

Cardiac Trauma

Traumatic injury to the heart occurs frequently in motor vehicle accidents. Cardiac tamponade and myocardial contusion can result. Myocardial contusions present like MIs.

Depending on the nature of the injury, the patient may be asymptomatic or may show symptoms of tamponade or MI.

The mechanism of injury is consistent with cardiac trauma. ECG and echocardiogram lead to a definitive diagnosis.

The first priority is to stabilize the patient. Surgical decompression may be necessary.

Cardiogenic Shock

Cardiogenic shock can occur in any pathological state that compromises cardiac output, including MI, tamponade, and pulmonary embolism.

The patient is frequently sleepy or confused, with cold, moist extremities that are typically pale and cyanotic. On exam, the patient's pulse is weak and rapid, and systolic blood pressure is less than 90 mm Hg. Tachypnea, engorged neck veins, and signs of pulmonary congestion are often present.

The clinical presentation, particularly in a patient with a known underlying disorder, suggests a diagnosis. Neck vein engorgement and pulmonary congestion suggest cardiogenic shock over other types of shock.

Treatment of the underlying cause will often reverse cardiogenic shock. Oxygen and ventilatory assistance, if necessary, are important initial steps. Norepinephrine or dopamine will reverse profound hypotension and preserve kidney function. Catheterization permits monitoring of the central venous pressure.

Life Support

Life support is divided into basic and advanced interventions.

Basic life support can be done immediately, using the ABC mnemonic:

A: Airway is opened by a head tilt and chin lift, but this procedure is contraindicated in spinal injury. In that setting, a jaw thrust alone is appropriate.

B: Breathing is restored by mouth-to-mouth resuscitation.

C: Circulation is restored by external cardiac compression.

Complications of basic life support techniques include rib fractures and liver and spleen lacerations.

Advanced cardiac life support adds a "D" to the list:

D: Definitive treatment consists of
1. Defibrillation,
2. Drugs (ordinarily lidocaine and epinephrine), and
3. Diagnostic aids (ECG).

3 Respiratory Disorders

Bronchospasm

Bronchospasm refers to a spasmodic muscular contraction of the bronchi that usually occurs in the context of asthma; however, occupational dust exposure, acute allergic reactions, and water inhalation may all result in bronchospasm in the absence of asthma.

Wheezing

Described as a whistling sound in the lungs during respiration, **wheezing** is most commonly caused by asthma. Other causes include foreign body obstruction (known as an "asthmatoid wheeze") and inflammation, as seen in pneumonia and bronchitis.

Pleurisy

Also known as pleuritis, **pleurisy** is a general term describing inflammation of the pleural lining. Multiple causes, including infectious diseases (e.g., pneumonia), neoplasms (e.g., metastatic cancer), and connective tissue disorders (e.g., systemic lupus erythematosus), may be involved. Pain resulting from pleurisy may be referred to the shoulder as a result of diaphragmatic irritation.

Upper Respiratory Infections

Acute Coryza

Also known as "the common cold," viral infections causing acute coryza result in inflammation of the upper airways, including the nose, sinuses, throat, and often the bronchi. Associated viruses include rhinoviruses, influenza, parainfluenza, and adenoviruses.

Patients complain of nasal or throat irritation, followed by sneezing, rhinorrhea (runny nose), and malaise. A hacking, productive cough may persist for 1–2 weeks. Bacterial complications, such as sinusitis, otitis media, and bronchitis, may develop. Viral URIs do not typically produce fever; a high fever may therefore suggest a bacterial infection.

Clinical signs and symptoms are adequate for diagnosis. A throat culture may be performed if streptococcal pharyngitis is suspected.

Rest, analgesics, and decongestants may be helpful. Aspirin should not be given to children as it is associated with an increased risk of **Reye's syndrome** (a highly fatal encephalopathy discussed in Chap. 15). Antibiotics are not helpful and may place the patient at risk for drug reactions and for future bacterial resistance.

Streptococcal Pharyngitis

Also known as "strep throat," a streptococcal pharyngitis infection is caused by group A beta-hemolytic streptococci, usually *Streptococcus pyogenes*.

Fever, sore throat, and a beefy, red pharynx with tonsillar exudate are characteristic but are not specific to streptococcal infections. Tender cervical lymph nodes may be present. In young children, rhinorrhea may be the sole manifestation.

The above symptoms suggest streptococcal pharyngitis. A streptococcal culture is diagnostic.

Spontaneous resolution will occur in about 10 days; however, untreated streptococcal infections may have severe sequelae, including rheumatic heart disease and acute glomerulonephritis. Penicillin significantly reduces this risk and should be given even if symptoms appear to be resolving.

Thrush

Also known as oral candidiasis, thrush occurs predominantly in individuals with increased susceptibility to infection, including infants, the chronically ill, the immunocompromised, corticosteroid users, and those receiving antibiotics. It is caused by the fungus *Candida albicans* and is usually benign in children. In adults, it may suggest the presence of an underlying immunocompromised state, such as AIDS.

The typical lesion is a patchy, creamy-white exudate on an erythematous tongue and buccal mucosa. The exudate is easily scraped off the affected areas.

Gram's stain or KOH mount shows typical yeasts and pseudohyphae.

Antifungals, such as nystatin, may be administered as topical agents or as a "swish and swallow" medication.

Influenza

Known as "the flu," influenza is caused by specific influenza viruses. Significant mortality is associated with the development of influenza in elderly and chronically ill patients.

Generalized malaise, arthralgias, myalgias, and headache are early symptoms, ordinarily followed by a sore throat, a runny nose, and a nonproductive cough. Fevers of up to 103°F (39.5°C) are common. Symptoms typically last for several days but may persist for weeks. Sequelae include severe hemorrhagic bronchitis and pneumonia.

Clinical signs and symptoms are generally sufficient. A definitive diagnosis with serological tests and viral culture is rarely necessary.

Rest and symptomatic treatment are generally adequate. Amantadine may be helpful in the early stages of influenza A and is given to elderly patients or patients with chronic infections.

Annual influenza vaccinations are recommended for people over age 65 and people with chronic respiratory or cardiovascular diseases. Influenza vaccination is described in more detail in Chap. 9.

Tonsillitis

Tonsillitis is an acute inflammation of the palatine tonsils that usually occurs as a result of streptococcal or viral infection.

Sore throat, pain with swallowing, and referred pain to the ears are common. Patients may also have high fever, malaise, headache, and vomiting. Young children may not complain of sore throat but are often unable to swallow food due to discomfort and obstruction. Examination reveals red, swollen tonsils with a purulent exudate. A white, thin membrane that peels away without bleeding may be present on the tonsillar surface.

The above history and symptoms are diagnostic. *Streptococcus* may be found on culture.

While treatment is symptomatic, penicillin may be given for streptococcal infections. Recurrent episodes of acute tonsillitis may require tonsillectomy.

Peritonsillar Abscess

The formation of an abscess near the palatine tonsils is rare in children but common in young adults. The most common organism is group A beta-hemolytic *Streptococcus,* but anaerobes such as *Bacteroides* may also be present.

Patients experience fever, severe pain on swallowing, and trismus (muscle spasm resulting in difficulty opening the mouth). The head may be tilted toward the affected side, while the uvula may be displaced to the opposite side. On exam, the palate is erythematous and the tonsils may appear asymmetric.

The above symptoms and visualization of the abscess suggest the diagnosis.

IV penicillin is administered over 24–48 hours. Incision and drainage may be required. Because these abscesses tend to recur, tonsillectomy after the acute infection is often indicated.

Sinusitis

Inflammation of the paranasal sinuses may be precipitated by viral URIs but is usually caused by *Streptococcus pneumoniae* and *Haemophilus influenzae*, as well as various other streptococci and staphylococci. The maxillary and frontal sinuses are frequently involved.

Pain over the involved sinuses is characteristic. Nasal membranes are red and swollen with yellow or green purulent discharge. Inability to transilluminate the sinuses indicates local fluid accumulation.

The history and physical exam suggest the diagnosis. X-rays show air-fluid levels or opacification of the sinuses. CT scan may aid diagnosis in difficult cases.

Antibiotics are necessary for at least 2 weeks. Nasal vasoconstrictors and decongestants may promote sinus drainage. Recurrent or chronic sinusitis may require surgery to improve drainage.

Acute Bronchitis

Acute bronchitis, inflammation of the trachea and bronchi, often arises following an acute viral or bacterial URI, but it may also occur in an occupational setting after exposure to dust or respiratory irritants. In nonsmokers, the most common bacterial etiology is *Mycoplasma pneumoniae*. In smokers, acute bacterial exacerbations of chronic bronchitis are caused by *S. pneumoniae* and *H. influenzae*.

A persistent cough following a URI is initially nonproductive but becomes productive of small amounts of sputum. Purulent sputum suggests a bacterial etiology. Fever and sore throat are also common complaints.

Symptoms suggestive of bronchitis are adequate for diagnosis. On exam, scattered rhonchi (moist, gurgling noises from the larger bronchi), crackles, and wheezing may be noted. Chest x-ray may be necessary to rule out pneumonia.

Most cases are viral and require only rest, fluids, and analgesics. Bacterial cases may be treated with antibiotics, but this is controversial.

Epiglottitis

Epiglottitis is a severe infection of the epiglottis and surrounding structures. It may become rapidly fatal as a result of sudden respiratory obstruction. The causative organism is typically *H. influenzae* type b, although streptococci are sometimes associated. This disease typically occurs in young children but can occur at any age.

Rapid development of sore throat, fever, muffled voice, dysphagia, and drooling are characteristic. The patient may lean forward with neck extended to improve breathing. Stridor (a harsh, high-pitched sound during inspiration) and retractions (inward movement of the intercostal and supraclavicular spaces with inspiration) may also be noted. Physical exam shows an inflamed pharynx with decreased breath sounds and rhonchi.

Lateral neck films show a classic "thumbprint sign." Visualization of a red, swollen epiglottis is diagnostic but must be done under controlled conditions to prevent airway obstruction. After an artificial airway is established, pharyngeal and blood cultures should be performed.

Epiglottitis is a medical emergency. Patients suspected of epiglottitis should be immediately hospitalized and intubated. An IV cephalosporin should be administered.

Infants older than 2 months of age may receive *H. influenza* type b vaccination. The vaccine need not be given after the age of 5 because most individuals have immunity by that age.

Laryngotracheitis

Also known as "croup," this disease of young children is usually caused by parainfluenza virus, but influenza and respiratory syncytial virus (RSV) may also be involved. This illness is often preceded by a URI, and seasonal outbreaks are common.

A barking, harsh cough accompanied by hoarseness and inspiratory stridor is characteristic. The patient's condition often worsens at night. On physical exam, decreased breath sounds, wheezes, and rhonchi may be noted. Chest retractions are common.

The above symptoms and exam are generally diagnostic, but lateral neck x-rays and visualization of the epiglottis are necessary to rule out epiglottitis.

Mild cases may be managed on an outpatient basis; more severe cases require hospitalization. Treatment involves supportive care, although inhalers and nebulizers may be helpful.

Lower Respiratory Infections

Bronchiolitis

Often occurring in epidemics, bronchiolitis, a viral disease of the bronchioles, primarily affects infants under 2 years of age. Bronchiolitis is usually caused by RSV and may progress to RSV pneumonia.

Children generally have 1–2 days of fever, rhinorrhea, and cough, followed by signs of respiratory distress, including circumoral cyanosis (blueness around the mouth), tachypnea, and retractions. A hacking cough and vomiting may develop. Physical exam reveals wheezing, crackles, prolonged expiration, and hyperresonance to percussion.

Chest x-ray shows hyperinflation of the lungs, interstitial infiltrates, and areas of atelectasis.

Outpatient treatment is usually adequate, and symptoms resolve within 3–5 days. Patients should be given supportive care, including adequate hydration and nebulizers if necessary. Hospitalization is necessary in severe disease.

Bronchiectasis

Bronchiectasis is a chronic destructive process that results in dilation of the bronchial tree. Bronchiectasis commonly occurs in patients with cystic fibrosis (CF), immunodeficiencies, lung infection, and foreign body aspiration.

Classic symptoms include cough productive of large quantities of sputum, dyspnea, and hemoptysis. Recurrent URIs and episodes of pneumonia are common. Chest exam is significant for moist rales and rhonchi over the affected areas. Clubbing of the fingers may be present.

Chest x-ray may show increased bronchial markings, "honeycombing," and areas of atelectasis; thin-section CT will detect more subtle disease. Sputum cultures should be obtained. Bronchography may show cylindrical or saccular dilatations of the bronchial tree but is no longer recommended for routine use due to its high morbidity.

Treatment consists of antibiotics, bronchodilators, postural drainage, and chest percussion, as well as further treatment of underlying conditions. Surgical resection is useful in patients with recurrent pneumonia who fail medical therapy.

Pneumonia

Pneumococcal Pneumonia

Caused by *Streptococcus pneumoniae*, pneumococcal pneumonia is the most common bacterial pneumonia seen in adults. It is an important cause of community-acquired pneumonia (occurring at home as opposed to in an institution or hospital). About half of normal adults harbor *S. pneumoniae* without accompanying symptoms. Those who develop pneumococcal pneumonia tend to have other underlying medical conditions (e.g., diabetes and cardiopulmonary disease).

Sudden onset of fever and chills, cough, and pleuritic pain are characteristic. The cough is typically productive of a red-brown "rusty" colored sputum that becomes yellow during resolution of the illness. Physical exam findings include rales, decreased breath sounds, dullness to percussion, and vocal fremitus (vibrations felt over areas of consolidation in the lung when the patient speaks).

Gram's stain of sputum reveals gram-positive diplococci and neutrophils. Chest x-ray typically shows lobar consolidation or patchy infiltrates, sometimes accompanied by a small pleural effusion.

Penicillin is the drug of choice for sensitive organisms. Cephalosporins and erythromycin are also effective.

One dose of pneumococcal vaccine (Pneumovax) is recommended for patients over age 65 or patients with chronic disease.

Haemophilus Influenzae **Pneumonia**

H. influenzae is a community-acquired bacteria that causes pneumonia primarily in patients with chronic obstructive pulmonary disease (COPD), in children, and in the elderly.

As in pneumococcal pneumonia, fever, chills, cough, and pleuritic pain are seen; however, onset is generally slower and young patients may experience upper respiratory symptoms, such as nasal congestion, before the onset of pneumonia. If pleural effusions develop, physical exam will reveal decreased breath sounds and mild dullness to percussion.

Since *H. influenzae* is commonly seen in the upper respiratory tract, Gram's stain of the sputum is not diagnostic, but it may show small gram-negative coccobacilli. Diagnosis may be established by culture of sputum, pleural fluid, or blood. Chest x-ray shows patchy bronchial infiltration or lobar consolidation.

Ampicillin is the drug of choice, but resistant strains require cephalosporins or trimethoprim-sulfamethoxazole.

The *H. influenzae* vaccine protects against pneumonia caused by type b but not against other strains of *H. influenzae*. The vaccine is given to children ages 2 months to 5 years.

Viral Pneumonia

The most common pneumonia seen in children, viral pneumonia is associated with a number of pathogens, including influenza viruses, parainfluenza, RSV, and adenoviruses. Cytomegalovirus (CMV) may be seen in immunocompromised patients.

Nonspecific symptoms, such as fever, headaches, and myalgias, arise first, followed by a cough productive of mucopurulent sputum. On exam, rales or pleural effusions may be present.

Specific identification of the causative virus is not necessary, except in suspected outbreaks. Gram's stain of the patient's sputum is normal. Chest x-ray shows patchy infiltrates. WBC count is normal or slightly elevated.

Supportive care is sufficient, and symptoms usually resolve within a few weeks. Amantadine may be helpful in early treatment of influenza A pneumonia.

Annual influenza vaccinations are recommended for persons over age 65 and those with chronic respiratory or cardiovascular diseases. Influenza vaccination is described in more detail in Chap. 9.

Klebsiella and Gram-Negative Pneumonias

Gram-negative pneumonias, seen primarily in alcoholics, are often caused by aspiration. The immunocompromised, the elderly, and infants are also at elevated risk for these community-acquired pneumonias. Gram-negative bacteria that may be involved include *Klebsiella, Escherichia coli,* and Enterobacteriaceae.

The course of illness is generally rapid. In *Klebsiella* pneumonia, typical pneumonia symptoms are present and often include a cough productive of reddish "currant jelly" sputum.

Gram's stain of the patient's sputum shows multiple encapsulated gram-negative bacilli. Blood and sputum cultures should be performed. Chest x-ray shows involvement of multiple lobes, especially the right upper lobe, with possible abscess formation.

Combinations of cephalosporins and aminoglycosides are recommended, but mortality rates may approach 50% in spite of treatment.

Staphylococcal Pneumonia

Staphylococcal pneumonia is seen in both community and hospital settings and may follow URIs. Infants, the immunocompromised, and the elderly are at elevated risk. Staphylococcal pneumonia may develop by hematogenous spread of a distant staphylococcal infection, such as endocarditis.

Symptoms resemble pneumococcal pneumonia and include fever, chills, productive cough, and pleuritic pain. Pink "salmon-colored" sputum may be seen.

Sputum Gram's stain shows gram-positive cocci in grapelike clusters. Chest x-ray shows patchy bronchial infiltration; in infants, pneumatoceles (benign, thin-walled, air-filled cysts) are pathognomonic for staphylococcal pneumonia.

Beta-lactamase–resistant penicillins, such as nafcillin, are recommended. Mortality rates of staphylococcal pneumonia approach 40%, but this rate may be partially attributable to concurrent illnesses.

Mycoplasma Pneumonia

Mycoplasma pneumonia is a community-acquired pneumonia that tends to occur among young people in close contact (e.g., in schools and the military). It is the most common pneumonia seen in teens and young adults. Its clinical and laboratory differences from pneumococcal pneumonia have led to its description as an "atypical" pneumonia.

Gradual onset with a nonproductive cough, fever, headache, and myalgia is typical. Cervical lymphadenopathy and small amounts of whitish sputum may also be seen. On physical exam, fine rales may be heard.

Because *Mycoplasma* has no cell wall, it is not visible on Gram's stain. *Mycoplasma* cultures are difficult and require 7–10 days for growth. Chest x-ray is usually diagnostic and includes patchy infiltrates, especially in the lower lobes, that often appear much more severe than symptoms suggest.

Antibiotics such as erythromycin and tetracycline are helpful, although many cases will resolve spontaneously.

Pseudomonas Pneumonia

Seen primarily in chronically ill and immunocompromised patients, *Pseudomonas* pneumonia is often a hospital-acquired pneumonia associated with ventilator use. Patients with cystic fibrosis are at increased risk for developing this type of pneumonia.

Symptoms are similar to those seen in other gram-negative pneumonias and include rapid onset and a productive cough.

A likely history of nosocomial infection and typical symptoms of *Pseudomonas* pneumonia suggest the diagnosis. Cultures provide the definitive diagnosis.

Since resistant strains develop rapidly, treatment should be based on specific sensitivities. Currently, an antipseudomonal penicillin combined with an aminoglycoside is recommended.

Legionella Pneumonia

Caused by *Legionella pneumophila*, *Legionella* pneumonia may develop in both community and hospital settings. Like *Mycoplasma* pneumonia, *Legionella* pneumonia is considered an atypical pneumonia due to difficulty in diagnosis with routine lab techniques and clinical differences from pneumococcal pneumonia. *Legionella* is typically seen in middle-aged men, who often have risk factors such as smoking, alcohol use, and immunosuppression. Outbreaks of *Legionella* are associated with aerosolized water, such as in air conditioners.

An incubation period of 2–10 days is followed by a cough productive of scanty nonpurulent sputum. GI symptoms such as nausea and diarrhea, as well as CNS symptoms such as confusion and ataxia, are common.

Gram's stain shows neutrophils but no bacteria. The definitive diagnosis can be made with fluorescent antibody tests of sputum and serum antibody titers during the convalescence phase. Chest x-ray reveals patchy infiltrates and possible lobar consolidation and pleural effusion. WBC counts may be mildly elevated.

Erythromycin is the treatment of choice.

Pneumocystis Carinii Pneumonia

Pneumocystis carinii pneumonia, commonly seen in AIDS and other immunocompromised patients, is considered an opportunistic protozoan. It is discussed in more detail in Chap. 10.

Tuberculosis

The systemic disease tuberculosis (TB) is caused by *Mycobacterium tuberculosis*, with pulmonary infection the most common site. Most cases arise from reactivation of dormant mycobacteria, usually in the upper lobes of the lung. Extrapulmonary manifestations include meningitis, pericarditis, and bone invasion (known as Pott's disease). Miliary TB refers to widespread dissemination of TB infection to multiple organs; "miliary" refers to the millet seed–like appearance of the lesions.

Symptoms include fever, a cough productive of blood-tinged sputum, weight loss, night sweats, chest pain, dyspnea, anorexia, and manifestations of extrapulmonary disease. Patients with dormant disease are asymptomatic.

Acid-fast staining of sputum may confirm mycobacterium infection, but *M. tuberculosis* is confirmed by culture. Patients may have positive tuberculin skin test (PPD) results, although false-negatives are common. Chest x-ray may show a Ghon complex, consisting of a calcified tubercular granuloma in the lung combined with a calcified regional lymph node. Primary lesions typically occur in the lower lobes, while reactivation lesions tend to occur in the lung apices.

PPD is a useful screening method for exposure to TB. Induration of 10 mm in nonimmunocompromised patients indicates infection. Because the test relies on a functional immune system, immunocompromised and TB-infected people may be anergic, showing a false-negative

response. Giving intradermal injections
dermal injection permits comparison in
sidered to be PPD-positive if the test

Respiratory isolation is important for
must be notified. At least two antitu
high rates of resistance, and prolon
rifampin, pyrazinamide, ethambutol

Chronic bronchitis is
disease are common
of chronic bronch
tis do not resol
emphysema

A produ
short

Chronic Obstructive

Emphysema

Seen almost exclusively in smokers, emp
destruction of alveoli and small airways. The chronic
results in the continual release of proteolytic enzymes from macrophages.
cause the pleural destruction. Along with chronic bronchitis, this disorder is known as
COPD.

One rare form of emphysema is seen in patients with congenital deficiency of alpha$_1$-antitrypsin. In this disorder, the individual is unable to neutralize the proteases that are released into the lung by macrophages, resulting in destruction of the alveolar walls. These patients typically develop emphysema by their 30s or 40s, independent of cigarette use.

Physical findings are highly variable but typically include prolonged expiration, lung hyperinflation, and pursed-lip breathing. On exam, decreased heart and breath sounds accompanied by rhonchi may be present. The two types of COPD patients, known as "blue bloaters" and "pink puffers," are described in more detail in the accompanying box.

The clinical picture, along with decreased pulmonary function tests (PFTs) and changes on x-ray, suggests the diagnosis. PFTs typically show a severely reduced FEV$_1$ (the amount of air that can be forced out of the lung in one second) and a reduced vital capacity (the maximum amount of air that can be expired after a full inspiratory effort). The FEV$_1$/FVC ratio in COPD patients commonly falls to less than 60% of normal values. Decreased PFTs in emphysema are due to the loss of elasticity of the airways (causing them to collapse on expiration) and subsequent air trapping. Chest x-ray reveals lung hyperinflation, a depressed diaphragm, and decreased vascular markings. Bullae (small fluid-filled vesicles) may be noted, although they are not specific to emphysema.

Smoking cessation is required in these patients. Patients are treated for their symptoms with antibiotics for bronchial infections and inhalers for improved airway tone. Patients with COPD should not receive sedatives or hypnotics, as these drugs may reduce respiratory drive. Patients with alpha$_1$-antitrypsin deficiency may receive enzyme replacement therapy, but there are few data supporting the clinical efficacy of this therapy.

almost always associated with smoking. Exacerbations of chronic [bronchitis are typicall]y caused by *S. pneumoniae* and *H. influenzae*. A less common type [of bronch]itis is seen in chronic asthmatics, in whom the symptoms of bronchi[tis persis]ve despite maximal asthmatic therapy. Together, chronic bronchitis and [emphysema] comprise COPD.

[produ]ctive cough, often with mild wheezing, recurrent respiratory infections, and progressive [shortn]ess of breath.

Diagnosis requires the presence of a cough productive of bronchial mucus secretion for 3 months a year over 2 years. The above signs and symptoms in a person at risk for developing the condition (e.g., a smoker or asthmatic) are suggestive.

DIAGNOSIS

Smoking cessation typically causes reversal of all symptoms. Recurrent URIs are treated with broad-spectrum antibiotics, such as tetracycline, amoxicillin, or trimethoprim-sulfamethoxazole. Bronchial dilators and corticosteroids are helpful in patients with asthmatic bronchitis.

TREATMENT

The terms "pink puffer" and "blue bloater" refer to two different extreme presentations of COPD. In reality, most patients lie somewhere between the two classifications.

Pink puffers are patients who primarily develop emphysema, rather than bronchitis. These patients do not tend to be as hypoxic as blue bloaters, and the development of their dyspnea is gradual. The patient is typically underweight with enlarged accessory respiratory muscles, and sputum production is scanty and mucoid. These patients usually suffer from a rapid worsening of their COPD late in the course of the illness.

Blue bloaters are patients who usually develop chronic bronchitis early in the course of COPD. Their cough is productive of copious, purulent sputum, and patients are often cyanotic as a result of retained CO_2. Weight loss is generally not significant. These patients tend to develop pulmonary hypertension and cor pulmonale.

Cystic Fibrosis

CF is an autosomal recessive disorder that is more frequent in Caucasian populations and is the result of a defect in the chloride-pumping mechanism of exocrine glands. The resulting secretions are viscid (gummy and sticky) and excessive. The classic triad of abnormalities includes COPD, pancreatic enzyme insufficiency, and high concentrations of sweat electrolytes.

Clinical course ranges from mild to severe, but newborns typically present with GI obstruction due to meconium ileus. Infants without meconium ileus may show inadequate weight gain. They present with malodorous steatorrhea and recurrent respiratory infections due to viscous lung secretions and lack of pancreatic enzymes. In adults, signs of right-sided heart failure may be present because of chronic lung obstruction.

Meconium may be analyzed for specific protein contents; however, some cases are missed with this method. The "sweat test," in which the electrolyte concentrations of the sweat are determined, is the most commonly performed test for CF.

Treatment is comprehensive and includes diet therapy, pancreatic enzyme replacement, expectorants, and antibiotic prophylaxis against respiratory infections. Gene therapy of CF is currently being studied but is not widely available.

Respiratory Tract Neoplasms

Laryngeal Carcinoma

Laryngeal carcinoma is typically squamous cell in origin and is associated with smoking and alcohol use.

The primary symptom is hoarseness, usually present for several weeks and often worsening gradually over time. Difficulty in swallowing may also be noted.

Laryngoscopy should be performed on any patient complaining of hoarseness lasting more than 2 weeks. Biopsy will reveal the presence of malignancy. A number of benign laryngeal tumors may also cause a similar presentation.

Radiation and surgery. Complete laryngectomy may be necessary in advanced cases. Rehabilitation after surgery may include training in "esophageal speech," which allows the individual to form words by expelling air from the esophagus.

Lung Cancer

Lung cancer is currently the most common cancer and the leading cause of cancer death in both men and women in the United States. Cigarette smoking is responsible for up to 90% of cases, but occupational exposures (such as asbestos) have also been implicated. Three major types of lung cancer include squamous cell carcinoma (accounting for 40–50% of cases), adenocarcinoma (about 35% of cases), and small-cell ("oat cell") carcinoma (about 25% of cases). Small-cell carcinomas sometimes produce hormones, resulting in paraneoplastic syndromes.

The lung is also a common site for bloodborne metastases of other primary cancers. The most common primary cancer sites associated with lung metastases are the breast, colon, prostate, and cervix.

The typical history consists of cough with bloody sputum, weight loss, and dyspnea. Later signs include pleuritic pain (due to pleural effusions), wheezing, and persistent infection. Other syndromes associated with lung cancer are listed in the accompanying box.

The history and chest x-ray findings of a mass suggest the diagnosis. The location of the tumor mass provides information regarding its histology. Squamous cell and small-cell carcinomas typically arise near the hilar region, while adenocarcinomas arise peripherally. Other x-ray findings associated with lung cancer include bronchial narrowing and atelectasis. Bronchoscopy may be used for visualization and biopsy.

Prognosis is generally poor, and few treatments are available. Circumscribed lesions may be surgically excised in a lobectomy, while radiation may be useful for controlling pain or compression of nerves. Five-year survival rates are less than 10%.

Syndromes associated with lung cancer are common. The following is a brief list of those seen most commonly in a clinical setting. Paraneoplastic disorders, associated with small-cell carcinoma, are described in Chap. 12.

Horner's syndrome results from the invasion of cervical sympathetic ganglia by an apical lung tumor (also known as a Pancoast's tumor). This condition results in the classic triad of miosis (pupillary constriction), ptosis (eyelid droop), and anhydrosis (lack of sweating) on the affected side. **Pancoast's syndrome** combines Horner's syndrome with pain in the arm and shoulder due to invasion of the brachial plexus.

Superior vena cava (SVC) syndrome involves obstruction of the venous drainage of the head and neck, resulting in swelling and CNS symptoms. SVC syndrome is seen in diseases other than lung cancer, including TB and other neoplasms.

Tobacco Use

Cigarette smoking has been identified as the single biggest cause of preventable morbidity and mortality in the United States. The majority of smoking-related deaths fall into three categories: atherosclerotic disease, cancer, and respiratory diseases.

Atherosclerotic disease is manifested in a number of ways, most of which have been strongly associated with cigarette smoking. The incidence of coronary heart disease, including angina and myocardial

(continued)

infarction, as well as strokes and peripheral vascular disease (e.g., intermittent claudication) are all significantly increased in smokers.

Numerous **neoplastic diseases** have also been associated with smoking. In addition to the most commonly known, such as lung, oral, and laryngeal cancers, other smoking-related cancers include esophageal, stomach, bladder, kidney, and cervical cancers.

The primary **respiratory illness** seen in smokers is COPD, which consists of emphysema and chronic bronchitis. Smokers are also more likely to develop upper respiratory infections and pneumonia than non-smokers, and they may experience more recurrences of tuberculosis as well.

Other smoking-related disorders include **GI disease** (e.g., peptic ulcer disease, gastritis, and esophageal reflux) and **complications of pregnancy**, including intrauterine growth retardation, stillbirth, spontaneous abortion, and placenta previa. Passive smoke exposure has also been associated with an increased risk of lung cancer, and passive exposure in children has been associated with increased incidence of URIs and asthma.

Currently, prevalence rates of smoking are decreasing in all age groups in the United States; however, for some age groups, rates are rising in specific ethnic groups, such as Asians. Smoking prevalence is also rising around the world. Changes in cigarette tar content have not been shown to reduce the risks of smoking, since individuals who use them appear to inhale more strongly than normal, thus increasing their tar exposure. Smokeless tobacco has also been promoted as an alternative to smoking but is associated with a greatly increased risk of oral cancer.

Allergy

Asthma

Asthma is characterized by reversible airway obstruction brought on by airway inflammation and increased airway sensitivity. Exacerbating factors include pollen, dust, smoke, and fumes; exercise and viral infections; and possibly aspirin and sulfites (found in red wine and beer). People with asthma often have a family history of asthma, allergies, or atopic dermatitis.

Occupational asthma may occur on exposure to specific particles or vapors. Symptoms in this setting may not be apparent until nighttime and will often resolve on weekends.

Wheezing, coughing, shortness of breath, and chest tightness are common. In severe attacks, patients may be cyanotic or unable to speak more than a few words. Sputum produced after the attack has resolved is white or yellow and has a rubbery quality. Physical exam reveals diffuse wheezing in the lungs, which may be audible without a stethoscope.

The above symptoms combined with pulmonary function testing provide the diagnosis. PFTs usually show decreased FEV_1 due to the constriction of the airways. Arterial blood gases reveal a respiratory alkalosis and low CO_2 early in the attack because the patient is hyperventilating. If the CO_2 rises to normal values, respiratory failure is imminent.

Most patients are managed medically. Beta-adrenergic inhalers are helpful for acute attacks. Theophylline, corticosteroids, cromolyn sodium, and anticholinergics such as atropine may also be useful. Severe, acute attacks may require oxygen and mechanical ventilation. Occupational asthma may require skin testing to diagnose the offending substance.

Rhinitis

Rhinitis is a common condition that occurs most frequently in association with a URI ("viral rhinitis"), but it may occur with bacterial infections and allergic reactions. Chronic rhinitis may be seen in syphilis and TB infections.

Nasal obstruction, purulent discharge, and occasional mild nasal bleeding are characteristic.

In acute cases, a history of symptoms is sufficient. Diagnosis of chronic rhinitis may require biopsy and culture of the causative organism.

Decongestants may be helpful. Bacterial rhinitis may require antibiotics.

Hay Fever

Hay fever is a seasonal form of allergic rhinitis that is usually precipitated by airborne pollens, which vary by location and season.

Itching, tearing eyes and clear nasal discharge are common. Coughing and wheezing may develop in severe cases. On exam, nasal membranes are erythematous and swollen, and conjunctiva are injected.

The history is generally adequate. The presence of eosinophils in nasal secretions also supports the diagnosis.

A variety of nonprescription and prescription medications may be helpful. Antihistamines, decongestants, nasal glucocorticoid sprays, and cromolyn sodium may be helpful in controlling and preventing symptoms. Long-term desensitization therapy is also recommended in some cases.

Accidents

Epistaxis and Facial Trauma

Epistaxis (nosebleed) is a common condition seen in people of all ages. Simple, unilateral epistaxis arises from the anterior nasal areas and can usually be controlled by holding the nostril closed. More complex nosebleeds can arise in elderly patients, especially those on antihypertensive or anticoagulation medications. These nosebleeds usually arise from the posterior nasal areas and may cause blood to enter the mouth and throat by leakage down the posterior pharynx. IV fluids and nasal packs are necessary for management.

Facial trauma may lead to nasal and maxillary injuries. The most common facial fracture is a broken nose. Symptoms include tenderness, swelling, bleeding, and crepitus (a crackling sensation). Treatment requires pressure and cold packs to reduce bleeding and swelling.

Pulmonary Aspiration

Aspiration of foreign materials into the airways may occur in a variety of contexts but occurs commonly in patients who are on mechanical ventilators, have a depressed level of consciousness, or are elderly. Three major types of aspiration include chemical pneumonitis (when toxic material such as gastric acid enters the lung), bacterial aspiration (seen in alcoholics and nosocomial settings), and mechanical obstruction (aspiration of foreign bodies).

One example of chemical pneumonitis occurring in the elderly is called "lipid pneumonia," in which castor oil and other mineral oils ingested by the patient become trapped in the lung. Bacterial pneumonitis occurs in individuals who aspirate gastric or oral secretions. Mechanical obstruction is seen commonly in children and is discussed in more detail in Chap. 18.

SIGNS & SYMPTOMS

Dyspnea, tachypnea, bronchospasm, and pink, frothy sputum are common manifestations. Symptoms depend on the severity and location of the aspiration.

DIAGNOSIS

Chest x-ray may reveal infiltrates, abscess formation, or a foreign body.

TREATMENT

If the aspiration is continuing (e.g., a vomiting patient), the patient should lie turned to the right, with the foot of the bed elevated, to minimize aspiration and to confine aspirated material to the right upper lobe. Large amounts of aspirated material may require suctioning. Pneumonia or abscesses that develop from bacterial aspiration should be treated with antibiotics.

Massive Hemoptysis

The condition of massive hemoptysis refers to the coughing up of more than 600 ml of blood within 24 hours. Hemoptysis must be differentiated from hematemesis (vomiting blood). Conditions in which massive hemoptysis might occur include trauma, pulmonary embolism, aortic aneurysm, and heart failure.

The signs are described above.

Bronchoscopy and x-ray may be helpful in localizing the source of bleeding. Clotting studies should be performed. Chest CT may be useful.

The primary aim in treatment is to stabilize the patient. The patient should be given IV fluids and must be monitored for the development of shock. To prevent asphyxiation, the patient should be encouraged to cough up as many clots as possible, and bronchoscopy may be used to clear clots that can potentially block an airway. Finally, the source of bleeding should be contained by surgical ligation or lobectomy. Narcotics should never be given because of their capacity for respiratory depression.

Hemothorax

Hemothorax describes the collection of blood in the pleural space, generally as a result of trauma, malignancy, TB, or pulmonary infarction. Thrombi that form may not be readily reabsorbed, and fibrosis or compromised respiratory function may result.

Signs and symptoms are similar to those of pleural effusion but include those of the underlying disorder.

Chest x-ray shows pleural effusion. Thoracentesis reveals blood.

Closed tube drainage removes blood from the pleural space. Other treatment and supportive care will depend on the underlying cause.

Pneumothorax

A collection of air in the pleural space, pneumothorax originates from rupture of part of the respiratory system, esophagus, or chest wall. **Spontaneous pneumothorax** most often occurs in 15- to 35-year-old males or in patients with chronic pulmonary disease. If the chest wall is intact, it is a closed pneumothorax; an open pneumothorax involves air passage through the chest wall. In a **tension pneumothorax**, pressure in the pleural space can displace the heart and diaphragm. The resulting respiratory compromise and compression of the vena cava constitute a surgical emergency. Microorganisms in the pleural space may produce gas, another potential source of pneumothorax. Iatrogenic causes include thoracentesis, subclavian or internal jugular catheter placement, lung or pleural biopsy, and other invasive procedures. Assisted ventilation may also create pneumothorax.

 Patients complain of dyspnea and chest pain that may be referred to the ipsilateral arm and shoulder. Decreased chest wall movement, decreased breath sounds, and increased resonance may be noted. Tension pneumothorax may be accompanied by a mediastinal shift away from the affected side.

 Chest x-ray shows space between the lung and the parietal pleura and may show a mediastinal shift toward the opposite side.

In a small, stable pneumothorax, air is reabsorbed and only expectant management is needed. Otherwise, closed tube drainage removes the air and allows the lung to re-expand. Thoracotomy is needed only when air leaks persist or recur.

Traumatic Injury to the Lung

Injury to the chest can result in numerous pulmonary complications, including hemothorax, pneumothorax, and flail chest. **Open pneumothorax** from penetrating chest injury occurs by the suction of air into the pleural space, forcing the lung to collapse. **Tension pneumothorax** can occur from blunt trauma. Tissue damage of the lung itself allows air to enter the pleural space and not escape. **Flail chest** describes the unstable condition that occurs after several ribs and the sternum are fractured.

 Reduced breath sounds and hyperresonance to percussion are noted. In open pneumothorax, air being sucked into the lung through the chest may be heard. In flail chest, the portion of the rib cage that has broken moves paradoxically in comparison to the rest of the chest during breathing.

 History of trauma combined with evidence of the above. Chest x-ray will show a mediastinal shift toward the opposite side in tension pneumothorax.

 Chest tube or valve placement may allow equalization of pressures and expansion of the lung in pneumothorax.

Interstitial Lung Disease

Sarcoidosis

A noncaseating granulomatous disease of unknown etiology, sarcoidosis may involve the lungs, liver, spleen, joints, skin, and bones. Many patients have spontaneous resolution of disease; however, one-third develop chronic disease. Sarcoidosis is much more common in blacks than in other races, with age of onset ranging from about 20 to 40.

Nonspecific symptoms of pulmonary infection are common, as are erythema nodosum (tender, red nodules on the tibia and arms), weight loss, fatigue, malaise, and enlarged lymph nodes. Occasionally, the symptoms include dyspnea, dry cough, and fever. Extrapulmonary manifestations include arthritis, cranial nerve palsies, and visual loss.

The above symptoms and x-ray findings suggest the diagnosis. On chest x-ray, the presence of bilateral hilar and paratracheal adenopathy is pathognomonic. Diffuse pulmonary infiltration is also present, which may have a diffuse, "ground glass" appearance or a more nodular character on x-ray. Laboratory exam reveals increased calcium in the blood and urine.

Spontaneous improvement is common. Steroids are often given, although the benefit is unproved except in cases with ophthalmologic disease or severe systemic compromise.

Asbestosis

Asbestosis, caused by chronic inhalation of asbestos fibers, is also associated with increased risks of lung cancer and malignant mesothelioma (carcinoma of the mesothelial cells of the pleura and peritoneum). Occupations associated with asbestos use include construction workers, shipyard workers, and automobile mechanics.

Gradual onset of dyspnea and reduced exercise tolerance are typical. Productive cough and wheezing are usually not associated with asbestosis.

History of exposure and characteristic chest x-ray are diagnostic. Chest x-ray typically reveals diffuse linear opacities in the lower lungs.

No effective therapy is available. Preventive measures to reduce asbestos exposure, such as masks, are useful. Smoking cessation is also associated with decreased severity of disease.

Silicosis

The oldest of occupational lung diseases, silicosis follows long-term silicon dioxide inhalation. Associated industries include metal mining, pottery making, soap production, and granite cutting. Required exposure times are generally 20–30 years, although high exposures can precipitate disease within 10 years. These patients also have an increased risk of developing TB.

SIGNS & SYMPTOMS

Many patients are asymptomatic; others complain of chronic cough and dyspnea. Later stages may show signs of congestive heart disease.

DIAGNOSIS

History of exposure and characteristic chest x-ray findings, which include multiple small nodules and calcification of the hilar lymph nodes, are diagnostic. Pulmonary function abnormalities include decreased lung volumes and diffusing capacity.

TREATMENT

No treatment is available. Effective dust control and protective measures such as facial hoods may prevent the development of silicosis.

Other Lung Disorders

Respiratory Failure

Respiratory failure refers to respiratory dysfunction that results in abnormalities in CO_2 elimination. It may result from a failure of ventilation, a failure of oxygenation, or a combination of the two.

SIGNS & SYMPTOMS

Dyspnea, headache, cyanosis, and tachypnea are common, often accompanied by delirium, restlessness, and anxiety.

DIAGNOSIS

Arterial blood gases usually show a PO_2 of 50–60 mm Hg and a PCO_2 of more than 45 mm Hg.

TREATMENT

Treatment depends on the underlying disorder causing the respiratory failure. For patients retaining CO_2 (Table 3-1), high levels of oxygen may suppress the respiratory drive and can be dangerous. COPD patients should receive low-flow oxygen, and oxygen saturation need not be raised above 90% in these patients. Non-CO_2 retainers can be given high-flow oxygen to raise PO_2. Patients with hypercarbia should be placed on mechanical ventilation as needed.

Table 3-1. Conditions associated with CO_2 retention

CO_2 retainers	Non-CO_2 retainers
COPD	ARDS
Cystic fibrosis	Pneumonia
Asthma	Aspiration
Chest wall trauma	Pulmonary edema
Neuromuscular diseases (e.g., Guillain-Barré disease)	
CNS depression/drug overdose	

Table 3-2. Differentiation of transudative and exudative pleural effusions

	Laboratory analysis	Common causes
Transudates	Pleural/serum protein ratio < 0.5 Pleural/serum LDH ratio < 0.6 Total protein < 3 g/dl	Congestive heart failure Nephrotic syndrome Cirrhosis
Exudates	Pleural/serum protein ratio > 0.5 Pleural/serum LDH ratio > 0.6 Total protein > 3 g/dl	Neoplasms Infections Collagen vascular disease

Pleural Effusion

Fluid collection within the pleural space may be serous, bloody, or lymphatic. **Transudative effusions** result from changes in normal hydrostatic or oncotic pressure, as seen in congestive heart failure and hepatic cirrhosis. **Exudative effusions** are protein-rich effusions that generally arise from inflammation, such as infections or neoplasms (Table 3-2). An effusion of blood (hemothorax) can also occur after trauma. Lymph may accumulate in the pleural space when the thoracic duct is ruptured or when drainage is blocked, as in mediastinal carcinomatosis. One-fourth of all effusions are associated with malignancies, and the level of suspicion for a malignancy should be high in a patient with bilateral effusions but with a normal-sized heart. **Meigs' syndrome** (pleural effusion accompanied by ascites) is associated with ovarian fibromas and other pelvic tumors.

SIGNS & SYMPTOMS

Patients may complain of chest pain, shortness of breath, fever, and weakness. On exam, diminished tactile fremitus, dullness to percussion, and decreased breath sounds may be noted. Egophony (increased resonance and change of voice to a high-pitched, bleating quality) may be noted with larger effusions.

DIAGNOSIS

Chest x-ray confirms the diagnosis, showing the effusion as a dulling of the costodiaphragmatic angles with fluid. Thoracentesis (aspiration of pleural fluid through the chest wall) provides a fluid sample for analysis, permitting transudates to be differentiated from exudates by comparing pleural protein and lactic dehydrogenase (LDH) levels with serum levels (Table 3-2). Frank pus indicates empyema, most often due to *Staphylococcus aureus*. High triglyceride levels reflect chylous effusions. Further evaluation may include cytology for malignant cells, pH, stains and cultures, and amylase levels (to assess pancreatitis or esophageal rupture). Pleural biopsy may be helpful to diagnose TB.

Thoracentesis or tube drainage allows for re-expansion of the lung, but this procedure can be complicated by pneumothorax, infection, or fluid loculation. In addition, the underlying cause of the effusion must be treated.

Pulmonary Edema

Pulmonary edema results from increased pulmonary venous pressure, causing congestion of the lung tissue. Common causes include left ventricular failure, myocardial infarction (MI), valvular heart disease, arrhythmias, and hypertensive crises. Acute pulmonary edema may be seen in adult respiratory distress syndrome (ARDS), discussed later in this chapter.

Dyspnea, tachypnea, and pleuritic chest pain are common manifestations. Cyanosis, orthopnea (difficulty breathing while supine), paroxysmal nocturnal dyspnea (sudden onset of breathing difficulty during sleep that requires the patient to sit upright), and pink, frothy sputum are also common. Physical exam findings include wheezing, rhonchi, gurgles, moist rales, and dullness to percussion.

Chest x-ray reveals the diffuse presence of fluid throughout the lung, resulting in indistinct lines and shadows. **Kerley B lines,** seen when the outer interlobular septa become waterlogged and fibrotic over time, are also noted. The cardiac silhouette may be enlarged if the edema is cardiac in origin.

Treatment is targeted to the underlying condition. Diuretics and salt restriction are useful for relief of symptoms. Acute pulmonary edema must be aggressively treated with oxygen, morphine, vasodilators, and rapid-acting diuretics, such as furosemide.

Pulmonary Embolism

Pulmonary embolism (PE), blockage of a pulmonary vessel, usually arises from a thrombus that has been dislodged from a large vein. The resulting increase in pulmonary artery pressure due to embolism increases the work of the right ventricle. This condition is particularly dangerous in a patient with preexisting heart disease. Most PEs arise from deep venous thromboses (DVTs) in the iliac and femoral veins. Virchow's triad of factors related to venous thrombosis include injury to the vascular endothelium, stasis, and increased coagulability of the blood. Therefore, risk factors for pulmonary thromboembolism include heart disease, immobilization, carcinoma, recent surgery, venous disease in the lower extremities, pregnancy, and administration of estrogens.

Symptoms vary, with dyspnea, tachypnea, and tachycardia most common. "Classic" signs are less common and include hemoptysis, pleural friction rub, gallop rhythm, cyanosis, chest pain, and chest splinting. Physical exam is often normal.

Arterial blood gases show increased P(A-a)O$_2$ and hypoxemia (see accompanying box). Electrocardiogram (ECG) may show sinus tachycardia with right heart strain or occasionally atrial fibrillation. Chest x-ray may be normal but may reveal atelectasis or small effusions; wedge-shaped peripheral infiltrates may be seen on later films.

Ventilation-perfusion ($\dot{V}/\dot{Q}$) lung scans show areas that are ventilated but not perfused. A negative $\dot{V}/\dot{Q}$ scan essentially rules out the diagnosis, whereas a positive $\dot{V}/\dot{Q}$ scan is sufficient grounds for diagnosis. An equivocal $\dot{V}/\dot{Q}$ scan requires pulmonary angiography, the "gold standard" of diagnosis.

Supportive care, thrombolytics, and immediate and prophylactic anticoagulation are the mainstays of treatment. Intravenous heparin is given until the partial thromboplastin time (PTT) is approximately 2.0–2.5 times the normal value. After a week, warfarin is added until the prothrombin time (PT) is maintained at 1.5 times normal. If recurrence is a problem, placement of a filter in the inferior vena cava is sometimes performed. Pulmonary embolectomy is only rarely necessary, in cases of massive embolisms.

The **alveolar-arterial (A-a) gradient** provides a measure that compares the oxygenation status of the blood with that of the alveolar environment. The formula for its calculation is:

$$\text{A-a gradient} = \left[(713 \text{ mm Hg}) (\text{FiO}_2) - \frac{(\text{PaCO}_2)}{(0.8)} \right] - \text{PaO}_2$$

FiO$_2$ refers to the fraction of oxygen in the inspired air. Room air has a value of 0.21; however, patients on oxygen supplementation may have values up to 1.0 (100% oxygen). PaCO$_2$ and PaO$_2$ refer to the arterial carbon dioxide and oxygen, which are obtained from the blood gas values.

The normal A-a gradient is 5–15 mm Hg. Increased values are seen in pulmonary embolism, diffusion defects (as in pulmonary edema) and right-to-left cardiac shunts.

Respiratory Distress Syndrome of the Newborn

Also known as hyaline membrane disease, respiratory distress syndrome of the newborn is seen predominantly in premature infants, especially those less than 37 weeks' gestation. Decreased production of pulmonary surfactant results in atelectasis of the newborn lung, causing severe breathing difficulty.

Within a few hours of delivery, the newborn develops rapid, labored breathing accompanied by grunting, intercostal retractions, nasal flaring, and cyanosis. Chest exam reveals crackles and decreased or absent breath sounds over the affected areas.

Diagnosis is based on history, physical exam, and arterial blood gas data demonstrating high CO_2 and low O_2 levels. Chest x-ray shows diffuse atelectasis, with loss of cardiac borders in severe cases.

Administration of artificial surfactant is the current treatment of choice. Oxygen supplementation and the use of continuous positive airway pressure (CPAP) are also helpful. Ventilator support may be necessary in severe cases.

Fetal lung maturity can be assessed prior to delivery by determining the concentrations of lecithin (L), sphingomyelin (S), and phosphatidyl glycerol (PG) in the amniotic fluid. An L/S ratio greater than 2 accompanied by the presence of PG shows fetal lung maturity. If fetal lung maturity has not yet occurred, the mother may be given steroids, such as beclomethasone, over 24 hours to hasten the production of pulmonary surfactant.

Adult Respiratory Distress Syndrome

ARDS describes acute lung injury that results in noncardiogenic pulmonary edema. Sepsis, major trauma, near-drowning, and drug overdose are common causes. Mortality is high, particularly when ARDS is associated with sepsis. The mechanism by which ARDS occurs is still unclear, but it may be related to vascular injury resulting in blood leakage into the lung.

Dyspnea is accompanied by rapid, shallow breathing within the first 24–48 hours following the causative illness or injury. Mottled or cyanotic skin and retractions may also be present. Physical exam may be normal or may reveal wheezing, rhonchi, or rales throughout the lung.

A presumptive diagnosis may be made by the presence of symptoms; the diagnosis is confirmed with arterial blood gases and a chest x-ray. Blood gases typically reveal an acute respiratory alkalosis, with low O_2 and low CO_2 (due to hyperventilation). Chest x-ray findings are typical of pulmonary edema but show diffuse infiltrates with a normal cardiac silhouette, since the edema is not cardiac in origin.

Maintenance of adequate oxygenation is crucial, and positive-pressure ventilation (PP) or positive end-expiratory pressure (PEEP) is generally used to accomplish this aim. Intravascular volume should be maintained as low as possible to decrease edema. Antibiotics are given when indicated.

Pulmonary Hypertension

Increased hydrostatic pressure in the pulmonary system may result from a variety of underlying diseases. **Primary pulmonary hypertension** is an uncommon diagnosis of exclusion that usually occurs in young women and is often fatal within a few years of diagnosis. Some causes of **secondary pulmonary hypertension** include pulmonary venous hypertension seen in valvular heart disease, left-to-right shunts, chronic hypoxemia as in COPD, and thromboembolic disease.

Dyspnea, fatigue, retrosternal pain, cough, and syncope are common. Physical exam may show cyanosis, clubbing of the fingers, and an accentuated P2 sound on cardiac exam.

Lab evaluation may show increased polycythemia, while ECG shows right ventricular hypertrophy. Chest x-ray reveals enlargement of the pulmonary artery and dilation of the right ventricle. Echocardiography, V̇/Q̇ scanning, and pulmonary angiography may assist in the diagnosis.

In secondary pulmonary hypertension, treatment of the underlying disease is most important. For primary pulmonary hypertension, supplemental oxygen, vasodilator treatment, anticoagulants, and lung transplantation are treatment options.

Hospital Interventions

Postoperative Pulmonary Complications

Respiratory complications are the single largest cause of postoperative morbidity. The five most common respiratory complications include atelectasis, pneumonia, aspiration, pneumothorax, and pulmonary embolism. **Atelectasis** (see below) occurs in more than 25% of patients undergoing abdominal surgery and is responsible for more than 90% of postoperative fevers. If atelectasis persists more than 72 hours, **pneumonia** is likely to develop and is associated with mortality rates of more than 20%. **Aspiration** of gastric contents may occur as a result of CNS depression during anesthesia, especially if the patient has eaten in the 12 hours prior to surgery; gastric fluid aspiration may also lead to pneumonia. **Pneumothorax** can occur as a result of positive-pressure ventilation or subclavian catheter insertion. **Pulmonary embolism** is especially common after abdominal, pelvic, or thoracic surgery and may be prevented with preoperative administration of small amounts of heparin to prevent deep venous thrombus formation. Postoperative patients should be mobilized early or given elastic stockings to promote blood flow.

Atelectasis

Atelectasis refers to localized collapse of the alveoli. Postoperative atelectasis is common, especially after abdominal surgery, due to anesthetic drugs and the accumulation of secretions in the bronchioles. Newborns may experience atelectasis as part of respiratory distress syndrome, due to a lack of pulmonary surfactant to help keep the alveoli open. Asthmatics may also experience patchy atelectasis. In a form of chronic atelectasis known as **middle lobe syndrome**, the right middle lobe collapses due to bronchial compression by surrounding lymph nodes. Poor drainage may result in infection and chronic pneumonitis. Finally, atelectasis commonly occurs after foreign body aspiration in children as a result of airway blockage.

Symptoms will depend on the speed at which the atelectasis occurs. Patients may be asymptomatic or may experience pain, dyspnea, and fever. Breath sounds are decreased over the affected lobes, which are also dull to percussion.

Diagnosis is based on the clinical findings as well as on the chest x-ray. X-ray typically shows an airless lung area with deviation of the heart and trachea toward the affected side. The hemidiaphragm of the affected side may be raised.

Severe atelectasis requires prompt intervention, including suctioning and chest percussion. Other measures include ambulation and encouragement of deep breathing with inspiratory spirometers. Newborns with atelectasis may be given artificial surfactant. Postoperative atelectasis should resolve within a few days.

Intubation and Tracheostomy

Intubation, insertion of a tube into the trachea, is usually done to maintain a patent airway and ventilate the lungs. The tube may be placed nasally or orally, but the oral method is preferred if the patient is unconscious. Careful visualization of the vocal cords is required to avoid damage. Once the tube is in the trachea, a balloon is inflated to create an airtight seal, and the patient can be ventilated. Intubation is associated with increased rates of infection and tracheal mucosal damage. If intubation is anticipated to exceed 3 weeks, a tracheostomy should be performed; less severe complications are associated with chronic ventilation through a hole in the trachea.

Assisted Ventilation

Ventilatory support is frequently required in the ICU and in the perioperative period. A variety of modes can be used, depending on the situation and condition of the patient. Absolute ventilatory control can be maintained only if the patient is paralyzed or heavily sedated. An intermediate level of ventilatory control allows the patient to initiate breaths but provides backup if a certain respiratory rate or volume is not achieved. The simplest level of assistance involves continuous pressure to help the patient overcome resistance provided by the endotracheal tube. Use of this level of assistance usually precedes extubation.

4

Endocrine Disorders

Thyroid Disorders

Thyroid Tests

Both thyroid hormones, T_4 and the more active T_3, are found in free and bound states in the serum. Only the free forms are biologically active. Variations in the quantity of thyroid-binding proteins can alter the total serum T_4 without changing the amount of free T_4 available. (This also applies to T_3, but free T_3 cannot be routinely measured.) For example, conditions that raise levels of thyroid-binding proteins, such as pregnancy, exogenous estrogen intake, chronic heroin use, and hepatitis, will cause the total T_4 to be elevated, although the free T_4 level remains normal. Thus, hypothyroidism, which results from excessively low levels of active T_3 and T_4, can be missed in these conditions by placing too much stock in "normal" total T_4 levels.

Thyroid-stimulating hormone (TSH) from the pituitary induces the thyroid gland to produce T_3 and T_4. Levels of TSH are low when the thyroid is hyperactive and high when the thyroid is hypoactive, assuming that the pituitary is functioning properly. Pituitary control over the thyroid gland is governed by a negative feedback loop (Fig. 4-1).

A thyroid scan uses small doses of radioactive iodine or technetium, which is taken up by the thyroid gland. This procedure makes it possible to visualize the gland and is useful in determining whether a nodule is "hot" (overactive) or "cold" (underactive).

Acquired Hypothyroidism

When thyroid hormone is deficient, hypothyroidism develops. The most common cause of acquired hypothyroidism is **Hashimoto's thyroiditis**, an autoimmune disorder typically affecting middle-aged women. Hypothyroidism can also be iatrogenic, caused by thyroid surgery, neck irradiation, chronic lithium therapy, and some types of iodine administration. Patients who are treated with ^{131}I for hyperthyroidism can develop hypothyroidism after many years. These patients' T_4 and TSH levels should be regularly monitored. Large doses of iodine in radiographic studies can actually inhibit the release of thyroid hormone, a phenomenon called the **Wolff-Chaikoff effect**. Hypothyroidism can develop in patients undergoing these tests.

SIGNS & SYMPTOMS

Common symptoms of hypothyroidism are lethargy, cold intolerance, constipation, weight gain despite reduced appetite, and irregular menses. Hair is coarse. Skin is dry and may show non-pitting edema in severe cases (myxedema). The relaxation phase of deep tendon reflexes may be slowed, and bradycardia may be present. In Hashimoto's thyroiditis, the thyroid is enlarged, nodular, and nontender early in the disease, but it eventually becomes small and fibrotic.

DIAGNOSIS

Serum T_4 (bound and free) is decreased. TSH is high in thyroid disease but low in hypothyroidism with pituitary or hypothalamic causes. In Hashimoto's disease, antithyroglobulin antibodies are found in the serum, and diagnosis is confirmed by finding lymphocytic infiltrates and fibrosis on needle biopsy of the thyroid.

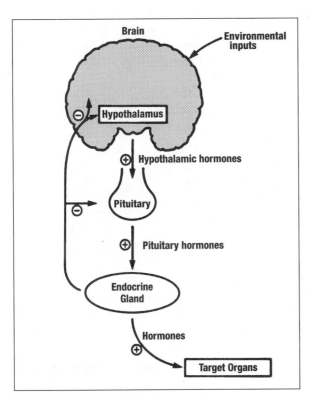

Fig. 4-1. Endocrine feedback loop.

Daily levothyroxine. Verify dose by monitoring free T_4 and TSH. Reduce dose if angina occurs or worsens.

Congenital Hypothyroidism (Cretinism)

Congenital hypothyroidism (cretinism) is a rare deficiency of thyroid hormone due to severe iodine deficiency, thyroid dysgenesis, or inborn errors of thyroid hormone synthesis. If left untreated, mental and growth retardation occur.

Infants have a hoarse cry, respiratory distress, cyanosis, poor feeding, jaundice, and retardation of bone growth.

Routine newborn blood testing reveals low T_4 and high TSH.

Levothyroxine must be started in the first week of life to minimize developmental delay.

Hyperthyroidism (Thyrotoxicosis)

Hyperthyroidism (thyrotoxicosis) is an excess of thyroid hormone. Specific etiologies are discussed below.

Symptoms reflect an overactive metabolism and include nervousness, sweating, hypersensitivity to heat, palpitations, weight loss despite increased appetite, insomnia, and frequent bowel movements. Signs include tachycardia, widened pulse pressure, tremor, warm skin, and occasional atrial fibrillation. Eye signs are found in Graves' disease only (see below).

Usually, both free T_4 and T_3 levels are elevated. Rarely, the T_3 will be elevated with a normal T_4 (called "T_3 toxicosis"). This presentation is generally an early manifestation of thyrotoxicosis, and T_4 will rise later in the disease. If the hypothalamic-pituitary axis is intact, TSH levels will be low.

Diagnosis and treatment are based on the etiology of the symptoms.

1. **Graves' disease,** an autoimmune disorder, is the most common type of hyperthyroidism. Antibodies bind to the TSH receptors in the thyroid, stimulating thyroid hormone synthesis. In addition to symptoms of hyperthyroidism, exophthalmos is typical. Pretibial myxedema is also characteristic but less common. Radioactive iodine uptake is high. Treatment is with surgery (subtotal thyroidectomy), radioactive iodine (contraindicated in pregnancy), or antithyroid medications (propylthiouracil [PTU] or methimazole).

2. **Subacute thyroiditis**, probably viral in origin, is characterized by a tender, enlarged thyroid gland. Symptoms of mild hyperthyroidism, neck pain ("sore throat"), and fever are common, though a period of hypothyroidism may follow the acute phase of the illness. Radioactive iodine uptake is decreased. Sedimentation rate is elevated. Treatment is with anti-inflammatory agents, including glucocorticoids, and beta blockers for symptom control. Thyroid replacement may be needed while the thyroid recovers.

3. **Silent lymphocytic thyroiditis** is a transient thyroiditis that is often found postpartum. There is no pain or fever, unlike in subacute thyroiditis. Radioactive iodine uptake is low, unlike in Graves' disease. Biopsy shows lymphocytic inflammation, similar to Hashimoto's thyroiditis. Treatment is symptomatic (beta blockade), and the disease is self-limited. Recurrences are common.

4. **Toxic adenoma** or **toxic multinodular goiter** occurs when one or more thyroid nodules begin to function autonomously. The condition is most common in older patients. The excess T_3 and T_4 depress pituitary TSH production, thereby causing hypofunction in the rest of the gland. Thus, thyroid scan shows one or more "hot spots" with a hypoactive background. Treatment is with surgery or radioiodine.

5. **Thyrotoxicosis factitia** occurs when exogenous thyroid hormone ingestion results in symptoms of hyperthyroidism without goiter. Treatment is obvious.

Thyroid Storm

Thyroid storm is a medical emergency characterized by the extreme effects of thyrotoxicosis. It may be triggered by surgery, illness, or other stress in a patient who is already thyrotoxic.

Diaphoresis, extreme restlessness, and fever are classic symptoms. Tachycardia may lead to congestive heart failure. Older patients may have myocardial infarctions.

 Elevated T_4 and T_3 concentrations and the presence of the classic signs and symptoms are diagnostic.

 Treatment options include beta-blockers, PTU, or methimazole and intravenous sodium iodine to block hormone release via the Wolff-Chaikoff effect. Glucocorticoids inhibit the conversion of T_4 to T_3, the more active form of the hormone.

Sick Euthyroid Syndrome

Sick euthyroid syndrome is a laboratory phenomenon found in acutely ill patients. Serum T_4 and T_3 levels are low because of changes in thyroid hormone metabolism, but TSH is not increased, indicating that true hypothyroidism is not present. Signs typically found in hypothyroidism (hypothermia, mental sluggishness) are frequently present in an acutely ill patient, but the diagnosis of hypothyroidism should not be made without an elevated TSH. Treatment for thyroid dysfunction is not necessary.

Goiter

Any enlargement of the thyroid gland that is not the result of a neoplasm is termed a goiter. Goiters can be associated with hyperthyroidism (Graves' disease, toxic nodular goiter), euthyroidism (iodine deficiency), or hypothyroidism (Hashimoto's thyroiditis). Thyroid enlargement may result from overstimulation with TSH or a TSH-like substance, or may be due to inflammation. Endemic goiter is present when a large proportion of a population has a goiter and is usually due to iodine deficiency.

Thyroid Nodule

The majority of thyroid nodules are benign, although malignancy must always be considered in the work-up. If benign, a nodule may produce appropriate or excessive amounts of thyroid hormone. Malignant tumors typically do not produce hormone and are therefore "cold" on thyroid scan. Risk of malignancy is increased by any of the following:

- The patient is male
- The patient is young
- The patient has had head or neck irradiation
- Vocal hoarseness is present
- The nodule is "cold"
- The nodule is solid (not cystic).

Considerable debate exists about how to best evaluate a thyroid nodule, but standard evaluation may include a thyroid scan, ultrasound, and fine-needle aspiration. Benign nodules require treatment (surgery or ^{131}I) only if symptoms of hyperthyroidism are present. Treatment for malignant nodules is discussed below.

Thyroid Carcinoma

There are four main types of malignancy found in the thyroid gland:

1. **Papillary carcinoma** is the most common and has the best prognosis. This slow-growing tumor often metastasizes to local cervical nodes (check for nodal enlargement).
2. **Follicular carcinoma** is more common in older patients. Prognosis of this tumor is not as good. Spread is via blood to bone, lung, brain, and liver.
3. **Anaplastic carcinoma** is less common. Prognosis is poor. Local invasion often causes hoarseness and dysphagia.
4. **Medullary carcinoma** is a malignancy of the parafollicular C cells, which produce calcitonin; thus, an elevated serum calcitonin is characteristic. Prognosis is poor. This tumor often occurs as a component of familial multiple endocrine neoplasia (MEN) type II.

The most common presentation is an asymptomatic nodule noted by the patient or physician. Cervical lymph node enlargement, hoarseness, and dysphagia may be present.

A nodule is evaluated as discussed above. Diagnosis is by biopsy.

Surgery, with subsequent ablation of remaining thyroid tissue using radioactive iodine, is the usual treatment. Thyroid hormone replacement therapy is necessary after surgery.

Disorders of Glucose Metabolism

Diabetes Mellitus (Type I)

Type I diabetes mellitus is also called juvenile-onset diabetes or insulin-dependent diabetes. Patients lose their ability to produce endogenous insulin. The mechanism is unknown, but it is thought to be autoimmune because patients generally have anti–islet cell antibodies. (Recall, insulin is produced in the islet beta cells of the pancreas.) Type I diabetes is associated with HLA-DR3, HLA-DR4, and HLA-DQ, and it may run in families. The average age of onset is 11–13 years.

Table 4-1. Effects of various types of insulin

Type	Peak effect (hours)	Duration of action (hours)
Regular	2.5–5.0	8
NPH	4–12	24
Lente	7–15	24
Ultralente	10–30	36

The classic triad of symptoms is polyuria (caused by osmotic diuresis from glucose dumping in the urine), polydipsia (to replenish water loss), and polyphagia (in a futile effort to increase available energy). Weight loss occurs because energy from glucose cannot get into the tissues. Accelerated fat breakdown leads to ketoacidosis, and patients may present with nausea and vomiting, air hunger, or coma (see below). In general, the onset of symptoms is rapid.

One of the following:
1. Elevation of random plasma glucose and classic symptoms of diabetes
2. Fasting plasma glucose >140 mg/100 ml on two separate days
3. Positive oral glucose tolerance test on more than one occasion (plasma glucose >200 mg/ 100 ml 2 hours after an oral glucose load)

Insulin injections are required. Insulin doses and combinations must be titrated to maintain optimal blood glucose levels (Table 4-1 and Fig. 4-2). Patients must be taught how to monitor their glucose level at home (finger-stick monitoring) and how to adjust diet and insulin accordingly. Note that type I diabetics often have a "honeymoon" period shortly after their diabetes is diagnosed, during which endogenous insulin levels rise. Therapy may not be needed for several months, but symptoms and insulin requirements inevitably return.

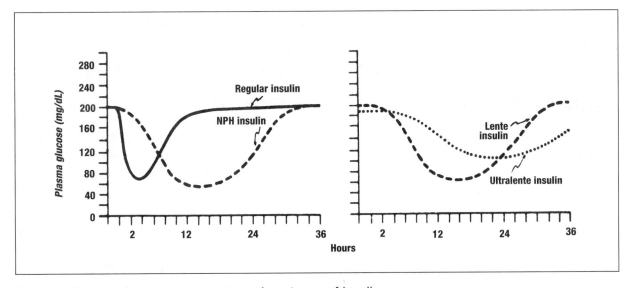

Fig. 4-2. Plasma glucose response to various types of insulin.

Diabetes Mellitus (Type II)

Type II diabetes mellitus is also called adult-onset diabetes or non–insulin-dependent diabetes. This type of diabetes arises when the body's response to insulin decreases and the tissues become increasingly resistant to insulin. Initially, the pancreas responds by increasing insulin production; however, the beta islet cells' capacity to produce insulin may diminish later in the course of the disease. Thus, depending on the stage of disease at the time of diagnosis, insulin levels may be high, normal, or low. Although patients may need insulin therapy (insulin-requiring non–insulin-dependent diabetes), endogenous insulin production is usually sufficient to protect against diabetic ketoacidosis. Obesity and a family history of diabetes are common, but there is no association with any human leukocyte antigen (HLA) type. Typical onset occurs after age 40.

Although the classic symptoms are the same as in type I, onset is more insidious, and ketoacidosis does not occur. Patients may complain of blurry vision, due to osmotic changes in the lens.

See diagnosis for type I diabetes.

- Diet should be low in concentrated sugar to minimize serum glucose fluctuations. The patient may be taught to monitor serum glucose with finger-sticks.
- Weight loss and exercise may increase insulin sensitivity in the tissues.
- Oral hypoglycemic agents, called sulfonylureas (tolbutamide, tolazamide, glipizide, glyburide), stimulate insulin secretion.
- Insulin injections are required in type II patients who do not respond to more conservative measures.

Chronic Complications of Diabetes

Most chronic complications of diabetes are due to microvascular disease. Development of complications is more severe in patients with poorly controlled diabetes and seems to be associated with chronic exposure to elevated levels of glucose, although the mechanism is unknown.

- *Retinopathy.* The effects of **nonproliferative** or **background retinopathy** include microaneurysms, blot hemorrhages, infarcts, hard exudates, and macular edema. Changes are seen early and do not usually cause visual loss until macular edema develops. In **proliferative retinopathy**, new vessels grow on the retinal surface (neovascularization). These vessels are fragile and prone to hemorrhage. Fibrosis occurs during healing and may put traction on the retina, leading to retinal detachment and visual loss. Laser therapy can slow the progression of proliferative retinopathy.
- *Renal disease.* The first sign of renal disease is proteinuria, with a subsequent decrease in creatinine clearance after 1–3 years. End-stage renal disease, requiring dialysis or transplant, typically occurs 3 years after that. Preventive measures include keeping strict control of plasma glucose, eating a low-protein diet, controlling hypertension—especially

with angiotensin-converting enzyme (ACE) inhibitors, avoiding contrast dye, and aggressively treating urinary tract infections.

- *Atherosclerosis.* Atherosclerosis, which causes coronary artery disease, stroke, and peripheral vascular disease (PVD), is more common in diabetics. PVD presents as intermittent claudication (leg pain with exercise due to ischemia) or nonhealing foot ulcers.
- *Neuropathy.* **Bilateral symmetrical sensory impairment** usually begins in the feet and progresses proximally. Patients may complain of pain or numbness. Foot ulcers may develop and become infected without the patient becoming aware of them, so diabetic patients should be trained to examine their feet regularly for ulcerations. **Autonomic dysfunction** can include impotence, orthostatic hypotension, constipation or diarrhea, and silent MI. **Mononeuropathy** is caused by infarction of a single nerve, frequently a cranial nerve. Pain is followed by a palsy, which usually resolves in several months.

Acute Complications of Diabetes

Ketoacidosis

Insulin normally inhibits peripheral lipolysis. When the insulin level is extremely low, triglycerides are degraded into free fatty acids, which are then converted to ketoacids by the liver. Diabetic ketoacidosis (DKA) occurs in type I diabetics who do not take their insulin. It also occurs when infection or MI has increased the body's insulin requirements. Type II diabetics usually produce enough insulin to protect against DKA.

The prodrome involves 12–24 hours of weakness, polyuria, polydipsia, and hyperventilation (in an attempt to compensate for the metabolic acidosis). A fruity, acetone odor may be smelled on the breath. Abdominal pain and vomiting are also common, but care must be taken to determine if gastrointestinal (GI) complaints are due to ketoacidosis or to a precipitating infection. As dehydration worsens, mental status changes can occur.

Serum glucose is 300–800 mg/100 ml (compare with hyperosmolar coma, below).

IV fluids and insulin. Potassium must also be given and monitored carefully. Insulin will cause potassium to enter cells, and if extracellular potassium is not replaced, hypokalemia can cause fatal cardiac arrhythmias.

Hyperosmolar Coma

Hyperosmolar coma, a complication of type II diabetes, usually occurs after many days of infection or other illness.

The symptoms of polyuria, polydipsia, and dehydration are similar to those of ketoacidosis; however, because some insulin is present, lipolysis and ketoacidosis do not occur. Therefore, there is no hyperventilation or acetone smell to the breath, but dehydration is profound and causes significant mental status changes. Dehydration may not be immediately apparent because urine output remains normal due to osmotic diuresis. Hemoconcentration may lead to stroke.

Serum glucose is 600–2,000 mg/100 ml.

Similar to that of ketoacidosis.

Hypoglycemia and Hyperinsulinism

There are several clinical entities that can cause hypoglycemia and hyperinsulinism. **Reactive hypoglycemia** is lowered blood glucose that occurs 2–4 hours after eating. A pancreatic islet cell tumor, or **insulinoma**, can produce excess insulin, causing hypoglycemia. **Iatrogenic hypoglycemia** can result from administration of too much insulin or, less frequently, from excessive oral hypoglycemics.

The symptoms of hypoglycemia fall into two categories. Faintness, weakness, tremulousness, palpitations, sweating, and hunger are the epinephrine-like symptoms. Presentation of these symptoms shows that endogenous, epinephrine-induced glycogen mobilization has begun. The other type of symptoms are CNS-related and includes headache, confusion, and personality changes.

Reactive hypoglycemia is diagnosed if hypoglycemia coincides with the occurrence of typical symptoms, which are then relieved by carbohydrate ingestion. Elevated insulin in the presence of hypoglycemia indicates insulinoma or an exogenous insulin source.

Frequent small meals improve reactive hypoglycemia. Surgery is required to treat insulinoma. For iatrogenic hypoglycemia, increased care should be used in monitoring glucose and administering insulin.

Parathyroid Disorders

Parathyroid hormone (PTH) is responsible for elevating serum calcium (Fig. 4-3). It mobilizes calcium stores from bone, increases reabsorption of calcium in the kidney, and increases the production of 1,25-dihydroxycholecalciferol, the vitamin D–based product that increases calcium absorption from the GI tract. PTH also decreases phosphate reabsorption in the renal tubules, lowering serum phosphate.

Primary Hyperparathyroidism

Primary hyperparathyroidism occurs when excess PTH is secreted by the parathyroid gland. A single, benign adenoma is responsible in 80% of cases. Hyperplasia of all four

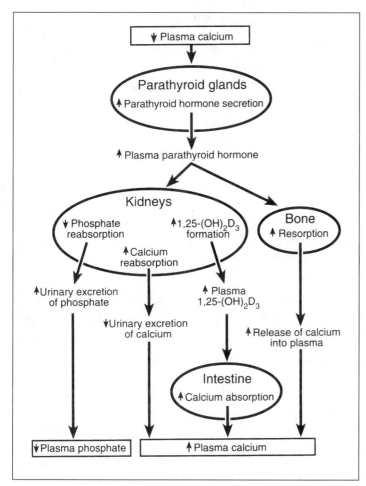

Fig. 4-3. Mechanism by which parathyroid hormone increases plasma calcium. (From RA Rhoades, GA Tanner. *Medical Physiology*. Boston: Little, Brown, 1995.)

glands accounts for most of the remaining cases. Parathyroid cancer is rare, comprising less than 2% of cases of primary hyperparathyroidism. Patients with primary hyperparathyroidism are usually older women.

SIGNS & SYMPTOMS

The disorder is often asymptomatic, but evidence of hypercalcemia (GI disturbances, muscle weakness, emotional lability), osteoporosis (bone pain if fracture has occurred), or renal stones may be present. Recall the mnemonic: "bones, stones, abdominal groans, and psychic moans."

DIAGNOSIS

Lab tests reveal high PTH, with the resulting high calcium and low phosphate.

TREATMENT

Treatment is surgical. Beware of postoperative hypocalcemia, as "hungry bones," freed from the power of PTH, take up the available calcium.

Secondary Hyperparathyroidism

Secondary hyperparathyroidism is parathyroid hypertrophy that develops in response to low serum calcium. Common causes of low serum calcium are vitamin D deficiency or malabsorption, renal tubular problems causing calcium loss (renal tubular acidosis, Fanconi's syndrome), and certain antiseizure medications that interfere with vitamin D metabolism (phenytoin, phenobarbital). Serum phosphate is low, unless there is renal insufficiency (see Chap. 5). The underlying disorder is treated.

Hypoparathyroidism

Hypoparathyroidism occurs when the parathyroid glands fail to develop (DiGeorge's syndrome), when they are removed by surgery, or when target tissues are not responsive (pseudohypoparathyroidism).

The ensuing hypocalcemia causes tingling of the lips and fingers and can lead to tetany. A positive Chvostek's sign occurs when a tap on the cheek causes facial muscle spasms. Trousseau's sign is present when a blood pressure cuff inflated on the arm for 3 minutes induces carpal spasm.

Low levels of parathyroid hormone, causing low calcium and high phosphate.

Calcium and vitamin D supplementation. Note that magnesium deficiency, common in alcoholics, causes hypocalcemia by decreasing PTH secretion and its effect on target organs. In this case, magnesium supplementation must be added to calcium and vitamin D.

Pituitary and Hypothalamic Disorders

Diabetes Insipidus

In diabetes insipidus, lack of antidiuretic hormone (ADH) secretion from the posterior pituitary causes excretion of large amounts of dilute urine. The etiology is most commonly head trauma, pituitary surgery, or an intracranial neoplasm. As long as the patient can drink enough fluid to replace losses (up to 15 liters per day!), dehydration, hypernatremia, and hyperosmolality will not occur. Treatment is with vasopressin or its analogues.

Syndrome of Inappropriate Antidiuretic Hormone Secretion

The syndrome of inappropriate ADH secretion (SIADH) occurs when excess ADH causes free water to be absorbed in the kidneys, resulting in hyponatremia and overly concentrated urine. The etiology can be a cranial lesion (trauma, tumor, infection), pulmonary

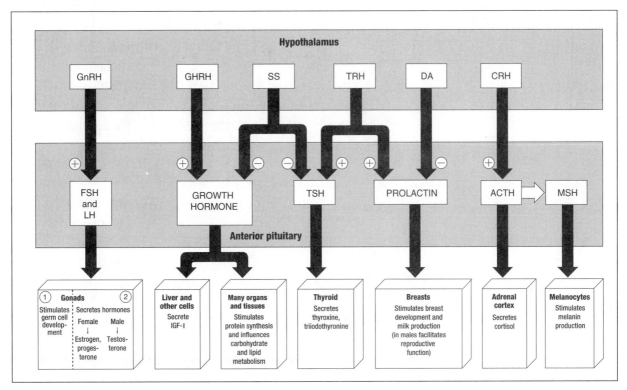

Fig. 4-4. Hormones of the hypothalamic-pituitary axis and their target tissues.

disease (tuberculosis, pneumonia, positive pressure ventilation), ectopic ADH production (usually from a lung tumor), and certain drugs. Fluid restriction will correct serum osmolality and serum sodium.

Panhypopituitarism

Panhypopituitarism is a deficiency of all pituitary hormones (Fig. 4-4). A variety of pituitary or hypothalamic lesions, including hypophysectomy from trauma, can cause this syndrome. Some hormones are stored in large quantities and other target glands maintain some autonomous function, so symptoms of deficiencies appear at varying times. Follicle-stimulating hormone (FSH) and luteinizing hormone (LH) levels are usually the first to decrease, with resulting menstrual irregularities and sexual organ atrophy. Adrenocorticotropic hormone (ACTH) and TSH decreases follow, leading to hypoadrenalism and hypothyroidism. Patients often seem depressed and apathetic. Treatment is with replacement hormones.

Acromegaly

Acromegaly, a condition in which continued bone growth results in a characteristically enlarged jaw, forehead, and hands, is caused by excess growth hormone produced by a pituitary tumor in adults. Soft tissues (tongue, heart, liver, kidneys) also enlarge.

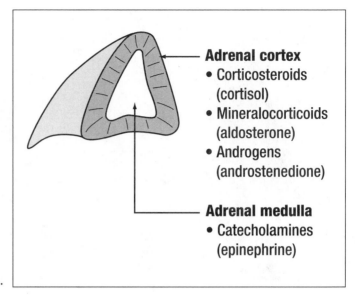

Fig. 4-5. Hormones of the adrenal gland.

Osteoarthritis is common, as is diabetes mellitus due to glucose intolerance caused by growth hormone. The offending pituitary tumor can cause visual disturbances and headaches if it becomes large enough. Treatment is via transsphenoidal surgery or radiation to destroy the tumor.

Adrenal Disorders

Primary Corticoadrenal Insufficiency (Addison's Disease)

Destruction of both adrenal glands results in a deficiency of mineralocorticoids (most important, aldosterone) and glucocorticoids (most important, cortisol) (Fig. 4-5). Etiology is usually autoimmune, infectious (TB, fungal), or hemorrhagic (usually due to anticoagulant therapy).

Symptoms are nonspecific, including fatigue, weakness, weight loss, nausea, and vomiting. A notable feature is hyperpigmentation of the skin, which develops because ACTH and melanocyte-stimulating hormone (MSH) are made from the same precursor (see Fig. 4-4). When ACTH production is increased in an attempt to stimulate cortisol production, MSH increases as well, causing darkening, especially of the folds of the skin.

Loss of aldosterone causes hyponatremia (with associated dehydration and orthostatic hypotension) and hyperkalemia. Eosinophilia is also characteristic.

Diagnosis is made by using the ACTH stimulation test, in which serum cortisol is assessed before and after ACTH is given. If serum cortisol does not increase when ACTH is given, the diagnosis is established.

Glucocorticoid and mineralocorticoid replacement. Glucocorticoid doses should be increased in times of stress and illness. (John F. Kennedy had Addison's disease, and he was healthy enough to become president only after cortisol was developed.)

Secondary Corticoadrenal Insufficiency

Secondary corticoadrenal insufficiency is due to a lack of ACTH. It most commonly occurs in patients who have received corticosteroids for more than 4 weeks. Exogenous steroids suppress ACTH, thus allowing the adrenal glands to atrophy. If steroid use is abruptly discontinued, the adrenals are not able to produce a sufficient supply of endogenous steroid. Because of this phenomenon, patients should be tapered off their steroid medication. Symptoms are the same as in primary disease, and a corticosteroid taper is sufficient treatment.

Acute Corticoadrenal Insufficiency Crisis (Addisonian Crisis)

Because patients with corticoadrenal insufficiency cannot make cortisol, the "stress" hormone, even a minor illness can cause profound weakness, shock, fever, and even coma. Treatment is with IV glucose, saline, and hydrocortisone.

Cushing's Syndrome

The excess of glucocorticoids in Cushing's syndrome can have several possible etiologies, discussed below.

Central obesity with a "buffalo hump" (think "cushion"), moon facies, and peripheral muscle wasting. Obesity in Cushing's syndrome is caused by cortisol, the "stress" hormone, mobilizing energy stores from the periphery to the body's core. Other symptoms include vertebral fractures from osteoporosis, atrophic skin with purple striae, easy bruising, hypertension, and psychiatric changes (depression or euphoria). In women, high adrenal androgens may cause hirsutism, acne, and menstrual irregularities. In men, cortisol may inhibit gonadotropin secretion by the pituitary, causing impotence and a loss of libido.

Dexamethasone suppression test. Dexamethasone is a potent glucocorticoid. In normal people, 1–2 mg dexamethasone, given at night, feeds back to inhibit ACTH release from the pituitary and results in lower serum cortisol levels the next morning. This serum cortisol suppression does not occur in people with Cushing's syndrome.

Treatment is based on the etiology of the symptoms.

1. **Cushing's disease**, caused by a pituitary adenoma, is one of several causes of Cushing's syndrome. The adenoma produces ACTH, which causes adrenal hyperplasia. ACTH levels may be normal or elevated. (Either is inappropriate, given the high levels of cortisol in blood.) High doses of dexamethasone (8 mg/day for 2 days) will suppress cortisol levels somewhat

because the pituitary still has some feedback regulation intact. Treatment is transsphenoidal removal of the pituitary tumor.

2. **Ectopic ACTH production** is usually associated with a lung tumor. This ACTH is not suppressible, even with high-dose dexamethasone. If the tumor is not resectable for cure, treatment is symptomatic and palliative.

3. An **adrenal cortical tumor** may produce high levels of cortisol. ACTH levels are suppressed, and cortisol production is not suppressible with dexamethasone. Treatment is with surgical resection of the tumor. Glucocorticoids must be given postsurgically while the atrophied adrenal gland recovers.

4. In **chronic glucocorticoid therapy** there are no symptoms of increased androgens. Other signs of steroid use (cataracts, glaucoma, hypertension) may be present. Elevated cortisol levels are not suppressible by dexamethasone. Exogenous steroids should be tapered if possible.

Adrenogenital Syndrome

Adrenogenital syndrome includes any condition in which high levels of adrenal androgens cause virilization (see the section on Hirsutism and Virilization in Chap. 6). Effects are more obvious in women and can include hirsutism, male-pattern baldness, acne, voice changes, amenorrhea, and clitoral hypertrophy. The condition can be congenital, in which an enzyme defect causes precursors of cortisol and aldosterone synthesis to be shunted to androgen synthesis. Later in life, adrenal hyperplasia, adenoma, or adenocarcinoma can increase androgen production and cause symptoms.

Hyperaldosteronism

Aldosterone is a mineralocorticoid secreted by the adrenal cortex. It acts on the distal renal tubules to increase sodium retention and potassium loss. Its release is stimulated by low sodium or low blood pressure (via the juxtaglomerular cell-renin-angiotensin system) and by hyperkalemia.

Primary aldosteronism (Conn's syndrome) is caused by adrenal hyperplasia or adrenal adenoma. Patients have hypertension and hypokalemia. Treatment is with the aldosterone antagonist spironolactone. Adenomas are surgically resected.

Secondary aldosteronism is caused by increased activity of the renin–angiotensin system. The most common cause is a decrease in the blood pressure perceived by the juxtaglomerular cells, as in congestive heart failure (CHF), cirrhosis, and nephrotic syndrome. The underlying disorder is treated.

Pheochromocytoma

Pheochromocytoma is a condition in which a tumor of the adrenal medulla or sympathetic ganglion secretes bursts of catecholamines, usually epinephrine. The increased sympathetic activity causes episodic hypertension, headaches, palpitations, and anxiety. Diagnosis is confirmed when 24-hour urine collection shows elevated levels of catecholamines and their metabolites. Treatment is surgical, though symptoms may be temporarily controlled with alpha and beta blockers.

Disorders of Lipid Metabolism

Cholesterol and triglycerides are carried in the blood by lipoprotein complexes. An elevated level of low-density lipoproteins (LDLs) is a risk factor for atherosclerosis and coronary artery disease (CAD), while an elevated level of high-density lipoproteins (HDLs) is protective against atherosclerosis. The risk associated with high triglycerides is debated. Serum lipid levels can be adversely affected by genetic disorders (see below), endocrine abnormalities (diabetes, hypothyroidism, Cushing's syndrome), medications (diuretics, beta blockers), high-fat diet, smoking, and obesity.

Primary Hypercholesterolemia

Familial hypercholesterolemia and **familial defective apoprotein B** are both common autosomal dominant diseases involving defective removal of LDLs from plasma. Homozygotes, though rare, show signs of CAD by adolescence. Women are less likely to show clinical disease, perhaps because of estrogen status or smoking history.

The classic clinical picture is CAD or an MI in a young man (average age of first MI is 41 years). Lipid deposits in the tendons (xanthomas) and eyelids (xanthelasma) are pathognomonic and are found most commonly in the Achilles tendon or the extensor tendons of the hand. Homozygotes may have xanthomas in childhood. Corneal arcus may occur.

Heterozygotes have plasma cholesterol of 300–600 mg/dl. Homozygotes have cholesterol levels of 600–1,200 mg/dl. Triglyceride level is normal or slightly increased.

Smoking cessation, a low-fat and low-cholesterol diet, and cholesterol-lowering medication (cholestyramine, nicotinic acid, lovastatin) may control effects of disease. Screening family members is advisable.

Primary Hypertriglyceridemia

Familial hypertriglyceridemia is a common autosomal dominant trait leading to enhanced hepatic triglyceride synthesis. Patients are not predisposed to CAD but may be more likely to develop pancreatitis. Serum triglycerides are elevated, with a normal LDL. Serum may appear milky if triglycerides are very high. These patients are unusually sensitive to other factors causing hypertriglyceridemia, such as alcohol, obesity, and certain medications (estrogen, diuretics, beta blockers, and glucocorticoids).

Primary Hyperlipidemia

Familial combined hyperlipidemia is an autosomal dominant trait. Affected individuals may have elevated cholesterol, elevated triglycerides, or both, at different times. CAD occurs early, as with familial hypercholesterolemia. There are no characteristic xanthomas. Diagnosis depends on examining family members.

Familial dysbetalipoproteinemia is a relatively rare disorder of the catabolism of lipoprotein remnants. Patients tend to have palmar or tuberous xanthomas and an increased risk of both peripheral vascular disease and CAD. Both cholesterol and triglycerides are elevated. Diagnosis can be established by using electrophoresis to demonstrate abnormalities of VLDL (very low-density lipoprotein).

Disorders of Mineral Metabolism

Hypercalcemia

Hyperparathyroidism and malignancy are the most common causes of hypercalcemia. Bony metastases and osteolytic tumors (multiple myeloma, lymphoma, leukemia) may raise calcium levels by increasing bone resorption. Bronchogenic tumors may produce a substance similar to PTH that acts on the PTH receptors to increase serum calcium. Prolonged bed rest may aggravate hypercalcemia in cancer patients. Other causes include increased intestinal absorption (sarcoidosis, hypervitaminosis A or D), increased renal reabsorption (thiazide diuretics, Addison's disease), and ingestion of large amounts of calcium carbonate and milk (milk-alkali syndrome).

SIGNS & SYMPTOMS

"Stones, bones, abdominal groans, and psychic moans." Renal stones may result in acute urinary tract obstruction. Polyuria occurs because the excess calcium blocks ADH receptor sites in the distal convoluted tubules.

LABS

A large proportion of calcium is bound to albumin in the serum. Patients with low albumin levels have low total calcium levels, although their free calcium level may be normal. To adjust for the effect of low albumin, the lower limit of normal for calcium should be shifted down by 0.8 mg/dl for every 1 g/dl of albumin below normal. For example, if the patient's albumin level is 2.5 (1 g below normal), a total calcium level of 7.6 mg/dl (0.8 mg/dl below normal) would still be considered normal.

TREATMENT

Aggressive, continuous hydration, followed by furosemide to promote calciuria after the patient is well hydrated. Pamidronate and calcitonin help to reduce bone resorption.

Hypocalcemia

Multiple etiologies include hypoparathyroidism, vitamin D abnormalities (deficiency, malabsorption, or impaired metabolism), renal tubular defects, and acute pancreatitis.

Tetany occurs in severe cases. Chvostek's sign (tapping the facial nerve in front of the ear elicits facial contraction) and Trousseau's sign (inflating a blood pressure cuff for 3 minutes causes carpal spasm) may be present.

Serum phosphate is high in hypoparathyroidism and renal failure but not in vitamin D deficiency.

IV and PO calcium. Magnesium if necessary.

Hemochromatosis

Hemochromatosis is a common autosomal recessive disease in which there is increased GI absorption of iron. Iron accumulation over time causes multiple organ damage. Clinical disease is much more common in men because women lose some of the excess iron during menses. Fifteen to 20% of patients develop hepatocellular carcinoma.

Classic triad is hepatic cirrhosis, diabetes mellitus, and bronze pigmentation of the skin. The last two characteristics give rise to the commonly used name "bronze diabetes." Testicular atrophy and cardiomyopathy (cardiomegaly, heart failure, and arrhythmias) also occur.

Serum ferritin (reflecting the body's iron stores) and transferrin saturation (the ratio of serum iron to total iron binding capacity) are increased.

Liver biopsy shows large iron stores.

Regular phlebotomy (removal of blood) is used to decrease iron stores. Deferoxamine, an iron-chelating agent, may also be given. Screening of family members may be helpful in early diagnosis.

Wilson's Disease

Wilson's disease is a rare autosomal recessive disease that involves impaired copper excretion into the bile, thereby resulting in copper retention.

Copper accumulation in the liver causes chronic hepatitis and cirrhosis. Copper in the CNS causes tremor, ataxia, psychoses, and dementia. All patients with neuropsychiatric signs have the characteristic Kayser-Fleischer rings, which are golden-brown or gray-green rings of pigment at the edge of the cornea.

Serum copper is low because of a deficiency of ceruloplasmin, the copper-binding protein. Urine copper is high.

Low serum ceruloplasmin and/or liver biopsy with increased copper stores.

Penicillamine chelates copper and reverses most of the disease process.

Multiple Endocrine Neoplasia Syndromes

Multiple endocrine neoplasia (MEN) syndromes are a group of autosomal dominant syndromes involving hyperplasia or neoplasms in more than one endocrine gland. All patients who have hyperplasia or neoplasms in one endocrine gland should be evaluated for these syndromes, and the family history should be thoroughly reviewed. **MEN type I** includes parathyroid hyperplasia or neoplasm (90% of those with the disorder), pituitary adenomas (65%), and pancreatic islet tumors (5%), which may secrete insulin, gastrin, somatostatin, ACTH, vasoactive intestinal polypeptide (VIP), serotonin, or prostaglandin. **MEN type II** includes parathyroid hyperplasia (90%), medullary thyroid carcinoma (90%), and pheochromocytoma (20%). **MEN type III** includes the same tumors as type II, but parathyroid tumors are much less common. In addition, most patients with type III have a marfanoid habitus and neuromas of the eyes, mouth, GI tract, and upper respiratory tract. Treatment of all the syndromes depends on the presentation and is frequently surgical.

5

Genitourinary Disorders

Disorders of the Bladder and Ureters

Cystitis

Bladder infections, or cystitis, are common in sexually active women. They are more rare in children, especially boys, and should prompt a search for congenital abnormalities or vesicoureteral reflux (described later), which can lead to renal scarring and insufficiency. Infections in the elderly have an equal gender distribution. *Escherichia coli* is the most common causative organism.

The classic symptoms are urinary frequency, urgency, dysuria, nocturia, and suprapubic pain. Pneumaturia is associated with a vesicoenteric fistula.

A urine specimen is obtained using a "clean catch" (midstream urine), urethral catheterization, or suprapubic bladder aspiration. WBCs in a centrifuged specimen or more than 100,000 bacteria/ml indicates infection. A voiding cystourethrogram is used to evaluate vesicoureteral reflux in children.

Trimethoprim-sulfamethoxazole or other appropriate antibiotics, based on culture results.

Dysuria

Painful urination is a symptom commonly associated with bacterial infections of the lower and upper urinary tract. If bacteria are not present and symptoms are persistent, other sources of inflammation, including neoplasms, must be ruled out.

Hematuria

Blood in the urine can be macroscopic or microscopic. If pain is also present, blood is often due to infection or a stone passing in the ureter. If no pain is present, blood may be due to a kidney or bladder tumor, renal cysts, or prostatic disease. Glomerulonephritis is indicated by the presence of red blood cell (RBC) casts in the urine.

Pyuria

White blood cells in the urine are prominent in urinary tract infections but may also be a nonspecific sign of inflammation. In particular, WBC casts in the urine indicate nephritis, which may or may not be infectious.

Obstruction

Obstruction of urine flow can occur at the kidney, ureter, bladder, or urethra. Possible causes include stones, tumors, fibrosis at sites of injury, and, in men, an enlarged prostate gland. The complications of

(continued)

obstruction include hydronephrosis and urinary stasis, leading to stone formation, infection, and loss of kidney function.

Oliguria and Anuria

Oliguria is the reduction of urine output to less than 500 ml per day, whereas anuria is the absence or severe reduction of urine output, generally less than 100 ml per day. These conditions may occur due to prerenal factors (bilateral renal artery occlusion), renal factors (acute renal failure), or postrenal factors (bladder outlet obstruction).

Azotemia

Azotemia is the accumulation of excess nitrogenous wastes in the blood in the form of urea, creatinine, ammonia, or uric acid. It is often a sign of kidney failure but may also be the result of increased protein digestion (e.g., during a gastrointestinal bleed) or increased protein catabolism (e.g., severe burns). Uremia is often used as a synonym for azotemia, but uremic syndrome is a separate clinical entity.

Urolithiasis

Most stones of the urinary tract contain calcium. Hypercalciuria predisposes to the formation of calcium stones. Patients with hypercalciuria should be worked up, as they may have a treatable disorder (e.g., primary hyperparathyroidism). More than half of the cases of hypercalciuria in people with urinary stones is due to a hereditary condition called **idiopathic hypercalcinuria**. Individuals with this condition can take preventive measures (outlined below) to avoid developing urinary stones. Struvite stones compose 10–15% of urinary tract stones and develop when a urinary tract infection (UTI) with a urea-splitting bacteria (e.g., *Proteus* or *Pseudomonas*) makes the urine basic enough to precipitate struvite (magnesium ammonium phosphate).

Severe pain, known as renal colic, results from the backup of urine that occurs when a stone blocks the urinary collecting system. The pain may be in the flank, abdomen, or groin and may be referred to the labia majora, testicle, or inner thigh, depending on the location of the blockage. The pain typically lasts 20–60 minutes. Dysuria, frequency, and nausea and vomiting may also be present. Hematuria occurs in some cases.

Abdominal x-rays will reveal calcium stones. IV urogram will show filling defects at the site of obstruction.

Narcotics are often necessary to relieve pain. Lithotripsy (ultrasound) can shatter small stones and allow them to be passed through the system. If lithotripsy is not possible and pain continues, surgery is indicated.

Drinking plenty of water and avoiding calcium reduce the risk of forming calcium stones. Thiazide diuretics lower urinary calcium in patients with idiopathic hypercalcinuria. Acidification of the urine and aggressive treatment of UTIs may help prevent struvite stone formation.

Ureteral Reflux

Reflux of urine into the ureter usually occurs because of a congenital defect in the connection between the ureter and the bladder. The increased pressure in the ureter can cause hydrostatic damage in the kidney and creates the potential for bacteria to ascend the ureter places the kidney at risk for infection as well.

Persistent UTIs in a child are the most common presentation.

A voiding cystourethrogram will demonstrate the reflux.

If the reflux is mild, the situation should be monitored because it may disappear with time. Infections should be aggressively treated. Surgical repair is necessary in severe cases.

Neurogenic Bladder

Bladder control requires intact sensation (to feel when the bladder is full), motor function (to initiate emptying the bladder), and cerebral control (to time it all correctly). Damage at any level of this complex loop results in neurogenic bladder.

An atonic, distended bladder with overflow dribbling occurs in acute spinal cord injury ("shock bladder") and when the sensory component of control is impaired, as occurs in diabetics. If the motor component is damaged, as in polio and some cases of tumor invasion, the patient can sense a full bladder but cannot initiate voiding. An autonomous bladder develops in spinal cord–injured patients after their acute recovery. The bladder fills and empties by reflex, and there is no cerebral control.

Evaluation includes urodynamic studies to assess bladder sensation, capacity, and sphincter control. Voiding cystourethrogram is used to identify obstruction and reflux.

Medications can be given to improve sphincter control, decrease detrusor spasticity, or increase autonomic stimulation. Regular catheterization can be done by the patient or an assistant. Surgical redirection of the urinary tract is also possible.

Enuresis

Nocturnal bedwetting is normal in the first several years of life. Thereafter, voluntary control can be expected. Nocturnal enuresis occurs in 30% of 4-year-olds and 10% of 6-year-olds. There is a familial tendency to late development of nighttime control, and boys are more commonly affected than girls. Only 1–2% of cases in children have an organic etiology, but any suspicious findings on history, exam, urinalysis, or urine culture should prompt further work-up. Treatment options include behavior modification strategies (e.g., awarding stickers for dry nights), enuresis alarms, and imipramine. Family therapy should be considered if stress seems to be a factor.

Bladder Carcinoma

Transitional cell carcinoma is the most common type of bladder cancer. Risk factors include smoking, schistosomiasis infection, and aniline dyes. Males are affected three times as often as females.

Hematuria is the most common finding. Frequency or dysuria may occur, especially as the tumor grows and occupies the bladder space or invades the bladder wall. A suprapubic mass may be palpable.

Urine cytology shows malignant cells, and IV urogram may reveal the presence of a mass. Cystoscopy and biopsy provide definitive diagnosis.

Surgical resection, radiation, and chemotherapy are used, depending on the stage of the tumor. Bladder tumors tend to recur, so patients should be carefully monitored.

Disorders of the Kidneys

Hydronephrosis

Dilation of the renal pelvis due to increased pressure in the urinary system can occur with or without accompanying dilation of the ureter, depending on the site of obstruction. If not corrected, this condition eventually leads to damage of the renal parenchyma and loss of renal function.

If chronic, hydronephrosis may be asymptomatic or associated with dull flank pain. Colicky pain is typical in acute cases. UTIs are common, and GI symptoms are particularly frequent in children with congenital ureteropelvic obstruction.

Ultrasound or IV urogram.

Temporary drainage via a nephrostomy tube will relieve acute symptoms. The underlying obstruction must be addressed, usually with lithotripsy or surgery.

Pyelonephritis and Pyelitis

Pyelonephritis (infection of the renal parenchyma) and pyelitis (infection of the renal pelvis) are clinically indistinguishable and are usually due to *E. coli*, which ascends from the lower urinary tract. Obstruction and urinary stasis predispose to infection.

Fever and chills, flank pain, nausea, and vomiting are the classic symptoms. There may be associated symptoms of a lower UTI (e.g., frequency, dysuria). On exam, there is costovertebral angle tenderness on the affected side.

Pyelonephritis can be distinguished from cystitis by the presence of WBC casts in the urine.

Many patients require hospitalization and IV treatment with a fluoroquinolone (ciprofloxacin) or third-generation cephalosporin for 1 or 2 days. After stabilization or in moderately ill patients, oral treatment with a fluoroquinolone for 2 weeks is standard.

Hypertensive Renal Disease

Hypertension is a frequent complication of renal disease and is usually due to salt and water retention. Hypertension can, in turn, worsen renal failure, so careful control of blood pressure is required to break the vicious cycle. Salt and water restriction and antihypertensive medications (calcium channel blockers or angiotensin-converting enzyme [ACE] inhibitors) are appropriate.

Renovascular Hypertension

Stenosis or occlusion of the renal artery causes hypertension via the renin-angiotensin system. The affected kidney receives less blood flow than normal and is fooled into "thinking" that there is systemic hypotension. It releases renin to increase blood pressure. This is the most frequent cause of curable hypertension, although it accounts for only a small percentage of all cases of hypertension. In the elderly, the most common cause of renovascular hypertension is atherosclerotic disease, whereas in young women, renal artery stenosis is due to fibromuscular hyperplasia of the artery wall.

Persistent hypertension is noted. A renal artery bruit is heard in the upper quadrant of the abdomen in half of patients.

Arteriography can demonstrate the lesion.

Angioplasty or renal artery bypass surgery are common options.

Uremic Syndrome

Symptomatic renal failure is termed uremic syndrome and usually does not develop until the glomerular filtration rate has fallen below 20 ml per minute. The wide variety of symptoms develops as a result of fluid and electrolyte imbalances, buildup of toxins, and depletion of necessary substances.

Neurologic symptoms begin to develop first and can include drowsiness, impaired mentation, asterixis (flapping tremor), encephalopathy, and seizures. Hypertension due to hypervolemia is common, and congestive heart failure may occur. GI manifestations are also quite common and include anorexia, nausea and vomiting, and an unpleasant taste in the mouth. The skin develops a yellow-brown color, and urea from sweat may crystallize on the skin, known as uremic frost. Peripheral neuropathy occurs only in chronic uremic syndrome.

A normochromic normocytic anemia results from decreased renal erythropoietin. Serum phosphorus is high and calcium is low, which may lead to renal osteodystrophy (see below).

Elevated serum urea (BUN) and creatinine in the presence of symptoms is usually diagnostic. A moderate metabolic acidosis due to impaired hydrogen ion excretion is present. Urine volume does not respond to changes in water intake, and urine osmolality is close to plasma osmolality because of the kidneys' inability to change the concentration of the urine.

Progression of renal disease can be slowed but generally not halted. Dietary intake of protein, water, and phosphate should be closely monitored, but dialysis or transplant may ultimately be necessary.

Renal Osteodystrophy

Renal osteodystrophy, which can include bony disorders such as osteitis fibrosa cystica, osteomalacia, osteoporosis, and osteosclerosis, develops in chronic renal failure. Because of poor renal function, phosphorus builds up in the serum and calcium is spilled in the urine.

Vitamin D metabolism in the kidney is also impaired, leading to decreased absorption of calcium in the GI tract. These factors lead to secondary hyperparathyroidism, and parathyroid hormone (PTH) draws calcium out of the bone to restore serum calcium levels to normal. If left untreated, bone pain and fractures occur. Dietary phosphorus restriction and calcium supplementation can halt the course of this disease by raising serum calcium and eliminating the need for PTH to release calcium from the bone.

Glomerulonephritis

Glomerular injury can arise in a variety of clinical situations. **Poststreptococcal glomerulonephritis** is an immune-complex–mediated disease that presents as acute glomerulonephritis. Group A beta-hemolytic streptococcal antigen-antibody complexes lodge in the glomerular capillary walls and trigger an immune response. This condition is usually preceded by several weeks with an upper respiratory tract infection and is most common in children over the age of 3.

Goodpasture's syndrome classically presents as a rapidly progressive glomerulonephritis. It is an antibody-mediated disease that, though rare, is most common in young men. Immunoglobulin (IgG) is deposited in the kidney and the lung, and the associated hemoptysis may be severe. **Diabetic glomerulosclerosis** is a chronic glomerulonephritis in which proteinuria gradually progresses to uremia.

There are several patterns in which glomerulonephritis can present. In acute glomerulonephritis, oliguria, edema, and hypertension are present in addition to the typical lab findings. In rapidly progressive glomerulonephritis, uremia develops within 3–9 months. In chronic glomerulonephritis, renal function is preserved for many years, but eventually hypertension and uremia develop.

The classic lab findings are hematuria, RBC casts, and proteinuria.

In poststreptococcal glomerulonephritis, antibiotics are only useful if the underlying infection has not resolved. Otherwise, supportive care is indicated, and steroids are ineffective. Goodpasture's syndrome is treated with high-dose corticosteroids, cyclophosphamide, and plasmapheresis to reduce the level of circulating antibodies. ACE inhibitors may forestall the development of diabetic glomerulosclerosis.

Lupus Nephritis

Renal disease is a frequent complication of systemic lupus erythematosus (SLE) and accounts for half of SLE fatalities. There are several types of disease, including mesangial, membranous, focal proliferative, and diffuse proliferative nephritis.

Patients may be asymptomatic or have signs and symptoms of nephritic or nephrotic syndrome.

Proteinuria with WBC and RBC casts on urine microscopy. Renal biopsy confirms diagnosis.

Corticosteroids or cyclophosphamide, an immunosuppressant, can improve survival of the kidney.

Nephrotic Syndrome

Nephrotic syndrome exists when there is proteinuria in excess of 3 g per day. It can be caused by any glomerular disease, but **minimal change disease** is the most common cause in children and **idiopathic glomerulonephritis** is the most common cause in adults. Albuminuria leads to hypoalbuminemia, which stimulates the liver to produce more proteins. In addition to albumin synthesis, lipoprotein synthesis also increases, leading to hyperlipidemia.

Generalized edema, pulmonary edema, ascites, pericardial effusion, and hypotension occur because of hypoalbuminemia.

Hypoalbuminemia hyperlipidemia, which causes the serum to appear milky.

Proteinuria greater than 3 g per day with the associated signs and symptoms.

High-protein low-salt diet, corticosteroids, and cyclophosphamide can be used. Prognosis is excellent for minimal change disease, though recurrences are common. End-stage renal disease occurs in slightly less than half of adults with idiopathic glomerulonephritis.

Toxic Nephropathy and Interstitial Nephropathy

Because of its rich blood supply, the kidney is susceptible to damage by substances that do not reach toxic concentrations in other areas of the body. Most often, these substances damage the renal tubules, causing **acute tubular necrosis** (ATN), but the interstitial cells of the kidney can also be damaged, causing **tubulointerstitial nephritis**. The list of potential toxins is enormous; it includes antibiotics (especially aminoglycosides and amphotericin B), analgesics (both acetaminophen and all nonsteroidal anti-inflammatory drugs), heavy metals, iodine-containing contrast dye, pesticides, and mushrooms. It may take good detective work to find the source of nephropathy in an individual patient. The offending agent should be removed and any available antidote given. Supportive care for acute renal failure is indicated.

Acute Renal Failure

Acute tubular necrosis is the most common cause of acute renal failure. It can be due to toxins (see above) or ischemic injury to the kidney (e.g., from shock, surgery, or rhabdomyolysis following a crush injury). Other causes of acute renal failure include tubulointerstitial nephritis, glomerulonephritis, and vascular disease.

The history may provide clues to the etiology of the renal failure. Uremic symptoms may be present, except peripheral neuropathy and renal osteodystrophy, which are only associated with chronic failure. Signs of allergy, such as urticaria and wheezing, suggest acute allergic interstitial nephritis.

Elevated blood urea nitrogen (BUN) and creatinine indicate a decreased glomerular filtration rate. Urinalysis and urinary sediment may help establish the etiology.

The patient may or may not be oliguric, but in either case, fluid intake and output must be carefully balanced to prevent fluid overload. Electrolytes should be monitored. Protein intake must be kept at a minimum to minimize azotemia. Dialysis may be necessary if conservative measures fail. Recovery usually takes several weeks.

Chronic Renal Insufficiency and Failure

The kidney has a great deal of reserve, and chronic renal insufficiency does not manifest symptoms until 90% of the nephrons have been destroyed. Thus, failure can develop over the course of many years. The most common causes of chronic renal failure are hypertension, diabetes mellitus, glomerulonephritis, tubulointerstitial disease, polycystic kidney disease, and obstructive uropathy. The problems of renal failure are related to the decreased glomerular filtration rate and the loss of tubular function.

Symptoms of uremia develop gradually.

Serum potassium is high and serum sodium may be low. The kidney is unable to metabolize vitamin D and is unable to absorb calcium and excrete phosphate, resulting in hyperphosphatemia and hypocalcemia. This leads to the development of renal osteodystrophy as the bones are broken down to maintain calcium levels. Anemia may be present due to decreased erythropoietin. A metabolic acidosis develops and the urine osmolarity is fixed at about 300 mOsm/liter.

Azotemia on a routine lab exam is usually the first finding. Abdominal x-ray or ultrasound typically shows small kidneys, except in polycystic kidney disease, amyloidosis, and diabetic nephrosclerosis.

Salt and protein intake should be restricted and metabolic disturbances corrected as much as possible. Dialysis and renal transplantation are indicated if symptoms are uncontrollable with conservative management.

Dialysis and Transplantation

The ultimate treatment for renal failure is dialysis or transplantation. Hemodialysis involves using a machine to filter the blood and redeliver it to the patient. Peritoneal dialysis involves infusing dialysis fluid into the peritoneal cavity via a permanent catheter. The peritoneum acts as the dialysis membrane, and substances in the blood diffuse into the dialysis fluid. This fluid is removed after 4–6 hours, and new fluid is infused. This procedure can be performed at home, which is often preferred by the patient. Infection is a danger with both methods, but peritonitis is a particular risk of peritoneal dialysis.

Kidney transplantation can be performed using a kidney from a living, related donor or from a cadaver. Donors are human leukocyte antigen (HLA) matched prior to transplantation, but graft rejection is the biggest concern. Cyclosporin and prednisone help suppress rejection. Despite the cost of surgery and immunosuppressive drugs, transplantation is still more cost-effective than long-term dialysis.

Inherited Disorders of the Kidney

Polycystic Kidney Disease

Polycystic kidney disease is an autosomal dominant disorder that causes multiple, bilateral renal cysts, resulting in large but poorly functioning kidneys. Some patients have associated intracranial aneurysms.

The disease is usually asymptomatic until adulthood. Chronic UTIs, episodic gross hematuria (due to ruptured cysts or dislodged stones), and, ultimately, uremic symptoms are characteristic. Hypertension is common, and 15% of polycystic kidney disease patients will have subarachnoid hemorrhages. In advanced stages, the kidneys may be palpable.

Proteinuria, hematuria, and pyuria are common.

Ultrasound or IV urogram shows large kidneys with multiple cysts.

Aggressive management of UTIs and hypertension extend kidney function. Dialysis or transplantation is required to treat kidney failure; however, familial donation of kidneys may be difficult, since half of family members will also have the disease. Genetic counseling should be provided.

Hereditary Nephritis (Alport's Syndrome)

Hereditary nephritis (Alport's syndrome) is an X-linked disorder of type IV collagen that affects the glomerular basement membrane. Affected males develop renal insufficiency in early adulthood.

Sensorineural deafness and renal insufficiency.

The signs and symptoms are usually diagnostic. Tissue analysis confirms the diagnosis.

Dialysis and transplantation are used when uremia occurs. Genetic counseling is advised.

Neoplasms of the Kidney

Renal Cell Carcinoma

Renal cell carcinoma, an adenocarcinoma, is the most common renal tumor in adults.

The classic triad is hematuria, flank pain, and an abdominal mass. Other symptoms include hypertension, fever, and weight loss.

Polycythemia due to erythropoietin activity is occasionally seen.

IV pyelogram, ultrasound, and MRI can help identify the extent of the tumor.

Surgery of localized disease is the only curative option.

Wilms' Tumor (Nephroblastoma)

Wilms' tumor (nephroblastoma) is the most common renal tumor in children, and most of these tumors occur in children under age 4. Bilateral tumors are present in 10% of patients.

Abdominal pain, hematuria, hypertension, or an abdominal mass may be present. Weight loss and fever may also occur.

Ultrasound and CT scan can define tumor extent and determine the presence of bilateral involvement.

Surgical resection and chemotherapy with vincristine and actinomycin-D are typically used. Radiotherapy may be appropriate in some cases. Prognosis is generally good, especially with younger children.

Electrolyte Metabolism

Hypernatremia

Blood sodium concentrations of more than 155 mEq/liter most commonly result from dehydration due to decreased fluid intake or increased skin (burns, sweating) or gastrointestinal (diarrhea and vomiting) fluid losses. Diabetes insipidus, in which there is a deficiency of antidiuretic hormone (ADH), causing the body to spill dilute urine even when severe dehydration is present, is another cause.

Clinical features include decreased urine output (except in the case of ADH deficiency), and CNS depression from neuronal shrinkage, leading to seizures, coma, and death.

Treatment involves the administration of free water. Patients with diabetes insipidus require ADH-analogues.

Hyponatremia

Hyponatremia refers to blood sodium concentrations of less than 135 mEq/liter and is most commonly due to renal retention of excess water. This type of hyponatremia occurs in diseases associated with edema (e.g., congestive heart failure, cirrhosis, and nephrotic syndrome), in the syndrome of inappropriate antidiuretic hormone (SIADH), and in patients taking thiazide diuretics (salt wasting causes hypovolemia, which stimulates ADH secretion). Osmotic hyponatremia can occur in patients with hyperglycemia. The excess glucose draws water into the extracellular volume, thereby diluting the sodium concentration. Because this will correct rapidly when the hyperglycemia is treated, the measured sodium level can be adjusted up by 1.6 mEq for every 100 mg/dl of glucose above normal levels.

True hyponatremia should be differentiated from **pseudohyponatremia,** which may be seen in the context of hyperlipidemia. In hyperlipidemia, a large proportion of the plasma volume is taken up by nonpolar lipids, and sodium is excluded from this volume because it is a polar molecule. When plasma electrolytes are measured, we assume that sodium is equally distributed throughout the volume, when in fact, the lipid-containing fraction contains little sodium. This faulty assumption leads to the diagnosis of hyponatremia, although the sodium concentration in the fraction of plasma that contains sodium may be normal.

SIGNS & SYMPTOMS

Sodium levels below 125 mEq/liter may lead to irreversible CNS damage due to cellular edema of the brain cells. If untreated, this condition eventually results in seizures, coma, and death.

TREATMENT

Treatment includes fluid restriction, salt-sparing diuretics, and hypertonic saline infusions. **Central pontine myelinolysis** is the destruction of CNS cells when hyponatremia is corrected too rapidly. It occurs most commonly in alcoholics, diuretic users, and patients suffering from malnutrition. Symptoms include progressive weakness of the face and extremities, resulting in a "locked-in" state, in which the patient can only communicate via eye movements. Prognosis is poor.

Hyperkalemia

Hyperkalemia is defined as serum potassium levels of more than 5.5 mEq/liter. It is often seen in metabolic acidosis, when hydrogen ions enter the cells, causing potassium to exit. The kidney is responsible for eliminating excess potassium from the body, so oliguria, potassium-sparing diuretics, and aldosterone deficiency can all result in hyperkalemia. Massive cell damage (e.g., crush injury, hemolysis, and burns) may release enough potassium to cause hyperkalemia as well.

Pseudohyperkalemia is due to hemolysis or release of potassium from blood cells and platelets after blood is drawn. To avoid this faulty measure, plasma potassium level should be measured immediately, and serum should be inspected for pinkish discoloration that signifies hemolysis.

SIGNS & SYMPTOMS

Clinical features include neuromuscular weakness and cardiac arrhythmias, which can be severe and fatal.

Treatment involves calcium (to antagonize cardiac effects) and sodium bicarbonate, glucose, and insulin (to stimulate potassium uptake by cells). Acute treatment may also include dialysis.

Hypokalemia

Serum potassium levels of less than 3.5 mEq/liter usually occur with GI or renal loss, although poor dietary intake can be a cause as well. GI loss occurs with vomiting, diarrhea, or chronic laxative use. Renal causes include adrenal steroid excess, potassium-wasting diuretics, osmotic diuresis, and renal tubular disease. Anise, found in European licorice, can mimic aldosterone and cause hypokalemia. In addition, insulin administration can cause acute hypokalemia because potassium accompanies glucose entering the cells.

The most significant symptoms are those of muscle weakness, which may lead to respiratory failure, and cardiac arrhythmias.

Treatment involves oral or IV potassium administration, usually in the form of potassium chloride.

Acid-Base Disorders

Acid-base disorders are easy. Really. It's true. All you need to do is approach each problem systematically. The approach described here will allow you to correctly solve virtually every acid-base problem presented on the USMLE Step 2. (Of course, real patients may be a bit more complicated than the problems you see on a multiple-choice exam, but this will give you a start.)

First, some basics. The pH of the blood is normally kept constant by a series of buffers and by the body's ability to excrete excess acid or base through the lungs and kidneys. The main buffer that we're interested in is the bicarbonate-carbonic acid buffer, which is described by the following reaction:

$$CO_2 + H_2O \rightleftharpoons H_2CO_3 \rightleftharpoons HCO_3^- + H^+$$

Disorders of acid-base balance occur when there is a buildup or depletion of CO_2, HCO_3^-, or H^+, driving the equilibrium of the reaction more in one direction or the other. (Does anyone remember Le Chatelier's principle?) There are four basic disorders, each caused by a variety of pathological processes (Fig. 5-1).

- In conditions causing **respiratory acidosis**, such as hypoventilation, CO_2 accumulates in the blood. This forces the above reaction to the right, resulting in an increased concentration of H^+ ions (a pH drop) and, hence, acidosis.
- The opposite occurs in hyperventilation. Rapid breathing causes the concentration of CO_2 to fall, the reaction is pulled to the left, and the concentration of H^+ ions drops (pH rises). This condition is called **respiratory alkalosis**.

(continued)

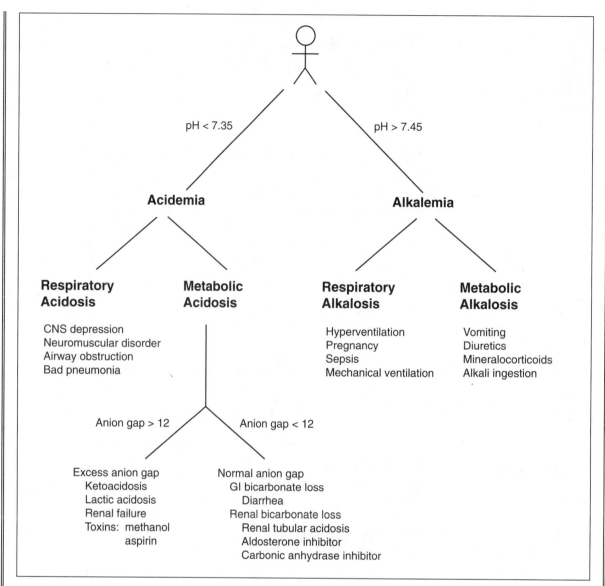

Fig. 5-1. Acid-base disorders.

- **Metabolic acidosis** can occur in two different ways. First, loss of bicarbonate can pull the reaction to the right, increasing the concentration of H^+. Second, there can be a direct increase in H^+ from another source, as is the case with diabetic ketoacidosis. Either way, H^+ concentration rises and pH falls.
- **Metabolic alkalosis** is usually caused by increased loss of H^+ from the kidneys, but it can also be due to alkali ingestion forcing the reaction to the left. The drop in H^+ concentration correlates to a rise in pH.

The lungs and kidneys adjust to try to compensate for these changes and keep the pH at its optimum level. It is important to realize that any compensation will not fully restore the pH to normal, and the direction of the abnormality of pH will always indicate the primary acid-base disorder.

And now for the practical stuff. To evaluate a patient's acid-base status, we start by measuring the pH and PCO_2 of arterial blood. The $[HCO_3^-]$ is then calculated from the Henderson-Hasselbalch equation. (Don't worry, this will be done for you.) The next step is to look at the pH to determine whether you're dealing

(continued)

Table 5-1. Lab values in acid-base disorders.

pH	Acidemia	<7.35–7.45<	Alkalemia
PCO_2	Respiratory alkalosis	<35–45<	Respiratory acidosis
$[HCO_3^-]$	Metabolic acidosis	<22–26<	Metabolic alkalosis

with an acidosis (low pH) or an alkalosis (high pH). You can then quickly determine the primary disorder by identifying which compound, PCO_2 or $[HCO_3^-]$, is altered in the same direction as the pH. Table 5-1 summarizes these relationships and provides normal values. Mastering this table will allow you to answer a large proportion of acid-base questions on the exam.

Take the example of a patient with pH = 7.5, PCO_2 = 57, and $[HCO_3^-]$ = 43. The pH shows that the patient is alkalemic. The PCO_2 is elevated, which would indicate a respiratory acidosis if it were the primary disorder. We know this isn't the case, because we already said that the patient was alkalemic. Therefore, the elevated $[HCO_3^-]$ is the primary disorder, and the patient has a metabolic alkalosis. The elevated PCO_2 is in the opposite direction as the pH (i.e., toward acidemia) and shows respiratory compensation. Note that the compensation did not fully restore a normal pH.

In a patient with metabolic acidosis, one final calculation must be made. The **anion gap** is the difference between the concentration of sodium, the main positive ion of the extracellular space, and the concentrations of chloride and bicarbonate, the main negative ions in the extracellular space. The formula for anion gap is as follows:

$$\text{Anion gap} = [Na^+] - ([Cl^-] + [HCO_3^-])$$

The overall ion balance in the extracellular space is neutral, but there are negative ions (anions) that we don't commonly measure. The anion gap quantifies the concentration of these unmeasured anions. Acidosis with a widened anion gap (>10–14) is due to the presence of an acid that dissociates into a H^+ and an anion that is neither Cl^- or HCO_3^-. The H^+ causes the acidosis, and the unmeasured anion is reflected in the increased anion gap. Acidosis with a normal anion gap is usually found in conditions in which a loss in HCO_3^- is compensated for by a rise in Cl^-, so the anion gap remains unchanged.

Now, believe it or not, you're ready to try a few problems! Figure out the primary acid-base disorder in each of the following and decide if compensation has occurred or not.

1. pH = 7.51, PCO_2 = 22, HCO_3^- = 16, Na = 138, K = 3.3, Cl = 108
2. pH = 7.30, PCO_2 = 31, HCO_3^- = 15, Na = 130, K = 5.0, Cl = 94
3. pH = 7.15, PCO_2 = 88, HCO_3^- = 22, Na = 139, K = 3.3, Cl = 107
4. pH = 7.25, PCO_2 = 27, HCO_3^- = 15, Na = 135, K = 3.1, Cl = 110

Answers:

1. The patient is alkalemic. The PCO_2 is abnormal in the same direction as the pH, indicating a primary respiratory alkalosis. The bicarbonate is low, indicating that metabolic compensation has occurred to try to bring the pH back down to normal. This is consistent with mechanical overventilation.

(continued)

2. The patient is acidemic. This time it's the bicarbonate that's off in the same direction as the pH, indicating a primary metabolic acidosis. The PCO_2 indicates that some respiratory compensation has occurred. Remember to calculate the anion gap! This is a metabolic acidosis with an elevated anion gap. Ketoacidosis can cause this picture.

3. This patient is also acidemic. The PCO_2 clearly indicates a respiratory acidosis, but this time the bicarbonate is normal, showing that no compensation has occurred. Airway obstruction would cause this picture.

4. This patient is acidemic, too. Working through the problem shows that this is a metabolic acidosis without anion gap. Diarrhea is a possible clinical cause.

And there you have it! Of course, in the real world, these disorders can occur simultaneously in the same patient, producing "mixed" disorders that we don't need to deal with here. From all reports, this is the scope of the acid-base problems on the Step 2 exam.

Disorders of the Male Reproductive System

Lower Urinary Tract Infections

With the exception of uncomplicated urethritis and prostatitis, UTIs are rare in males and should prompt a search for underlying abnormalities, such as congenital anomalies, obstructions, and stones. An intravenous urogram is a good first step.

Diagnosis of the specific location of infection is made using lower-tract localization cultures. After cleaning the prepuce, the patient urinates 10 ml into one container (the urethral specimen). A sample of the next 200 ml goes into another container (the bladder specimen). The physician then massages the prostate, and any expressed drops are collected for prostatic culture. Finally, the patient voids 10 ml into the last container (the prostatic specimen). The specimens are cultured, and the quantitative bacterial colony counts are compared to establish the diagnosis.

Urethritis

Urethritis in males is most commonly caused by *Neisseria gonorrhoeae* or *Chlamydia trachomatis* and is classified as "gonococcal" urethritis and "nongonococcal" (chlamydial) urethritis.

SIGNS & SYMPTOMS

Purulent urethral discharge is seen in gonorrhea, and thin, white, mucoid discharge is seen in chlamydia. Dysuria, frequency, and urgency may also occur.

DIAGNOSIS

Gonorrhea is diagnosed by finding gram-negative cocci within WBCs on Gram's stain or by a positive Thayer-Martin culture. Chlamydia is presumed if the Gram's stain is negative.

Ceftriaxone (for gonorrhea) and doxycycline or tetracycline (for chlamydia) are used together because of the high incidence of coinfection. If left untreated, urinary strictures can develop.

Prostatitis

Bacterial infection of the prostate can be acute or chronic. Gram-negative GI organisms are most commonly involved. Nonbacterial prostatitis is more common than bacterial but is less well understood.

Low back and perineal pain are accompanied by urinary frequency, urgency, and pain on urination. Acute prostatitis may cause chills and fever. The hallmark of chronic prostatitis is recurrent UTIs. Rectal exam usually reveals a tender, warm, boggy prostate.

Bacterial counts from prostatic specimens of lower-tract localization cultures are high. Prostatic secretions from nonbacterial prostatitis have WBCs but no bacteria.

Trimethoprim-sulfamethoxazole is used due to its ability to achieve high concentrations in prostatic secretions.

Epididymitis

Epididymitis is inflammation of the epididymis, which is the coiled tube continuous with the vas deferens that lies posterior to the testis. Epididymitis is often caused by urinary reflux, prostatitis, or urethral instrumentation.

Induration and intense tenderness of the spermatic cord. Supporting the testis relieves pain somewhat.

Urinalysis reveals bacteria and WBCs.

Tetracycline.

Torsion of the Testis

Torsion of the testis is caused by the twisting of the spermatic cord, cutting off blood supply to the testis. This condition occurs most commonly in adolescent boys.

Exquisitely tender, swollen, and superiorly displaced testis. Supporting the testis does not relieve pain (compare with epididymitis, above). Sometimes a knot can be felt in the spermatic cord above the testis. Nausea, vomiting, and fever may also be present.

If the diagnosis is in doubt, a testicular scan may be used.

Emergency surgery to restore blood supply to the testis and prevent gangrene is required within several hours (this is no time for long ER waits!). Bilateral orchiopexy (attachment of the testes to the scrotum) is then performed to prevent recurrence.

Hydrocele

If a painless scrotal lump can be transilluminated, it is most likely an accumulation of sterile fluid called a hydrocele. No treatment is necessary unless the cystic mass becomes large and symptomatic. A congenital hydrocele results when the processus vaginalis remains in open communication with the abdominal cavity. This condition may resolve spontaneously, but if it doesn't, the child is at risk for developing indirect inguinal hernias.

Varicocele

A varicocele is a collection of veins that occurs most often in the left scrotum. A "bag of worms" can be palpated when the patient is standing, but it is absent when patient lies down. Varicocele is associated with infertility, presumably because of increased temperature in the testes, inhibiting sperm production. Surgical treatment may be helpful if infertility or pain is a problem.

Cryptorchidism

One or both testes may lie in the abdominal cavity (true cryptorchidism) or in the inguinal canal (incomplete descent). If not surgically lowered, the affected testicle will not be able to produce sperm. The undescended testis will have a higher potential for the later development of testicular carcinoma. Unfortunately, this risk does not seem to diminish, even with corrective surgery. Retractile testes descend into the scrotum at times but then retract into the inguinal canal. This condition requires no treatment and usually resolves by adolescence.

Scrotal sac without a testicle, even in relaxed situations such as a hot bath.

Surgery to place the testicle in the scrotal sac is required prior to age 5 if the potential for spermatogenesis is to be maintained. If it is discovered later in life, cryptorchidism should be treated with orchiectomy to avoid the risk of testicular cancer.

Testicular Neoplasms

Of the several types of testicular neoplasms, seminomas are the most common and have the best prognosis. This is the most common neoplasm in men under age 30. Men who have a history of undescended testes are at increased risk.

A painless testicular mass that does not transilluminate (i.e., no light passes through it when it is lit from behind). Symptoms of metastasis, such as lymphadenopathy, may be present.

Transillumination and ultrasound localize the tumor to the testis. Biopsy is diagnostic.

Orchiectomy and irradiation are used to treat seminomas. Chemotherapy is helpful with other types of tumor. Five-year survival rates of patients with seminomas are greater than 80%, and cure is possible even if disease is metastatic.

Benign Prostatic Hyperplasia

Benign adenomatous hyperplasia of the prostate gland is common in older men. Because the hyperplasia is usually periurethral, varying degrees of bladder outlet obstruction occur. Bladder distention, UTI, hydronephrosis, and altered renal function may develop.

Symptoms of urinary obstruction include hesitancy, straining, decreased stream, dribbling, sense of incomplete emptying, and urinary retention. Irritative symptoms, including frequency, urgency, nocturia, and urge incontinence, may be the result of incomplete bladder emptying or UTI.

Digital rectal exam may reveal a large, fleshy prostate, but transrectal ultrasound is a more sensitive test. Measurement of urinary flow rate can document urinary obstruction.

Alpha blockers (prazosin, terazosin) inhibit contractions of the urinary bladder sphincter. If symptoms cannot be controlled medically, surgical treatment is indicated. The most common intervention is transurethral prostatectomy (TURP).

Prostate Carcinoma

Adenocarcinoma of the prostate is the most common non-skin cancer found in men. Its incidence increases with age. In contrast to benign prostatic hyperplasia, prostate cancer usually develops in the peripheral regions of the prostate. Prognosis is good if treated early.

Patients are often asymptomatic. On exam, the prostate is firm, nodular, or irregular. Symptoms occur late in disease and include bladder outlet obstruction, hematuria, and pyuria. Many patients present with back pain from bony metastases.

Serum acid phosphatase and prostate-specific antigen (PSA) are elevated.

Ultrasound and biopsy. Bone scan will show bony metastases.

Radical prostatectomy and radiation are both used. In late-stage disease, antiandrogen therapy may prolong life for several years. Older men with well-differentiated tumors may choose to delay treatment ("watchful waiting"), because tumors tend to progress quite slowly.

PSA is frequently used as a screening test for prostate cancer; however, false-positives are common, since patients with BPH may also have elevated PSA levels.

Hypospadias

Hypospadias is a congenital displacement of the urethral opening, usually to the underside of the penile shaft. Other malformations, such as a "dorsal hood" (incomplete foreskin) and chordee (ventral curvature of the penis), are commonly associated with this defect. Early surgical correction can prevent later urinary and sexual disability.

Urethral Stricture

Congenital strictures usually result from a thin diaphragm across the urethra. Acquired strictures may result from trauma, instrumentation, or infection (especially gonorrhea). Symptoms include dysuria, weak or spraying urine stream, urinary retention, or UTIs. Retrograde urethrogram demonstrates the location of the stricture. Treatment is by surgical incision.

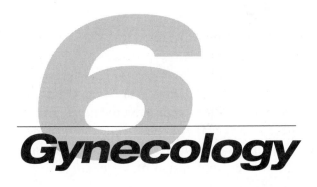

Gynecology

Physiology and Endocrinology

Menstruation and Ovulation

The normal ovulatory cycle consists of a follicular phase and a luteal phase (Fig. 6-1). The **follicular phase** begins on the first day of menses and is characterized by the development of the ovarian follicle. Follicle-stimulating hormone (FSH) secretion from the pituitary gland increases, stimulating growth of the ovarian follicle, which then secretes estradiol. Estradiol (in the absence of progesterone) drives the proliferation of the endometrium. Thus, the follicular phase of the ovary corresponds to the proliferative phase of the uterus. Luteinizing hormone (LH) secretion from the pituitary begins to increase after a lag of several days. As ovarian estradiol levels rise, a positive feedback loop develops, and the increasing estradiol enhances LH and FSH levels. This process culminates in the mid-cycle LH and FSH surge that precipitates ovulation.

The **luteal phase** begins with the LH surge and its accompanying ovulation and ends with the onset of menses. After ovulation, the follicle is called the corpus luteum. The corpus luteum continues to secrete estradiol and begins to secrete progesterone. After the LH surge, a negative feedback loop is re-established and the elevated estradiol and progesterone levels then suppress LH and FSH secretion. The elevated estradiol and progesterone levels also cause the endometrial lining to develop secretory ducts. Thus, the luteal phase of the ovary corresponds to the secretory phase of the uterus. The endometrium is then prepared to accept a fertilized egg. If no egg is fertilized, the decreased LH level allows the corpus luteum to regress, leading to a decline in progesterone and estradiol levels. This decline results in ischemia and sloughing of the endometrial lining (menstruation). The decrease in estradiol and progesterone allows FSH to increase, driving follicular growth in the next cycle.

If fertilized, the egg will implant in the endometrium. The early placental tissue secretes human chorionic gonadotropin (hCG), which acts like LH to maintain the corpus luteum. The corpus luteum continues to secrete progesterone, which maintains the uterine lining until about week 6 of pregnancy, when the placenta begins to produce its own progesterone for this purpose.

Spermatogenesis

The production of mature sperm occurs continuously throughout a man's life. The diploid precursors of sperm cells are able to divide, producing a renewable source of sperm. When a precursor cell undergoes meiosis, four sperm cells are formed. Sperm generation occurs in the seminiferous tubules of the testis. As the sperm travels to the epididymis, it gains motility and nutrients to prepare for its further journey. The development process takes about 70 days.

Ovigenesis

In contrast to spermatogenesis, the number of diploid precursors of ova in girls is fixed before birth. The precursor cells are stuck in the first meiotic division until the girl enters puberty. Each month, FSH causes a group of follicles to begin maturation. One follicle will dominate, complete the first meiotic division, and be expelled from the ovary (ovula-

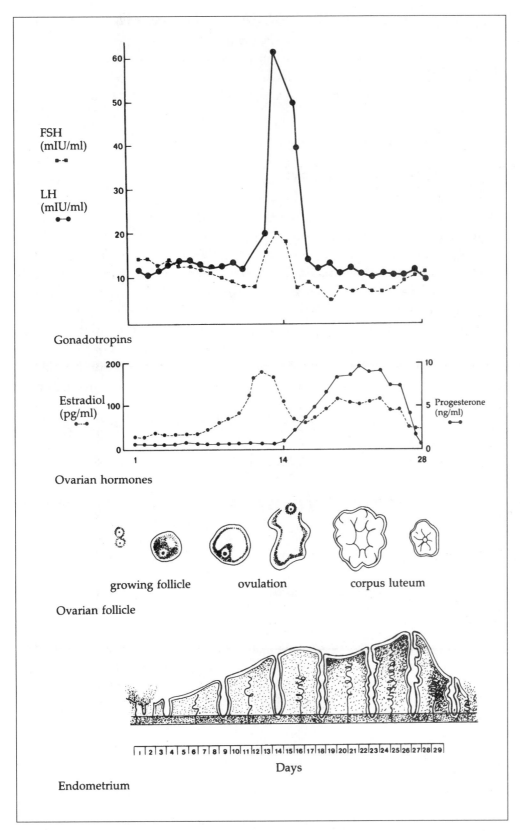

Fig. 6-1. Physiology of the normal ovulatory menstrual cycle. (FSH = follicle-stimulating hormone; LH = luteinizing hormone.) (From SJH Emans, DP Goldstein. *Pediatric and Adolescent Gynecology*, Third Edition. Boston: Little, Brown, 1990.)

tion). The second meiotic division, which results in the mature ovum, occurs after fertilization but before the sperm and egg nuclei actually fuse. Unlike spermatogenesis, in which each precursor develops into four equal sperm cells, each ovum precursor develops into one ovum and three smaller polar bodies. Because of the long interruptions in the process, ovum development can take as long as 45 years.

Intercourse, Orgasm, and Ejaculation

The sexual response cycle is usually described in four phases: desire, excitement, orgasm, and resolution. During the desire phase, vasocongestion causes vaginal lubrication and erection of the penis and clitoris. During the excitement phase, stimulation of the autonomic nervous system causes increases in breathing and heart rate. The inner two-thirds of the vagina expand, forming a depression that can receive sperm. During orgasm, both men and women experience rhythmic, involuntary contractions. In men, this leads to ejaculation of semen. The pleasurable sensation of orgasm is mediated by the central nervous system, so patients with spinal cord injuries may continue to be orgasmic. During the resolution phase, the changes of the previous phases are reversed. Resolution may take as long as an hour.

Human sexual behavior is remarkably varied, and it is unwise to assume anything about the sexual activities of patients. Both homosexual and heterosexual individuals may enjoy vaginal, oral, and anal sex, and monogamy may or may not be a part of a patient's chosen life-style. Questions about risk factors for sexually transmitted diseases and about sexual satisfaction should be posed in a direct and sensitive manner.

Sexually Transmitted Diseases

Trichomonas Vaginitis

Trichomonas vaginitis is caused by the protozoan *Trichomonas vaginalis* and is generally transmitted by sexual intercourse.

SIGNS & SYMPTOMS

Vaginal discharge is yellow-green, copious, thin, and bubbly. Pruritus and burning may be mild or severe. A few patients have the classic vaginal or cervical petechiae or "strawberry patches."

DIAGNOSIS

Saline wet mount shows the pear-shaped, flagellated, motile organism.

TREATMENT

Metronidazole.

Bacterial Vaginosis

Gardnerella vaginalis is the most common cause of symptomatic vaginal bacterial infection.

A heavy, malodorous discharge is the primary symptom. Vaginal or vulvar irritation is usually absent.

On a saline wet mount, characteristic "clue cells" (epithelial cells with intracytoplasmic coccobacilli) are observed. A fishy odor is released when 10% KOH is added to the discharge (the "whiff" test).

Metronidazole for both the patient and her sexual partner.

Chancroid

Caused by the gram-negative rod *Haemophilus ducreyi*, chancroid is a highly contagious venereal disease seen primarily in tropical and subtropical climates.

Within 3–10 days of inoculation, a small papule develops on the vulva or penis. The papule then ulcerates, forming a painful ulcer with a gray base and undermined borders. Inguinal lymphadenopathy occurs in half of cases and can be severe.

Gram's stain of material from the ulcer edge may show the gram-negative rod. Gram's stain and culture of inguinal node aspirates may also be diagnostic.

Erythromycin or ceftriaxone.

Chlamydia

Chlamydia trachomatis is an obligate intracellular organism that invades only columnar epithelium. This organism may account for half of the cases of nongonococcal urethritis in men. Homosexual males may develop chlamydial proctitis. Half of all patients with gonorrhea have coinfection with chlamydia.

Most women are asymptomatic, but urethritis or cervicitis with a mucopurulent discharge may be present. Men have a thin, mucopurulent urethral discharge.

Immunofluorescence of the discharge. Gram's stain is not useful.

Doxycycline (erythromycin during pregnancy). Sexual partners should be traced and treated. Salpingitis leading to tubal obstruction, ectopic pregnancy, and infertility is a potential complication of untreated disease. Infants born of infected mothers are at risk for chlamydial conjunctivitis and pneumonia.

Condyloma Acuminata

Also known as venereal warts, sexually transmitted lesions of condyloma acuminata are caused by human papilloma virus (HPV) 6 and 11. These subtypes are not associated with cervical cancer risk.

Lesions appear on the external genitalia, perineum, anus, or cervix, and may be small and discrete or large and cauliflower-like.

Inspection is usually sufficient for diagnosis.

Cryosurgery, electrocautery, or laser ablation.

Gonorrhea

Neisseria gonorrhoeae can cause acute infection of the cervix, urethra, rectum, and pharynx, depending primarily on sexual practices. Disseminated gonococcal infection is the most common cause of septic arthritis among young people.

Symptoms depend on the location of the infection and typically begin 1–3 weeks after inoculation. Cervicitis may be asymptomatic or may be associated with a purulent discharge. Urethritis is also associated with a purulent discharge and dysuria. Whereas rectal infection is frequently asymptomatic in heterosexual women (who may or may not have engaged in anal intercourse), it is associated with a bloody discharge and pain in homosexual males. Pharyngeal infection, also more common in homosexual men and heterosexual women, is frequently asymptomatic.

Gram's stain showing gram-negative intracellular diplococci or culture is usually diagnostic.

Ceftriaxone. Doxycycline is also given for presumptive coinfection with chlamydia. Untreated disease may cause salpingitis or pelvic peritonitis in women and urethral strictures in men.

Herpes Genitalis

Herpes simplex virus (HSV) is transmitted in oral or genital secretions. Herpes genitalis infection is most frequently caused by HSV type 2. After the primary infection, HSV DNA remains in the sensory ganglia and may reactivate at any time. During recurrences, new virus particles travel down the nerve to the skin and produce active lesions. Patients should avoid sexual contact while lesions are present due to the risk of transmission.

Symptoms of initial infection usually appear within a week of exposure. Patients with primary infections often have generalized malaise, inguinal lymphadenopathy, and a low-grade fever. Clear vesicles appear, rupture, and form painful ulcers. Lesions recur in half of infected individuals and are usually preceded by 24 hours of itching, tingling, or burning in the region. Secondary lesions are less severe, smaller, and of shorter duration than primary lesions.

The clinical presentation is usually diagnostic, but a Tzanck smear or a culture of vesicular fluid will reveal multinucleated giant cells with intranuclear inclusion bodies.

Acyclovir is not curative but may shorten the duration of the episode. Long-term acyclovir treatment may be used in patients with frequent outbreaks.

Molluscum Contagiosum

Caused by a mildly contagious virus, molluscum contagiosum is a benign syndrome that is spread only by direct contact.

Asymptomatic, umbilicated nodules ranging up to 1 cm in diameter are visible on the genitalia.

Inspection is sufficient for diagnosis.

Removal of the papules with a curette and cauterization of the base of the lesions.

Syphilis

Syphilis is caused by the spirochete *Treponema pallidum*.

Approximately 3 weeks after exposure, a chancre develops. A chancre is a papule that later becomes a painless ulcer with rolled edges and a punched-out base. There may be associated rubbery adenopathy. The chancre heals spontaneously in 6–9 weeks if left untreated. Secondary syphilis develops as the chancre heals. It involves condyloma lata (flat, coalescing papules containing spirochetes) on moist areas of the skin, generalized rubbery lymphadenopathy, a maculopapular rash on the palms and soles, and constitutional symptoms (malaise, headache, anorexia). If still untreated, tertiary syphilis may later develop and can include gummatous syphilis (granulomatous reactions in any tissue of the body), cardiovascular syphilis (endarteritis of the vasa vasorum leading to injury of the large arteries, and occasionally resulting in dilation of the aortic root with aortic insufficiency), and neurosyphilis (meningitis, cerebral atrophy caused by spirochetes in the parenchyma, and tabes dorsalis, which involves damage to the posterior columns causing multiple impairments and general paresis).

Serologic tests such as rapid plasma reagin (RPR), the Venereal Disease Research Laboratory (VDRL) test, and fluorescent treponemal antibody absorption (FTA-ABS) are commonly used to establish diagnosis. *T. pallidum* can be isolated from cutaneous lesions and viewed with dark-field microscopy.

Penicillin G.

Pelvic Inflammatory Disease

Pelvic inflammatory disease (PID) can include endometritis, salpingitis, tubo-ovarian abscess, and peritonitis. It is often caused by *N. gonorrhoeae*, but *Chlamydia, Bacteroides, E. coli,* and streptococci are other frequent players. Risk factors include multiple sex partners, prior episode of PID, current or past IUD use, and cervical instrumentation. Long-term complications of PID include chronic pelvic pain, infertility, and ectopic pregnancy.

Low abdominal pain often starts within a few days of menses, in which flow may be heavier than normal. Nausea, vomiting, fever, and chills may be severe, and there may be purulent discharge from the cervix. If the urethra is involved, the patient may have dysuria, frequency, and urgency. Abdominal exam reveals uni- or bilateral lower quadrant tenderness and occasionally an abdominal mass; guarding and rebound tenderness are present if the peritoneum is inflamed. Bimanual exam reveals characteristic cervical motion tenderness.

Leukocytosis with neutrophilia and an elevated erythrocyte sedimentation rate (ESR) are characteristic.

Diagnosis is frequently based on presentation, but a culdocentesis yielding pus is diagnostic. Gram's stain of cervical discharge may reveal gram-negative intracellular diplococci. A negative serum pregnancy test rules out ectopic pregnancy, but a positive pregnancy test does not exclude coexisting PID.

Broad-spectrum antibiotic combinations are started immediately. Patients should be hospitalized if they have fever higher than 38°C, are pregnant, or are not able to tolerate oral intake.

Infections

Candida Vulvovaginitis

Most "yeast" infections are due to *Candida albicans*, although other *Candida* species may be involved. Predisposing risk factors include oral contraceptive use, antibiotic use, pregnancy, and diabetes mellitus.

Intense pruritus and a "cottage cheese" discharge are the primary symptoms. The vulva is tender, red, and swollen. The pH of the discharge is low (4–5).

A KOH wet mount shows pseudohyphae and spores. Sabouraud's medium can be used to culture *Candida,* if necessary.

Vaginal antifungal medication (miconazole, clotrimazole). Consider screening for diabetes.

Urinary Tract Infections

The vast majority of urinary tract infections (UTIs) are due to *E. coli*. The remainder are caused by other gram-negative organisms. *C. trachomatis* may cause urethritis.

Dysuria, frequency, urgency, and suprapubic pain are the typical symptoms. Fever, chills, and costovertebral angle tenderness indicate that the infection has ascended to the kidneys.

Urinalysis showing positive leukocyte esterase, centrifuged urine with white blood cells and bacteria, and urine culture with more than 100,000 bacteria/ml are indicative of UTI. Persistent pyuria without bacturia may indicate chlamydial infection.

Trimethoprim-sulfamethoxazole or, if *Chlamydia* is suspected, doxycycline.

Bartholin's Gland Abscess

An abscess often occurs from secondary infection of a Bartholin's cyst, the most common vulvar tumor.

The cyst presents as a unilateral swelling in the lateral posterior introitus, and is otherwise asymptomatic. The abscess is tender and inflamed.

Cysts do not need treatment, but they can be drained if they are troublesome to the patient. Sitz baths should be used to treat an abscess. If the abscess does not resolve, incision and drainage are performed. For a recurrent abscess, marsupialization is suggested.

Toxic Shock Syndrome

The multisystemic condition toxic shock syndrome (TSS) is caused by the exotoxin from certain strains of *Staphylococcus aureus*. Most frequently associated with tampon use, it has also resulted from prolonged use of intravaginal contraception and from nasal packing, septic abortions, and postpartum infections.

Patients usually present with sudden high fever, an erythematous rash, and a constellation of symptoms that may mimic a viral infection, including diarrhea, vomiting, sore throat, and headache. Hypotensive shock develops within several hours. Desquamation of the palms and soles occurs approximately 10 days into the illness.

The clinical presentation suggests the diagnosis. Culture of the vagina (or other site of infection) may reveal *S. aureus*.

Remove any foreign bodies. Aggressively treat hypotension with fluids, transfusions, and dopamine, as necessary. Penicillinase-resistant penicillins will not affect symptoms but will reduce recurrences.

Disorders of Pelvic Support

Pelvic Relaxation

The pelvic organs are supported by the muscles of the pelvic floor and their ligaments. Pelvic relaxation is a weakness of these ligaments resulting in prolapse of pelvic organs.

Uterovaginal prolapse is the descent of the uterus through the urogenital diaphragm into the vagina. **Cystocele** is the descent of the bladder into the upper anterior vaginal wall. **Urethrocele** describes the bulging of the urethra into the lower anterior vaginal wall without urethral dilation. A **rectocele** involves prolapse of the rectum into the lower posterior vaginal wall, while an **enterocele** is the prolapse of a loop of intestine into upper posterior vaginal wall. Enteroceles are almost always due to herniation of the pouch of Douglas.

Cystocele may be associated with urinary urgency, frequency, incontinence, and, rarely, retention. Symptoms of lower posterior wall prolapse include difficulty emptying the rectum.

Vaginal examination is required for the diagnosis of pelvic relaxation. If prolapse is not apparent, having the patient strain may precipitate it.

Asymptomatic pelvic relaxation does not require any intervention. For symptomatic cases, treatment is primarily surgical, although perineal exercises and pessaries may be helpful.

Urinary Incontinence

Involuntary loss of urine is a common complaint, particularly of postmenopausal women. **Stress incontinence** occurs when intra-abdominal increases in pressure (e.g., coughing, sneezing, or exercise) cause leakage of usually small amounts of urine. **Urge incontinence**, also called detrusor instability, generally involves the loss of large amounts of urine immediately following the urge to void.

A detailed history about the incontinent episodes, including precipitating factors, should be obtained. In addition, the presence of dysuria, frequency, nocturia, and enuresis should be ascertained. Physical exam involves the "Q-tip test," which measures the angle of the urethra at rest and during a Valsalva maneuver. If the urethra moves significantly, an anatomic defect is present.

The history is generally diagnostic, but cystometry and urethral pressure studies may be useful.

Kegel exercises may improve stress incontinence. Both behavior modification, with biofeedback and bladder retraining, and anticholinergic agents are useful in urge incontinence. Estrogen replacement therapy in postmenopausal women will improve both types of incontinence. Surgery is available if an anatomic defect is present.

Gynecologic Neoplasms

Vulvar Neoplasms

Malignant tumors of the vulva usually occur after menopause. The vast majority are squamous cell carcinomas.

Lesions may be pruritic but are otherwise asymptomatic until late in disease.

Biopsy.

Surgical excision with lymph node dissection. Unfortunately, many women wait several years before seeking medical attention, so prognosis is generally poor.

The **squamocolumnar junction** is the junction between the columnar epithelium of the endocervix and the squamous epithelium of the ectocervix and vagina. Throughout life, this junction moves progressively closer to the os, eventually moving into the endocervical canal. The **transformation zone**, the site most likely to show cervical dysplasia and neoplastic transformation, is the area between the new squamocolumnar junction and the original junction.

Cervical Dysplasia

Cervical dysplasia, or cervical intraepithelial neoplasia (CIN), is a preinvasive phase of cervical cancer and can be diagnosed by Pap smear. If left untreated, 10–15% of mild and moderate dysplasias will progress to invasive cancer. Infection with HPV types 16, 18, or 31 is a strong risk factor for cervical dysplasia. Other risk factors are consistent with a sexual mode of transmission (multiple sexual partners, early age at first intercourse, etc.).

Dysplasia is asymptomatic.

During a Pap smear, both the ectocervix and the endocervical canal should be sampled. Lesions can also be visualized by culposcopy because they turn white following the application of acetic acid. Biopsy provides definitive diagnosis.

Superficial ablation is appropriate if the entire transformation zone is visible and invasive disease has been excluded. Techniques available include local excision, laser ablation, cryosurgery, and electrocautery. For more extensive carcinoma in situ, a cone biopsy can be curative.

Cervical Cancer

Cervical cancer is a direct progression from cervical dysplasia, so risk factors for developing the disease are the same as for dysplasia. Due to widespread cervical cancer screening in the United States, which detects the disease in a more treatable stage, mortality from cervical cancer is quite low. Histologically, 85% of cervical cancer is squamous cell carcinoma, while the remainder is adenocarcinoma.

Patients with cervical cancer are most often asymptomatic, but some may present with post-coital bleeding or bloody discharge.

An abnormal Pap smear suggests the diagnosis, and biopsy confirms it.

Treatment of cervical cancer is primarily surgical (hysterectomy and pelvic node dissection), though chemotherapy and radiation may be used in advanced disease.

Uterine Myoma

Fibroids are extremely common, benign masses comprised of smooth muscle tissue. They are hormonally responsive, growing only in the reproductive years.

Many fibroids are asymptomatic. Symptoms may include menorrhagia, metrorrhagia, a sensation of pelvic heaviness, urinary frequency, infertility, and spontaneous abortion. The mass may be felt on bimanual or abdominal exam.

Anemia due to excessive bleeding is common.

Exam, ultrasound, and hysterosalpingography are used to establish the presence of a uterine mass. Biopsy may be necessary if the diagnosis is in doubt.

Treatment is not necessary for asymptomatic, slow-growing masses. Myomectomy or hysterectomy are surgical options.

Endometrial Cancer

Endometrial cancer is strongly correlated with high estrogen states. Risk factors include unopposed exogenous estrogen, obesity, early menarche, nulliparity, late menopause, anovulatory cycles, diabetes, and hypertension.

Vaginal bleeding is the most common presenting symptom. Any postmenopausal woman with vaginal bleeding must be evaluated for endometrial cancer.

Endometrial biopsy.

Hysterectomy is curative if the tumor has not spread. Radiation, hormone therapy, and chemotherapy may be used in more advanced disease.

Ovarian Neoplasms

Ovarian cancers have a large variety of histologic types and, taken together, they make up almost one-fifth of all gynecologic neoplasms. They occur most often in middle-aged women. Most ovarian neoplasms are diagnosed after the disease has spread beyond the confines of the ovary, traveling initially by direct extension and by lymphatics to regional lymph nodes, and eventually by hematogenous dissemination to the liver and lung.

Ovarian tumors are asymptomatic until late in disease. The earliest symptoms are often related to mild GI distress or abdominal discomfort. Later, ascites, pain, anemia, and cachexia develop. Early bimanual exam may reveal an enlarged ovary, which later becomes fixed and nodular.

Work-up may involve an ultrasound and a laparotomy, with lymph node dissection if appropriate.

In a young patient with low-grade disease, a unilateral oophorectomy may be sufficient treatment. More extensive disease may require radical surgery, radiation therapy, and chemotherapy.

Disorders of the Breast

Breast Cysts

Solitary breast masses are either solid or cystic, which can be established by ultrasound. If cystic, a fine-needle biopsy is indicated. If clear fluid is found, no further surgical intervention is necessary, as fluid-filled cysts are generally benign. If, however, bloody fluid is found or there is residual thickening after the fluid is drawn off, excisional biopsy is indicated.

Fibrocystic Change of the Breast

Fibrocystic change of the breast is a common condition of premenopausal women, and it is found postmenopausally only in women who take exogenous estrogens.

Multiple, bilateral masses that are tender and fluctuate in size are typical. Minor discomfort frequently increases during the premenstrual period.

Although the term **fibrocystic disease** is often used as an umbrella term for mastalgia, breast cysts, and breast lumpiness, the diagnosis is histologic. Fibrocystic disease involves hyperplastic changes of the ductal epithelium, lobular epithelium, and/or breast connective tissue. Only if cellular atypia is present is there an increased risk of breast cancer.

Women over age 25 with fibrocystic disease should have a baseline mammogram to rule out carcinoma. Fine-needle biopsy of suspicious cystic lesions is indicated, as this disorder can be indistinguishable from carcinoma. Progesterone or tamoxifen therapy is useful in patients with relative or absolute increased estrogen levels. Diuretics and decreased salt intake may relieve premenstrual, edema-associated mastalgia, and bromocriptine may be useful in the treatment of general mastalgia. The role of decreased caffeine consumption is controversial, but many women report that decreasing caffeine intake relieves their symptoms.

Abscess of the Breast

Peripheral breast abscesses are typically due to streptococci or to *S. aureus*. Subareolar abscesses are usually due to anaerobes. More than 50% of subareolar abscesses are secondary to mammary duct ectasia, an inflammation and thickening of the large mammary ducts.

A red, swollen, painful mass in the breast.

Clinical presentation.

Incision, drainage, and appropriate antibiotics, such as clindamycin, are used for treatment. Most peripheral breast abscesses do not recur, but subareolar abscesses may reappear. Recurrent abscesses may cause fistula formation, and excision of the large duct system may be necessary for cure.

Fibroadenoma

Fibroadenomas are the most common benign breast tumors. Although they can occur in women of any age, they are most common before age 30. Pregnancy may stimulate their growth, and they often regress and calcify after menopause.

These tumors present as sharply circumscribed, mobile masses that are usually solitary.

Excisional biopsy for histologic evaluation.

Surgical excision, which also provides tissue for diagnosis. Fibroadenomas frequently recur.

Breast Cancer

Breast cancer accounts for approximately one-third of female malignancies and is the most common malignancy in women. There are a number of associated risk factors (Table 6-1). Invasive ductal tumors comprise approximately 90% of breast cancers, with the remaining 10% primarily arising in the breast lobules. Nonspecific infiltrating ductal carcinoma is by far the most common type of invasive ductal tumor, and it is responsible for about 80% of all breast cancers.

The typical early presentation is a hard, painless breast lump. A bloody or serous nipple discharge may be present (although this is more commonly a sign of the benign intraductal papilloma). The mass may be freely mobile, but with progressive growth it affixes to the deep fascia and becomes immobile. Nipple retraction secondary to ductal involvement or skin retraction and dimpling secondary to skin invasion may be present. Peau d'orange (lymphedema and skin thickening from obstruction of skin lymphatics) may also be observed. Axillary or supraclavicular lymphadenopathy may indicate tumor spread.

Table 6-1. Breast cancer risk factors

Category	Risk factor
Genetic	Family history in a first-degree relative
Hormonal	Nulliparity
	First pregnancy after age 35
	Early menarche
	Late menopause
	Older age
Dietary	High fat intake
Morphologic	Cancer of the other breast
	Cancer of the ovary or endometrium
	Fibrocystic change with cellular atypia

Mammography and open biopsy are used for diagnosis. Fine-needle aspiration (FNA) can precede open biopsy, but a negative FNA requires a follow-up open biopsy due to the high rate of false-negatives with this procedure (20%). Chest x-ray may show pulmonary metastases.

Modified radical mastectomy (total mastectomy plus axillary dissection) and partial mastectomy with subsequent irradiation are standard surgical options. Endocrine therapy may be used in tumors positive for estrogen and progesterone receptors. Chemotherapy appears to delay recurrence, but there is no evidence that it will cure patients who do not respond to radiotherapy or mastectomy. Better prognosis is seen in older patients and those with estrogen receptor-positive tumors. Involvement of the axillary lymph nodes is the most important negative prognostic indicator.

Most early breast cancers are found by patients. Monthly self-exams of the breast should be encouraged. All women should have a clinical breast exam once a year, and women over the age of 50 should have annual mammography.

Paget's Disease of the Breast

Occurring in only about 3% of breast cancer patients, Paget's disease of the breast is an intraductal carcinoma that involves the main excretory ducts of the breast. It presents as a crusting erosion of the nipple with or without discharge. The tumor is apparent on palpation in only two-thirds of patients. Diagnosis is made by biopsy of the nipple, and treatment is similar to that of other breast tumors. Prognosis depends on the extent of disease at diagnosis.

Menstrual and Endocrinologic Disorders

Primary Amenorrhea

Primary amenorrhea is the absence of menarche by age 16 in a woman with otherwise normal secondary sexual characteristic development or the absence of both menarche and secondary sexual characteristics by age 14. The keys to diagnosis often lie in a careful history and physical exam and in appropriate laboratory studies. Pregnancy, the most common cause of amenorrhea, should generally be ruled out regardless of the history.

The patient should be asked about growth and development, exercise and dietary habits, and family history of genetic anomalies. The patient should be questioned about symptoms of hyperandrogenism (e.g., excess hair growth), thyroid dysfunction, and galactorrhea. A history of medications may also be important. On exam, breast development and pubic hair growth should be assessed. Pelvic exam should check for the presence of a normal vaginal orifice, vagina, uterus, and ovaries.

Appropriate studies may include beta-hCG to rule out pregnancy, thyroid function tests, prolactin levels to rule out prolactinoma, and FSH levels to assess the hypothalamic-pituitary axis.

The etiologies of primary amenorrhea include:

- **Anatomic abnormalities**. These may include imperforate hymen, transverse vaginal septum, vaginal agenesis, and müllerian dysgenesis (congenital absence of the uterus and of the upper two-thirds of the vagina).
- **Ovarian failure**. These disorders are associated with low levels of estradiol. FSH and LH are elevated (hypergonadotropic hypogonadism) in enzyme defects of the estradiol synthesis pathway and in ovarian dysgenesis (which may be related to the XO karyotype of Turner's syndrome).
- **Pituitary defects**. A prolactinoma of the pituitary may cause amenorrhea by unclear mechanisms. Galactorrhea is a common symptom. Bromocriptine inhibits prolactin secretion and is the treatment of choice. This may also be the cause of secondary amenorrhea.
- **Hypothalamic amenorrhea**. Low levels of FSH and LH are associated with hypogonadotropic hypogonadism, which can be caused by anorexia nervosa, excessive exercise, and emotional stress. These factors may also cause secondary amenorrhea.
- **XY karyotype.** Testicular feminization is caused by an insensitivity of the tissues to androgens, causing female genitalia to develop in a genetically male child. There is no uterus, and the undescended testicles should be surgically removed to eliminate the risk of testicular cancer.

Secondary Amenorrhea

Secondary amenorrhea includes the absence of menses for at least 6 months in a woman with previously regular menses and the absence of menses for at least 12 months in a woman with a history of oligomenorrhea. Once again, pregnancy must be ruled out.

Galactorrhea may indicate a prolactinoma, whereas hirsutism suggests polycystic ovarian disease (PCO).

The first step in establishing a diagnosis is a progestin challenge, in which oral progestin is given; the test assesses whether or not the patient bleeds within 2 weeks. If bleeding occurs and the patient is hirsute, PCO is likely. If the patient is not hirsute, mild hypothalamic dysfunction is the likely etiology. If the patient does not bleed, an FSH level should be measured. Low FSH indicates severe hypothalamic dysfunction (usually due to extreme weight loss or exercise), whereas high FSH indicates gonadal failure.

PCO and mild hypothalamic dysfunction may be treated with cyclic progestin. Ovarian failure may be treated with estrogen replacement therapy. The cause of severe hypothalamic dysfunction should be sought and treated.

Premenstrual Syndrome

Premenstrual syndrome (PMS) occurs only in ovulating women and is independent of the presence of a uterus. After hysterectomy, cyclic symptoms continue if the ovaries are preserved. While most menstruating women experience some adverse symptoms prior to menses, 5–10% of women suffer from severe PMS that interferes with daily living. A specific etiology for PMS has not yet been identified.

Typical physical symptoms are abdominal bloating, edema and consequent weight gain, breast swelling and tenderness, headache, pelvic ache, altered bowel habits, and decreased coordination. Common psychological complaints are irritability, depression, anxiety, fatigue, and a change in sleep, appetite, or libido.

Supportive evidence for the diagnosis of PMS includes a worsening of symptoms with age, the regular occurrence of symptoms at the same time in each cycle, onset well after menarche, a positive family history, postnatal depression, and improvement with drugs that inhibit ovulation. When applicable, organic disease should be excluded.

The main treatment options are NSAIDs, oral contraceptive pills, and progestins.

Primary Dysmenorrhea

Primary dysmenorrhea, a common symptom of cyclic pain associated with menses, frequently begins in adolescence. Prostaglandins ($PGF_{2\alpha}$ and PGE_2) probably mediate the pain, which may be associated with uterine contractions and ischemia.

A crampy pain is typical, usually strongest over the lower abdomen and back. The dysmenorrhea usually starts a few hours before the onset of menstruation and may last several days. Nausea, vomiting, fatigue, headache, and diarrhea may be associated.

The history is usually diagnostic, but further evaluation may be indicated if the symptoms are severe and cannot be controlled with medication.

NSAIDs and oral contraceptive pills may be used alone or in combination.

Secondary Dysmenorrhea

Secondary dysmenorrhea is an acquired disorder that is due to an identifiable underlying pathology and typically occurs in young and middle-aged women. The symptoms may not correlate as well as in primary dysmenorrhea with the first day of menstrual bleeding. Endometriosis is the most common etiology, but pelvic inflammation, adenomyosis and uterine fibroids, ovarian cysts, uterine polyps, cervical stenosis, and pelvic congestion should be considered.

Signs and symptoms vary according to underlying etiology but may include dyspareunia, abnormal bleeding, and infertility.

Laparoscopy is required to diagnose endometriosis. Hysterosalpingogram or ultrasound may be useful to diagnose other etiologies.

The underlying disorder is addressed.

Abnormal Uterine Bleeding

Normal menstruation occurs every 21–35 days and generally lasts 3–7 days. Abnormal uterine bleeding involves a change in menstrual frequency, duration, or volume. A wide variety of gynecologic and nongynecologic diseases can lead to abnormal uterine bleeding, including uterine fibroids, cervical or endometrial polyps, cervical or endometrial carcinomas, disorders of the hypothalamic-pituitary-ovarian axis, and blood-clotting disorders. Diagnosis depends on thorough history, physical, and laboratory testing.

Endometriosis

Endometriosis is the presence of endometrial tissue outside the uterine cavity. It is estimated that 25–50% of infertile women have endometriosis.

Cyclical symptoms are produced when the ectopic endometrial tissue undergoes the same changes during the menstrual cycle as normal endometrial tissue. Progressive dysmenorrhea, dyspareunia, and infertility are the most common complaints. Examination may be normal or reveal visible lesions on the genitalia or cervix.

If no lesions are visible, laparoscopy is required for definitive diagnosis.

Medical treatment attempts to minimize ovarian stimulation of endometrial tissue. Continuous birth control pills, androgens, and gonadotropin-releasing hormone (GnRH)-agonists may be used. Surgical treatment includes laparoscopic ablation of endometrial tissue, which preserves reproductive potential. Postsurgery fertility rates range from 40% to 70%, depending on the severity of initial disease. Radical surgery involves a hysterectomy and bilateral salpingo-oophorectomy.

Hirsutism and Virilization

Androgens are produced in the adrenal glands and the ovaries. Hirsutism and virilization are the clinical manifestations of increased androgen effects. One cause is congenital adrenal hyperplasia, in which a defect of an enzyme in the steroid synthesis pathway (21-hydroxylase, 11-beta-hydroxylase, or 3-beta-hydroxy steroid dehydrogenase) leads to the overproduction of androgens. Cushing's syndrome, polycystic ovary syndrome, adrenal neoplasms, and ovarian neoplasms are other possible etiologies.

Hirsutism is defined as excess body hair in a male hair pattern and is often accompanied by acne and oily skin. Virilism occurs in severe hyperandrogenism and is characterized by the development of increased body hair, muscle bulk, and a deepening voice in a female. Clitoromegaly may be present. In the most severe form of congenital adrenal hyperplasia, the deficiency leads to ambiguous genitalia in female neonates and to life-threatening salt wasting.

A pattern of serum hormone level elevation is helpful in diagnosis.

Glucocorticoid replacement treats congenital adrenal hyperplasia. Surgical treatment of neoplasms is typical. Treatment of Cushing's syndrome depends on the specific etiology (see Chap. 4).

Polycystic Ovary Syndrome

Polycystic ovary syndrome affects 1–4% of women of reproductive age. It is characterized by a constellation of androgen excess, chronic anovulation, and, frequently, obesity. Hyperandrogenism is typically secondary to androgen overproduction by both the ovary and the adrenal gland. Excess androgen is peripherally converted to estrogen which, when unopposed by progesterone, can cause endometrial hyperplasia or carcinoma. Increased estrogen also stimulates excess ovarian androgen production. Chronic anovulation occurs because of both chronic, mild suppression of FSH release and the androgen's antagonism of the follicle's response to FSH.

Hirsutism and menstrual irregularity are present in 90% of patients, infertility in 75%, obesity in 50%, and virilism in 15%.

A progestin challenge test results in vaginal bleeding within 2 weeks. Serum LH is high.

Clomiphene, an orally active antiestrogen, is useful in patients who wish to conceive. It allows FSH levels to rise normally, thereby permitting the stimulation of follicular maturation. Otherwise, use oral progestin monthly to induce periodic sloughing of the endometrium. Steroid contraceptives are not necessary but are useful in treating patients with hirsutism and acne.

Menopause

The average age of menopause is 51 years, with a range of 45–55 years. The ovarian response to FSH and LH is reduced, resulting in decreased production of estrogen and progesterone. Without the negative feedback of estrogen, the circulating FSH and LH levels rise substantially.

Premature menopause is defined as ovarian failure before the age of 40. Smoking, chemotherapy, exposure to radiation, and surgery that limits the ovary's vascular supply are all associated with premature menopause. Artificial menopause arises from ovary removal or pelvic irradiation.

Symptoms of menopause include hot flushes and sweating, which arise from vasomotor instability; intermittent dizziness, palpitations, tachycardia, and paresthesias; insomnia, fatigue, irritability, and nervousness; nausea, flatulence, diarrhea, and constipation; and myalgias and arthralgias.

Long-term symptoms associated with menopause are related to the low-estrogen state and include urogenital atrophy (with associated vaginal dryness, dyspareunia, and urinary frequency and urgency), osteoporosis, and cardiovascular disease.

The history is frequently diagnostic, but an elevated FSH is confirmatory.

Estrogen replacement therapy (ERT) will relieve acute symptoms. In addition, ERT reduces the risk of cardiovascular disease by increasing the level of high-density lipoprotein (HDL), the "good" cholesterol, and reducing the level of low-density lipoprotein (LDL), the "bad" cholesterol. Osteoporosis is prevented with ERT taken for more than 5 years. If the patient's dietary calcium intake is insufficient, calcium supplementation is recommended. Cyclic progestin must be given with ERT to reduce the risk of endometrial cancer in all patients with a uterus. Absolute contraindications to estrogen replacement include a history of estrogen-dependent endometrial or breast neoplasms, a history of thromboembolic disease or thrombophlebitis, and severe liver disease. Symptomatic treatment of vaginal atrophy includes estrogen creams and the use of lubricants during intercourse.

Postmenopausal Bleeding

Postmenopausal bleeding is always abnormal, and malignancy must be excluded. Exogenous estrogens are the cause of 30% of postmenopausal bleeding, but bleeding in this context should only occur during the hormone withdrawal period. Atrophic endometritis or vaginitis is responsible for another 30% of postmenopausal bleeding. Fifteen percent of cases are caused by endometrial cancer. The remaining 15% are caused by uterine polyps or endometrial hyperplasia.

Infertility

Infertility is generally defined as the failure to conceive after 1 year of regular intercourse without contraception. It affects 15% of all couples and 20% of American women above the age of 35 who are attempting to conceive. Abnormalities fall into the following four categories:

- **Male factor:** Semen analysis assesses sperm morphology, semen volume (>1 ml), concentration of sperm (>20 million/ml), and sperm motility (>50%). A golden hamster assay is performed when the semen is tested for the ability to fertilize a hamster egg. Major causes for decreased semen viability are congenital, chromosomal, and hormonal (e.g., hyperprolactinemia) etiologies and varicoceles (incompetent vein valves). Abnormal tests should be repeated to rule out normal variability.
- **Cervical mucus:** Functional sperm must be able to interact properly with cervical mucus in order to travel to the egg. This interaction can be tested by evaluating the postcoital cervical mucus on the day before ovulation. If numerous immobile sperm are seen in the mucus, the sperm may have been destroyed by an overactive immune response. Antibody tests are appropriate for both partners.
- **Tubal factor:** Scarred fallopian tubes can often lead to infertility. A history of damage, such as with PID, STDs, IUD use, previous ectopic pregnancy, or previous tubal

surgery, suggests a tubal factor. A hysterosalpingogram can assess tubal patency. Surgery may be curative.

- **Ovulatory factor:** Most women who menstruate regularly are ovulating, but this can be evaluated by monitoring the basal body temperature (BBT), which should rise by 0.4°F at ovulation. Sufficient progesterone levels in the luteal phase also indicate ovulation. Abnormal BBT or a history of spontaneous abortion may indicate an inadequate luteal phase, even if ovulation is occurring. This can be evaluated with an endometrial biopsy, which is dated histologically and in relationship to menses. If these dates differ by more than 2 days, a luteal phase defect is present and should be treated with cyclic progesterone. Treatment with clomiphene citrate may enable certain anovulatory women to conceive.

7

Obstetrics

Physiology and Endocrinology of Normal Pregnancy

Conception and Implantation

For effective conception, an egg and a sperm cell must meet and implant in the endometrium. Spermatozoa must undergo capacitation by the acrosome reaction to be capable of fertilization. When a sperm cell enters the egg, which is a secondary oocyte at this point, the zona reaction creates a barrier around the egg and prevents additional sperm from entering. The ovulated egg then undergoes another meiotic division and gives rise to the ovum. The sperm and ovum nuclei are finally able to fuse and form the zygote.

Fertilization typically occurs in the fallopian tube within 12 hours of ovulation. Cleavage of the zygote produces a solid morula and then a hollow blastocyst. The blastocyst reaches the uterine cavity about 3 days after ovulation, and on day 6 or 7 the developing embryo implants. At this time, the trophoblastic cells, which will develop into the placenta, invade the endometrial lining and begin to produce beta-human chorionic gonadotropin (β-hCG). The syncytiotrophoblasts, the cells closest to the endometrium, form lacunae that will fill with maternal blood for exchange of oxygen and nutrients. By 17 days after fertilization, fetal and maternal blood vessels function, and a placental circulation exists.

Endocrinology of Normal Pregnancy

The fetoplacental unit controls the majority of the endocrinologic changes of pregnancy. The hormones most involved are discussed below.

- **β-hCG** is secreted by the placental trophoblasts. This hormone is responsible for maintaining the corpus luteum and its progesterone production until the eighth week of pregnancy, when the placenta begins to produce progesterone itself.
- **Androgens** are produced by the fetal adrenal cortex during pregnancy. Since the placenta cannot directly convert progesterone to estrogen, it uses androgens as its precursors for **estrogen** synthesis, particularly estriol. In a male fetus, the testes also secrete androgens, especially testosterone, in response to β-hCG. Testosterone drives the development of the male external genitalia.
- **Cortisol** is produced by both the fetal adrenal gland and the placenta. This hormone aids lung maturation by promoting the production and release of surfactant.
- The placenta makes **human placental lactogen (hPL)**, which maintains fetal glucose levels. Levels of hPL increase until the last 4 weeks of pregnancy, parallel to increasing placental weight.
- **Prolactin** production in the maternal anterior pituitary increases in response to increased maternal estrogen levels. Prolactin stimulates milk production. Fetal prolactin stimulates fetal growth during the second half of gestation, and it may also act in fetal fluid and electrolyte balance.

Maternal Physiology

The mother must provide oxygen, nutrients, and a safe environment for the developing fetus. These demands are a tremendous stress on the maternal system. Average maternal weight gain is 12.5 kg (28 lb), and less than half is due to the weight of the fetus and placenta. Adaptations occur in many organ systems:

Cardiovascular Adaptations

Plasma volume increases to 50% above nonpregnant levels. Despite an associated red blood cell mass increase, hematocrit falls slightly due to dilution. By the second half of pregnancy, cardiac output increases 40%, heart rate increases 12–18 beats per minute, and stroke volume increases 25%. These changes then plateau until delivery. A systolic murmur and an audible S3 are normal in pregnant women.

Blood pressure, particularly the diastolic component, decreases slightly in the first half of gestation. The pressure then rises slowly and returns to normal prepregnancy values by 40 weeks.

The normal hypoalbuminemia of pregnancy promotes generalized edema, and compression of veins by the uterus causes dependent edema.

Respiratory Adaptations

Total body oxygen consumption increases during pregnancy. Tidal volume increases by about 40% in response to the respiratory stimulating effects of progesterone. The respiratory rate, however, remains unchanged in normal pregnancy.

Renal Adaptations

Increased estrogen and progesterone levels promote increased secretion of renin, which causes levels of angiotensin and aldosterone to rise. These elevated levels contribute to the retention of water necessary for the increased plasma volume. The kidneys dilate, and the glomerular filtration rate increases by about 40%.

Metabolic Adaptations

During the first half of gestation, the actions of insulin dominate, and fasting glucose levels are low. Later in pregnancy, hPL antagonizes the effects of insulin, and insulin resistance appears. Glucose levels are elevated long after meals, and pregnant women are at an increased risk for ketoacidosis. Fasting triglyceride levels are dramatically increased.

Fetal Circulation

Fetal gas exchange occurs in the uteroplacental circulation. Fetal hemoglobin has a higher affinity for oxygen than maternal hemoglobin, so it is able to withdraw oxygen from the maternal blood. The fetal umbilical artery brings deoxygenated blood to the placenta, and the umbilical vein carries oxygenated blood from the placenta to the fetal portal system. Some of the blood from the umbilical vein passes through the liver and then into the inferior vena cava. The rest enters the ductus venosus, which leads directly from the umbilical vein into the vena cava. As the oxygenated blood enters the right atrium, one-third crosses the foramen ovale directly into the left atrium and travels via the aorta to the brain and upper body. Two-thirds enters the right ventricle, mixes with deoxygenated superior vena caval blood, and passes into the pulmonary trunk. Most of this blood bypasses the lungs via the ductus arteriosus, which leads to the descending aorta. While some of this blood supplies the lower body, the majority enters the umbilical arteries and returns to the placenta.

Prenatal Care

Prenatal Visits

The goals of prenatal care are to prevent, detect, and manage conditions that can cause adverse outcomes in pregnancy. Prenatal visits require careful assessment of risk factors for premature labor and delivery, intrauterine growth retardation, diabetes, hypertension, perinatal infections, and post-term pregnancy. Some important historical points include previous pregnancy outcomes, smoking and drug use, and medical history. Measurements taken at each prenatal visit include the following:

- **Maternal weight** should be measured because inadequate weight gain is associated with premature labor and intrauterine growth retardation (IUGR), and excessive weight gain is associated with gestational diabetes and, in the third trimester, preeclampsia.
- **Urinalysis** can identify urinary tract infections; glucosuria, which may indicate diabetes; and proteinuria, which may indicate preeclampsia.
- **Blood pressure** should be monitored for the development of preeclampsia.
- **Fundal height** should be measured at each visit to estimate proper fetal growth, and after 28 weeks, the fetal position can be assessed using Leopold maneuvers.

Prenatal Lab Tests

A variety of tests are commonly performed to assess the health of the mother in the prenatal period and to identify any sources of potential complications.

- A **Pap smear** should be done if the woman has not had one recently.
- A **complete blood count** (CBC) can detect anemia.
- **Urinalysis** is done to rule out bacteria, proteinuria, and glucosuria.
- **Rhesus factor** (Rh) should be documented so that Rh-negative women can be appropriately managed.
- A **syphilis test** is mandatory because early treatment can reduce perinatal mortality.
- A **rubella antibody screen** should be done, but nonimmune women cannot be immunized until after delivery.
- A **glucose screen** should be done between 24 and 28 weeks to screen for gestational diabetes.
- A **tuberculin skin test** should be performed on all pregnant women. If active tuberculosis (TB) is found on further evaluation, isoniazid (INH) is given postpartum.

Table 7-1. Genetic disorders

Autosomal dominant	Autosomal recessive	X-linked recessive
Achondroplasia	Cystic fibrosis	Androgen insensitivity
Ehlers-Danlos syndrome	Gaucher's disease	Duchenne's muscular dystrophy
Huntington's chorea	Phenylketonuria	Hemophilia A and B
Intestinal polyposis	Sickle cell anemia	Lesch-Nyhan syndrome
Marfan's syndrome	Tay-Sachs disease	
Neurofibromatosis	Wilson's disease	
Adult polycystic kidney disease	Most enzyme diseases	
Von Willebrand's disease		

- A **hepatitis B surface antigen test** will determine if the mother is a chronic carrier of the hepatitis B virus. If so, the newborn must be treated with hepatitis B immune globin (HBIG) and the hepatitis B vaccine to reduce the high risk of developing a chronic infection.

Human Genetics

Every pregnancy has a 3–4% risk of a genetic disorder or a structural congenital anomaly. Congenital and hereditary disorders include chromosomal abnormalities (e.g., Down's syndrome, with trisomy 21), autosomal dominant disorders (e.g., adult polycystic kidney disease), autosomal recessive disorders (e.g., cystic fibrosis), X-linked disorders (e.g., fragile X syndrome), and multifactorial disorders (e.g., spina bifida, anencephaly). Table 7-1 includes some of the most important genetic disorders. A personal or family history of any of these disorders suggests the need for counseling prior to a pregnancy. If a patient decides to become pregnant or has her first visit while she is already pregnant, prenatal testing and pregnancy options must be discussed.

Fetal Evaluation

Many fetal abnormalities can be detected prenatally using a number of diagnostic tests. Common indications for a prenatal work-up include women older than 34 (who have an increased risk of fetal chromosomal abnormalities), a history of several spontaneous abortions, a history of neonatal mortality, a history of exposure to teratogens during the current pregnancy, and any maternal conditions (such as diabetes) that are associated with an increased fetal risk of congenital abnormalities. Frequently used tests include the following:

- **Maternal serum alpha-fetoprotein** (MSAFP) is a blood test performed between the fifteenth and twentieth week of gestation. Elevated MSAFP suggests neural tube defects (e.g., spina bifida), ventral abdominal wall defects, multiple gestation, fetal demise, or inaccurate estimated age of gestation. Low MSAFP indicates a possibility of Down's syndrome. Subsequent ultrasound can rule out all but some neural tube defects and Down's syndrome, and amniocentesis is then used to determine the amniotic fluid AFP level (to rule out neural tube defects) and the fetal karyotype (to rule out Down's syndrome).

- **Amniocentesis** is performed between gestational weeks 16 and 20. Amniotic fluid is withdrawn through a needle placed in the abdominal wall. Amniocentesis assesses the amniotic fluid AFP content and the fetal karyotype, so it identifies both neural tube defects and chromosomal disorders with high accuracy. This test has a 1 in 200 risk of spontaneous abortion.
- **Chorionic villus sampling** (CVS) is a more invasive test performed transcervically between 9 and 12 weeks of gestation. It permits first-trimester identification of chromosomal abnormalities and genetic disorders that have biochemical markers (e.g., Tay-Sachs disease). It carries a 1% risk of spontaneous abortion in the first trimester. CVS cannot measure AFP levels, however, so patients using CVS should also have serum screening for this marker.
- **Percutaneous umbilical blood sampling** (cordocentesis) is typically performed between 10 and 22 weeks of gestation. This test involves withdrawing blood from the umbilical vein, and risk to mother and fetus is minimal. This test is useful in identifying some genetic disorders, particularly in patients who present late for prenatal care. It also permits a rapid karyotype if ultrasonography suggests a chromosomal disorder.
- **Ultrasonography** is used at any stage of pregnancy and can be used to identify fetal structural abnormalities. It presents no associated risk and is the most common diagnostic device used to assess the effects of teratogens on fetal development. Structural abnormalities that may be detected include anencephaly, spina bifida, gastrointestinal defects, renal anomalies, and congenital heart defects.

Medical Complications of Pregnancy

Hyperemesis Gravidarum

Severe nausea and vomiting occasionally arise during pregnancy. This is more frequent in nulliparas, in caucasians, and in patients with recent stressful experiences. Patients with gestational trophoblastic disease also have a high rate of this syndrome, which has been correlated with an elevated β-hCG. Severity of symptoms parallels levels of β-hCG, which peak in the first trimester and then decline.

SIGNS & SYMPTOMS

A history of intractable nausea and vomiting typically accompanies signs of weight loss and decreased skin turgor.

DIAGNOSIS

Diagnosis is based on the clinical presentation, after other GI complications have been ruled out. The presence of ketonuria and electrolyte disturbances, including hypokalemia, hyponatremia, and hypochloremic alkalosis, must be monitored.

TREATMENT

Patients should have frequent, light meals of solid food. Rehydration, correction of electrolyte disturbances, and antiemetics are also useful.

Gestational Diabetes Mellitus

Gestational diabetes mellitus (GDM) refers to glucose intolerance beginning or newly recognized during pregnancy. The insulin-antagonist hormones produced by the placenta may be responsible, or the stress of pregnancy may unmask a subclinical abnormality in insulin activity. GDM is associated with multiple pregnancy complications, including macrosomia and its associated risks for traumatic delivery, delayed fetal lung maturity and respiratory distress syndrome of the neonate, congenital abnormalities, and intrauterine fetal death. The pregnant diabetic mother is also prone to complications, including preeclampsia, polyhydramnios, hypoglycemia, ketoacidosis, diabetic coma, and the typical end-organ involvement of diabetes. Also, up to half of women with GDM will develop diabetes later in life.

GDM is often asymptomatic. Risk factors include obesity, maternal age greater than 25 years, family history of diabetes, and personal history of a macrosomic baby, polyhydramnios, stillbirth, congenitally deformed baby, or recurrent abortions.

Since half of all women who develop GDM do not have an associated risk factor, glucose screening between 24 and 26 weeks is mandatory for all patients. Screening involves measuring a fasting glucose level followed by measuring glucose levels recorded at 1 and 2 hours after a glucose load. A true diagnosis of GDM can be made only if a postpartum glucose tolerance test returns to normal.

Strict metabolic control during pregnancy decreases perinatal morbidity and mortality. Appropriate diet, insulin, and exercise can maintain normal glucose levels. Oral hypoglycemic agents are contraindicated, however, since they can cross the placenta and cause fetal and neonatal hypoglycemia.

Ultrasound, fetal electrocardiogram, and maternal serum alpha-fetoprotein measurement in the first half of gestation can exclude many congenital abnormalities. Periodic fetal monitoring, including a nonstress test, ultrasonography, and a biophysical profile, is indicated. Given the association with birth trauma, macrosomic babies are sometimes delivered by cesarean section.

Preeclampsia

Also known as pregnancy-induced hypertension, this multisystem disease involves the development of hypertension, proteinuria, and edema. Its cause is not completely understood. It develops at least 20 weeks' postpartum and affects 5% of pregnancies. Preeclamptic patients are almost always primiparous. Other risk factors include preexisting hypertensive states, advanced maternal age, multiple gestation, and other vascular disease.

Most signs and symptoms are due to endothelial injury and vasoconstriction; these include hypertension, proteinuria, and edema, in addition to headache, blurred vision, scotomata, epigastric pain, and oliguria. The HELLP syndrome is a highly morbid complication consisting of *h*emolysis, *e*levated *l*iver enzymes, and *l*ow *p*latelets. Complications include abruptio placenta, disseminated intravascular coagulation (DIC), acute renal failure, pulmonary edema, and encephalopathy. Fetal complications from vasoconstriction and platelet aggregation include intrauterine growth retardation.

Hypertension, nondependent edema, and/or greater than 1+ albuminuria, with onset during the second half of pregnancy, is diagnostic of preeclampsia. Hypertension during pregnancy requires a 30-mm Hg rise in systolic pressure or a 15-mm Hg rise in diastolic pressure during the course of the pregnancy. If baseline values are not known, an alternate definition requires pressure at or above 140/90 mm Hg after 20 weeks of gestation. Pressure must remain elevated at a second measurement at least 6 hours after the initial elevated reading.

Therapy attempts to control symptoms, minimize complications, and avoid progression to full-blown eclampsia. The definitive cure is delivery, and the patient returns to baseline pressures within 1–2 days.

For mild preeclampsia, increased water intake and bed rest are appropriate. IV magnesium decreases hyperreflexia and the risk of seizures and may decrease blood pressure. Blood pressure, proteinuria, weight gain, and other symptoms must be carefully monitored.

For severe preeclampsia, the mother's condition should be stabilized with IV rehydration and magnesium and the baby delivered. If urinary output does not increase, hydralazine or other anti-hypertensives should be used. Even when antihypertensive treatment is effective, blood pressure must be maintained above 130/80 mm Hg to ensure adequate uterine perfusion. Vaginal delivery within 4–6 hours is preferable, and cesarean section is performed only if needed. Antihypertensive medications and seizure prophylaxis should continue for at least 24 hours postpartum.

Eclampsia

Eclampsia is defined as the presence of seizures in a preeclamptic patient, and it can be fatal if left untreated. Seizures in this context are diagnostic of eclampsia only if underlying seizure disorders can be excluded.

Treatment of eclampsia is similar to that of severe preeclampsia. The patient must be stabilized and then delivered. Antihypertensives may be given to lower blood pressure. In addition, IV diazepam helps to control the seizures. Again, vaginal delivery is preferable.

Late Transient Hypertension

Also known as gestational hypertension, late transient hypertension is difficult to differentiate from preeclampsia. It involves hypertension during the second half of gestation or in the first day postpartum in the absence of proteinuria or edema. It is a retrospective diagnosis only, made after delivery, when proteinuria never appears and renal disease has been ruled out.

Chronic Hypertension

Patients with known hypertension or with high blood pressure detected prior to the twentieth week of pregnancy have chronic hypertension. This includes primarily long-standing, clinically recognized disease, but the physiologic stress of pregnancy is also capable of exacerbating a previously subclinical hypertensive disorder. Methyldopa, beta-blockers, and hydralazine can be used throughout the pregnancy, but diuretic use is generally discouraged. Blood pressure should be monitored closely.

Cardiac Disease in Pregnancy

The 40% increase in cardiac output that accompanies pregnancy requires significant increased work by the heart. This stressor can exacerbate existing cardiac abnormalities.

Congenital heart disease is the most common source of preexisting cardiac disease. Increased cardiac dysfunction usually arises during the period of maximal increase in cardiac output, which occurs at 18–24 weeks of gestation, but it may begin during labor, delivery, or immediately postpartum.

Rheumatic heart disease in pregnancy, now rare, is associated with an increased incidence of heart failure, pulmonary edema, thromboembolic disease, and subacute bacterial endocarditis. Most often, rheumatic heart disease leads to mitral stenosis. Severe mitral stenosis predisposes to atrial fibrillation, which, in pregnancy, almost always leads to congestive heart failure.

TREATMENT

Patients should avoid excessive weight gain and strenuous physical activity and should take supplemental iron. During labor, cardiac output increases an additional 50% from its prelabor levels, but the increase may be lessened by sedation and epidural anesthesia. Prophylactic antibiotics against subacute bacterial endocarditis should be administered at the onset of labor and continued through the first 2 days postpartum.

Immediately postpartum, the normal contraction of the uterus adds half a liter of blood to the effective blood volume. This increase can overload a diseased heart, so the patient's legs should be kept below the level of the heart, and Pitocin and uterine massage should be avoided.

Obstetric Complications of Pregnancy

Ectopic Pregnancy

In ectopic pregnancy, the fertilized ovum implants outside of the uterus. The usual site of implantation is the fallopian tube, most commonly in the ampulla. Rupture of an ectopic pregnancy can cause severe and sometimes life-threatening intra-abdominal hemorrhage. Implantation in the fallopian tube is generally related to prior tubal infection and scarring. Other risk factors for ectopic pregnancy include history of IUD use, prior tubal surgery including tubal ligation, prior ectopic pregnancy, and any risk factors for sexually transmitted diseases, including multiple sex partners.

SIGNS &
SYMPTOMS

Patients are often unaware of their pregnancy, and ectopic pregnancies may rupture and reabsorb without causing clinical symptoms. With an unruptured ectopic pregnancy, signs of early pregnancy (amenorrhea, nausea) may accompany light vaginal bleeding ("spotting") and/or crampy lower abdominal pain. The patient may report that her last menstrual period was not entirely normal. Physical exam shows abdominal tenderness, adnexal tenderness, and an adnexal mass in 50% of patients. A ruptured ectopic pregnancy usually presents during weeks 6–8 of gestation, with sudden, sharp abdominal or pelvic pain. Rapid intra-abdominal hemorrhage may result in hypotension and shock.

An elevated urine or serum β-hCG level confirms the pregnancy, but it does not confirm that the pregnancy is ectopic. β-hCG levels are, however, useful in differentiating ectopic pregnancy from other diseases with similar clinical manifestations, such as appendicitis, ruptured cyst, and torsion of an ovarian cyst. During an ectopic pregnancy, β-hCG levels do not rise as rapidly as in normal pregnancies, in which β-hCG should double every 48 hours. When the β-hCG titer reaches 6,500 mIU/ml, a gestational sac is normally visible on transvaginal or transabdominal ultrasound. Its absence at high β-hCG levels strongly suggests ectopic pregnancy. Ultrasound can also show hemoperitoneum, consistent with rupture. Laparoscopy confirms the diagnosis, if necessary.

Treatment options for an unruptured ectopic are either surgery or methotrexate, which is used only for early presentations. A ruptured tubal ectopic is treated with immediate fluid resuscitation and surgery. With surgical treatment of ruptured or unruptured cases, evacuation of the products of conception should be performed with maximal conservation of the fallopian tube.

Spontaneous Abortion

Commonly called "miscarriage," spontaneous abortion (SAB) is the loss of the products of conception prior to 20 weeks' gestation. It is a frequent complication, occurring in up to 20% of all pregnancies despite attempts at medical intervention. The vast majority of SABs occur during the first trimester, and fetal causes (e.g., chromosomal abnormalities) are generally responsible. Second-trimester SABs are generally due to maternal causes, such as infections, cervical abnormalities (e.g., incompetence), uterine abnormalities, medical disease, and cocaine use. In these late abortions, a more organized placenta increases the risk of bleeding, and more advanced fetal bone formation increases the risk of uterine perforation. The different types of SABs are discussed below:

- **Threatened abortion** refers to any uterine cramping or bleeding in the presence of a closed cervix during the first 20 weeks of pregnancy. In addition to inspection of the cervix, diagnosis requires ultrasonography to identify cardiac activity in a viable fetus. In its absence, or if the sac is empty, uterine evacuation should be performed. If the fetus appears viable, maternal bed rest and pelvic rest are the only available treatment. At least one-fourth of threatened abortions will progress to complete abortion.
- **Inevitable abortion** involves uterine bleeding or pain when the cervix is beginning to efface or dilate. Prevention of the abortion is not possible. Dilatation and curettage (D & C) are usually performed to ensure that no products of conception are retained.
- **Incomplete abortion** is the term used to describe the passage of part of the products of conception through the cervix. The cervix is dilated, and fetal tissue may be visible on exam. Bleeding from the uterus is present and may be severe. Again, D & C will remove any remaining products of conception from the uterus.

- **Complete abortion** refers to passage of all of the products of conception, with subsequent closure of the cervix and return of the uterus to its normal size.
- A **missed abortion** refers to the death of a fetus and its retention in utero for 4 weeks or longer. This condition is discussed in detail later in this chapter.

Therapeutic Abortion

Elective termination of a pregnancy may be performed during the first and second trimesters. First-trimester elective abortions are currently legal throughout the United States, although the practice is controversial. D & C or vacuum curettage are the primary methods used, as RU486 is not yet an option in this country. Limitations on second-trimester abortions are determined by the individual states. The most common procedure used for second-trimester abortions is dilatation and evacuation, similar to D & C. Otherwise, prostaglandins or intra-amniotic saline injection are used to induce labor. Bleeding, infection, retained products of conception, and mechanical damage to the uterus or cervix are the major complications.

Septic Abortion

Septic abortion refers to infection of the uterine contents before, during, or after an abortion. It may be caused by an improperly performed therapeutic abortion.

Patients present with acute infection, involving fever, chills, septicemia, and peritonitis. A threatened or incomplete abortion may be evident. In severe cases, septic shock can occur, with hypotension, hypothermia, oliguria, and respiratory distress.

History and clinical presentation. Leukocytosis is present.

Stabilization, vigorous antibiotic treatment, and evacuation of the uterus are indicated.

Intrauterine Fetal Death

Intrauterine fetal death is defined as death of a fetus after 20 weeks' gestational age but prior to onset of labor. Common etiologies include placental and umbilical cord complications, hypertensive states, erythroblastosis fetalis, congenital anomalies, infections, and autoimmune diseases.

A uterus small for gestational age, absence of fetal movements, and absence of fetal heart tones may be noted by the mother and on exam.

Real-time ultrasonography confirms the absence of heart activity and fetal movement.

Management varies depending on gestational age. Fetal demise before the twenty-eighth week of pregnancy can be treated by induction of labor (usually by vaginal suppository) or, more often, by waiting for spontaneous labor to begin. Spontaneous labor occurs within 3 weeks of fetal death in 80% of cases. Fetal death after 28 weeks of gestation is generally treated by induction of labor with oxytocin. If labor is not induced, weekly fibrinogen, hematocrit, and platelet counts are important for early detection of DIC, which occurs in a minority of patients.

Polyhydramnios

Polyhydramnios, excess amniotic fluid volume, may develop gradually during pregnancy with several possible causes. Fetal anomalies (e.g., duodenal atresia, tracheoesophageal fistula, or anencephaly) can lead to decreased swallowing and therefore decreased resorption of fluid. Pulmonary system anomalies (e.g., cystic malformations of the lung) can also lead to polyhydramnios via excessive secretion. Imbalanced passive water absorption can also occur, as in some diabetic pregnancies. Other risk factors include multiple gestation, isoimmunization, and fetal hydrops.

This complication is usually asymptomatic. Preterm labor may be the initial presentation.

Ultrasonography can confirm polyhydramnios and exclude hydrops or malformations. The mother should be tested for diabetes, anti-Rh antibody, hemoglobinopathies, and viral titers.

Rest and tocolytics may be of value for preterm labor. In an acute presentation due to multiple gestation, induction of labor may be necessary.

Oligohydramnios

Oligohydramnios is a severe deficiency of amniotic fluid volume. Most cases are associated with IUGR and with a poor outcome. Fetal stress may promote oligohydramnios because the fetal stress hormones increase fetal swallowing of amniotic fluid. Renal agenesis, pulmonary hypoplasia, and other malformations can result in insufficient fluid secretion.

Decreased amniotic fluid in the first trimester can lead to structural abnormalities, such as facial distortion, limb reduction, and defects in the abdominal wall. In the third trimester, oligohydramnios can produce fetal hypoxia due to umbilical cord compression. Meconium in the decreased volume of amniotic fluid can also compromise fetal respiration.

Usually asymptomatic, although evidence of growth retardation or fetal distress may be present.

Oligohydramnios is confirmed by ultrasound, and fetal abnormalities may be visualized.

The underlying cause must be identified and addressed, if possible.

Rh Isoimmunization

Rh blood group incompatibility arises when an Rh-negative woman conceives an Rh-positive fetus. RBCs from the fetus can enter the woman's circulation, during pregnancy or, more commonly, during birth, stimulating the production of maternal antibodies against the Rh factor. Spontaneous or induced abortions of an Rh-positive fetus can also result in isoimmunization. In subsequent pregnancies, transplacental transmission of the maternal anti-Rh antibody leads to hemolytic anemia in the fetus or neonate. The resulting disease, called **erythroblastosis fetalis**, may be fatal. Unless a woman was previously sensitized by transfusion, a first pregnancy rarely leads to erythroblastosis fetalis.

After birth, bilirubin levels in the neonate can increase dramatically due to the hemolytic anemia. This causes **kernicterus,** characterized by decreased tone, poor feeding, apnea, seizures, and death. Survivors of kernicterus can be left with mental retardation, choreoathetosis, and hearing loss.

High maternal anti-Rh antibody titers, checked at the first prenatal visit and at week 26, suggest sensitization of the mother. Amniocentesis showing high bilirubin levels suggests impending fetal death.

If bilirubin levels are elevated, intrauterine transfusions to the fetus can be performed at 2-week intervals. Delivery should be minimally traumatic, and the placenta should not be manually removed. In the neonate, hyperbilirubinemia may necessitate phototherapy or an exchange transfusion.

At the first prenatal check-up, all patients should be screened for Rh type. If the patient is Rh-negative, maternal Rh antibody titers should be repeated at the twenty-sixth week of gestation. A previously unsensitized mother will not normally produce anti-Rh antibody until after delivery, when mixing of the maternal and fetal blood occurs. Rh isoimmunization can be prevented by injecting the mother with anti-Rh immunoglobulin (RhoGAM) within 3 days of delivery. IgG binds the fetal Rh factor and prevents the mother from developing anti-Rh antibodies. Anti-Rh IgG should be given at the termination of each pregnancy, whether a delivery, ectopic pregnancy, or

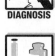

abortion. If no Rh sensitization has occurred, Rh-negative mothers should receive an additional dose of anti-Rh antibody at the twenty-eighth week of gestation.

Multiple Gestation

Dizygotic twins arise through fertilization of two eggs by two sperm, resulting in two amnions and two chorions. Monozygotic twins develop through abnormal division of one fertilized egg. If the division takes place within 3 days of fertilization, two amnions and two chorions develop. If division occurs between days 3 and 8 after fertilization, two amnions but only one chorion will develop. Division of the fertilized egg after 8 days leads to twins sharing one amnion and one chorion.

Multiple gestation has a higher risk of complications and higher rates of morbidity and mortality. The average gestational age at delivery is 35 weeks in twins versus 39 weeks in singletons. Prematurity confers a high risk of respiratory distress syndrome, which is responsible for about half of the perinatal mortality of twins.

SIGNS & SYMPTOMS

Signs of multiple gestation include large "size for dates" (i.e., the uterus is larger than expected for the gestational age) and the auscultation of more than one fetal heart.

DIAGNOSIS

A family history of multiple gestation or a history of fertility drug use raises clinical suspicion. Diagnosis is established by ultrasound. Separate gestational sacs are visible from week 6 of gestation.

TREATMENT

Antepartum management can prolong gestation, decrease perinatal mortality, and decrease perinatal and maternal morbidity. Weekly visits starting after week 20 allow evaluation of cervical changes to detect preterm labor and blood pressure measurement to detect preeclampsia. Monthly sonography is useful to assess fetal growth and amniotic fluid volume.

Aggressive treatment of preterm labor is appropriate. Vertex-vertex presentations are most common and can be delivered vaginally. Otherwise, delivery is usually by cesarean section.

Third-Trimester Bleeding

Prior to 20 weeks' gestation, bleeding is referred to as a threatened abortion. After 20 weeks, the term third-trimester bleeding is used, although the third trimester does not actually begin until week 26. Third-trimester bleeding complicates about 5% of pregnancies. **Placental abruption** and **placenta previa** are the most common causes of life-threatening hemorrhage and are discussed in detail below. Less severe third-trimester bleeding results from many extrauterine sources, such as cervical trauma, cervical inflammation or infection, cervical dilatation, coagulation disorders, and vaginal, vulvar, or rectal lesions. The most common cause of bleeding late in pregnancy is called "bloody show" and is due to the normal extrusion of the cervical mucus.

Abruptio Placenta

Early separation of a normally implanted placenta can cause severe hemorrhage because this area is so highly vascularized. Risk factors for placental abruption include trauma, hypertension, cigarette smoking, cocaine use, and a history of prior abruption.

Symptoms depend on the degree of placental separation, the location of the placenta, and the subsequent loss of blood. Retroplacental bleeding leads to cervical bleeding and external hemorrhage in 90% of cases. In the remainder, the blood collects in the retroplacental space and can be detected incidentally from postpartum examination of the placenta. The patient may complain of unremitting uterine or low-back pain, associated with a tender and tonically contracted uterus. Maternal shock, DIC, and fetal distress or death may occur.

Abruptio placenta is primarily a clinical diagnosis, as ultrasonography shows the separation in less than one-half of patients. Vaginal exam should not be performed unless the diagnosis of placenta previa has been firmly ruled out (see below). The amount of vaginal bleeding gives minimal indication of the total blood loss. Check labs to rule out possible complications.

If the abruption does not threaten fetal or maternal well-being, bed rest may reduce the bleeding. If the hemorrhage does not improve or if fetal or maternal well-being are compromised, an immediate cesarean section should be performed.

Placenta Previa

In placenta previa, implantation of the placenta occurs over or near the cervical os. In total previa, the placenta completely covers the internal os. In partial previa, the os is partially covered. Placenta previa is not uncommon early in pregnancy, but most cases resolve spontaneously as the placenta and uterus enlarge. Risk factors include multiparity, advanced maternal age, previous cesarean section, history of abortions, and uterine fibroids.

Painless, bright-red vaginal bleeding begins suddenly, usually early in the third trimester. The amount of blood loss varies from "spotting" to severe hemorrhage. It often resolves spontaneously, with another, heavier episode a few days later.

Transabdominal ultrasound demonstrates the placement of the placenta in 95% of cases. Manual vaginal examination is contraindicated, since it can precipitate greater hemorrhage.

For minor bleeding early in pregnancy, bed rest is recommended. Tocolytics can be given to reduce uterine contractions, if present. Delivery must be by cesarean section for complete previa. For severe bleeding, stabilization of the mother is critical, followed by cesarean delivery of the infant. Preterm delivery results in the high perinatal mortality associated with this complication.

Gestational Trophoblastic Disease

Molar pregnancies are neoplasms of trophoblastic cells, the cells that form the placenta. Gestational trophoblastic disease ranges in severity from the benign hydatidiform mole (the great majority of cases) to malignant and metastatic choriocarcinoma. Locally invasive disease also occurs. Since excessive placental tissue develops, levels of β-hCG increase.

Hydatidiform Moles

SIGNS & SYMPTOMS

Hydatidiform moles usually present with heavy or irregular painless uterine bleeding during the first half of pregnancy. Preeclampsia in the first half of pregnancy is pathognomonic of hydatidiform mole. A uterus that is large for dates and hyperemesis gravidarum are also common clinical presentations. On exam, expulsion of vesicles that resemble a "bunch of grapes" may be evident. There is no fetal movement or heart tones.

DIAGNOSIS

Higher than normal β-hCG titers are a suspicious finding. Ultrasound provides definitive diagnosis, showing a "snowstorm" pattern with no sac or fetus. A chest x-ray is important to rule out metastases to the lung.

TREATMENT

A hydatidiform mole is removed by suction evacuation and curettage. Serum β-hCG is assayed weekly after evacuation and should decline within 3–4 months to undetectable levels. Patients with persistent β-hCG titers should be worked up for metastases, started on chemotherapy, and monitored. If β-hCG levels do not fall to a normal level, a hysterectomy is indicated and is usually curative.

Gestational Choriocarcinoma

Half of gestational choriocarcinomas arise in the context of a molar pregnancy. The remainder are seen following a normal, ectopic, or aborted pregnancy. Choriocarcinomas may metastasize through the circulation to the lungs, vagina, brain, GI tract, liver, and kidneys.

SIGNS & SYMPTOMS

Choriocarcinoma generally presents after metastasis has occurred, and the diagnosis may be missed unless onset follows a molar pregnancy. Vaginal bleeding, dyspnea, cough, hemoptysis, CNS findings, and rectal bleeding are possible signs of metastases and should prompt an evaluation of β-hCG levels in any woman who has recently been pregnant.

DIAGNOSIS

High β-hCG levels and a "snowstorm" on ultrasound indicate gestational trophoblastic disease. To evaluate for metastasis, CT scans of the abdomen, pelvis, and head and a cerebrospinal fluid β-hCG titer are necessary.

TREATMENT

Chemotherapy and radiation are used. Frequent follow-up β-hCG titers confirm remission in the majority of patients.

Labor and Delivery

Endocrinology of Normal Labor and Delivery

Although hormonal actions may initiate labor, the hormones responsible have not yet been identified. Levels of prostaglandins increase during labor, particularly prostaglandins E_2 (PGE_2) and $F_{2\alpha}$ ($PGF_{2\alpha}$). These are synthesized by the myometrium and endometrium and can elicit uterine contractions. $PGF_{2\alpha}$ is more potent than PGE_2 for uterine contraction, but PGE_2 is more critical for ripening the cervix.

Oxytocin is not released from the posterior pituitary until the first stage of labor has already begun. Its release is evoked by distention of the birth canal, as well as by mammary stimulation. Although oxytocin does not appear to initiate normal labor, it does induce uterine contractions.

Stages of Normal Labor and Delivery

During the last 1–2 months of pregnancy, Braxton-Hicks ("false") contractions may be noted. These contractions are irregular, usually painless, and not associated with progressive cervical effacement and dilation.

Normal labor should begin between gestational weeks 38 and 42. It occurs in four stages. The first stage extends from the onset of labor to complete dilation of the cervix. The second stage is from cervical dilation until the birth of the infant, and the third stage lasts until delivery of the placenta. The fourth stage extends from the end of placental delivery until the mother is stable, which typically takes about 6 hours.

The **first stage of labor** consists of a latent and an active phase. During the **latent phase**, the cervix softens and effaces, but it dilates only minimally. The latent phase lasts up to 12 hours in primiparas but is shorter in multiparous women. The **active phase** of labor begins when the cervix has dilated to 3–4 cm and the uterus has begun contracting regularly. Descent of the fetal head and complete dilation of the cervix occur over about 6 hours (Fig. 7-1). The rate of cervical dilation increases during the active phase of the first stage, with minimum normal rates for primiparous and multiparous women of 1 and 1.2 cm/hour, respectively.

The **second stage of labor** typically lasts 30 minutes to 3 hours in primiparous women and 5–30 minutes in multiparas. The mother's desire to bear down during the regular uterine contractions permits her to increase her abdominal pressure and deliver the infant.

The **third stage of labor** involves separation of the placenta from the uterus, which occurs 5–10 minutes after birth of the child. Signs of separation include sudden blood flow from the vagina, lengthening of the umbilical cord, and rising and firming of the uterine fundus.

The **fourth stage of labor** involves a risk of hemorrhage, particularly in the first hour after delivery. Close observation of the patient's uterine blood loss and vital signs is important.

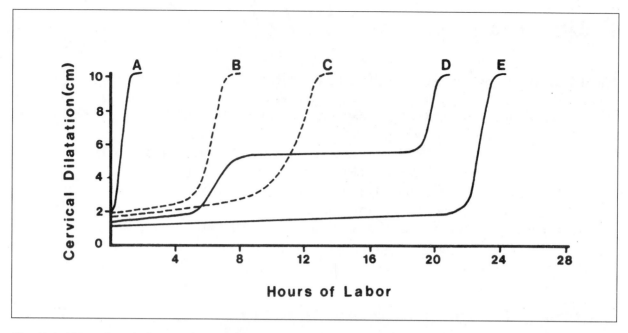

Fig. 7-1. Normal and abnormal labor curves. A. Precipitate labor. B. Normal multiparous labor. C. Normal primigravida labor. D. Protracted active phase due to arrest of dilatation. E. Prolonged latent phase. (From DR Coustan, RV Haning, Jr, DB Singer. *Human Reproduction: Growth and Development*. Boston: Little, Brown, 1995.)

Normal Movements of Delivery

Six movements of the fetus characterize its descent through the maternal pelvis (Fig. 7-2):

- **Descent** progresses continuously.
- **Flexion** permits the fetus to enter the birth canal with the part of its head that has the smallest diameter.
- **Internal rotation** means that the occiput rotates anteriorly toward the symphysis pubis from its oblique or transverse diameter.
- **Extension** of the head allows it to project through the vaginal outlet. Crowning is the point at which the largest diameter of the head extends through the vulvar ring.
- **External rotation** involves the realignment of the just-delivered head with the upper body.
- **Expulsion** occurs as the anterior shoulder delivers under the symphysis pubis, the posterior shoulder delivers over the perineal body, and the baby's body rapidly follows.

Fetal Monitoring

Intrapartum Fetal Stress

Fetal distress may be caused by the stress of labor. During uterine contractions, the fetal blood supply is repeatedly interrupted. Since the oxygen reserve of a healthy fetus will last 1–2 minutes, a normal fetus does not become hypoxic. A fetus with a decreased supply of oxygen, however, may become hypoxic during labor. Results of stress are demonstrated by

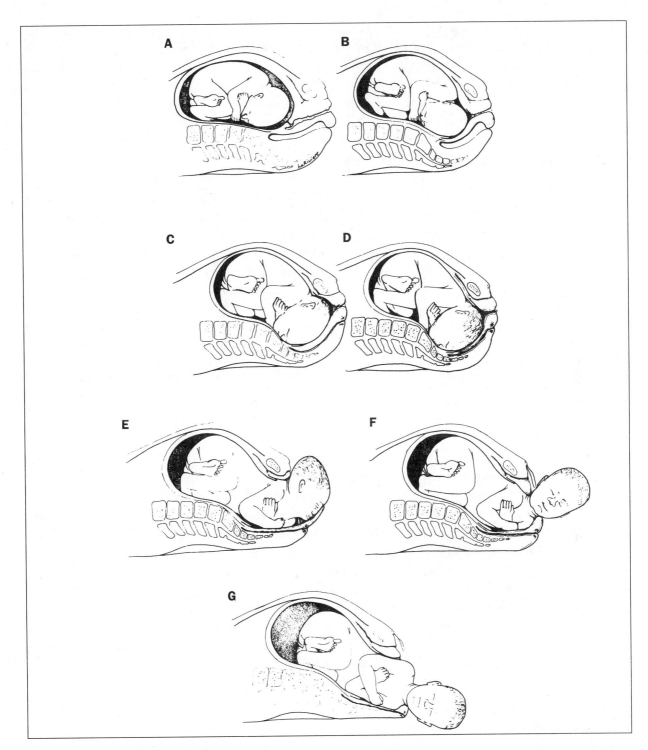

Fig. 7-2. The cardinal movements of labor. A. Floating head prior to the onset of labor. B. Descent. C. Flexion. D. Internal rotation. E. Extension. F. External rotation. G. Expulsion. (From DR Coustan, RV Haning, Jr, DB Singer. *Human Reproduction: Growth and Development*. Boston: Little, Brown, 1995.)

periodic fetal heart rate decelerations, detected by fetal heart rate auscultation or monitor, and by decreases in fetal blood pH, detected by fetal scalp blood samples.

Meconium in the amniotic fluid is another sign of fetal distress and is associated with poor outcome. Heavy meconium may be detected in the amniotic fluid when the membranes rupture. Neonates with heavy meconium should be aggressively managed. (See Meconium Aspiration in Chap. 8.)

Fetal Heart Rate Monitoring

The normal fetal heart rate at term is 120–160 beats per minute (bpm). Tachycardia (>160 bpm) may result from maternal or fetal infection, fetal anemia, hypoxia, or medications. Bradycardia (<120 bpm), often caused by medications, congenital heart block, or fetal hypoxia, is only threatening if it is associated with decreased variability. Normal beat-to-beat variability is about 5 bpm and reflects proper autonomic function. Increased variability may occur during mild hypoxia. Decreased variability is seen with fetal sleep, prematurity, some drugs, and hypoxia.

Fetal heart rate accelerations are generally reassuring signs of fetal movement or uterine contractions. However, an accelerated heart rate may be the first indication of fetal distress, occurring sometimes with partial occlusion of the cord. At least 2 accelerations, with an increase of 15 bpm lasting at least 15 seconds, should occur every 20 minutes.

Decelerations are transitory episodes of a decreased fetal heart rate. There are three types (Fig. 7-3):

- **Early decelerations** occur synchronously with contractions. They arise because of head compression and do not suggest fetal distress.
- **Late decelerations** begin more than 30 seconds after onset of a uterine contraction and do not end until well after the contraction has stopped. They may indicate fetal hypoxia, especially if a loss of variability or an altered baseline fetal heart rate is associated. They are usually due to chronic placental insufficiency, venacaval compression, maternal hypotension, or uterine hyperactivity. Scalp sampling for fetal blood pH can confirm fetal hypoxia and acidosis.
- **Variable decelerations** are not consistent in intensity, duration, or onset relative to the contraction of the uterus. They are secondary to transient umbilical cord compression and suggest fetal distress only if variability has also decreased. If the woman changes position, cord compression is often relieved.

Intrapartum Care

Successful labor requires appropriate coordination of "the three Ps": *p*ower (the strength and regularity of uterine contractions), the *p*assenger (the fetus), and the *p*assage (the pelvis). Whenever a difficult delivery arises, these aspects must be assessed.

Management of Normal Labor and Delivery

During the first stage of delivery, fetal heart rate and uterine contractions are monitored. Manual vaginal exams are minimized through the latent phase to prevent additional risk

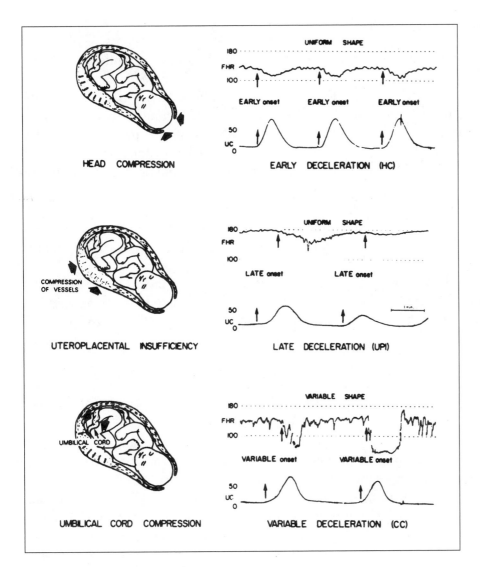

Fig. 7-3. Fetal heart rate decelerations. (FHR = fetal heart rate; UC = uterine contractions.) (From E Hon. *An Introduction to Fetal Heart Rate Monitoring.* Los Angeles: University of Southern California, 1973.)

of infection and discomfort to the patient. During the active phase, regular exams assess the progress of labor, including cervical dilation and fetal descent.

In the second phase, all postures except the supine position are acceptable for bearing down. Monitoring of the fetal heart rate and fetal descent should continue. Delivery of the fetus may require episiotomy during crowning to prevent vaginal trauma.

Following delivery of the placenta, uterine massage and oxytocin will reduce excessive uterine bleeding. The placenta should be examined to verify that it is normal and that no placental fragments have been retained in the uterus.

Perineal lacerations are then repaired. First-degree lacerations involve the perineal skin or vaginal mucosa. Second-degree lesions extend into the submucosal tissue of the perineum or vagina. Third-degree lacerations involve the anal sphincter, and fourth-degree lacerations involve the rectal mucosa. Following repair, digital rectal exam is performed to rule out any additional rectal tears and any possibility that repair itself has penetrated the rectal mucosa.

Anesthesia and Analgesia

Medical analgesia during labor can be provided by local, inhaled, or systemic medications.

- The most commonly used local technique is the **epidural**, in which anesthetics are injected into the epidural space between L3 and L4. If administered during latent phase, an epidural can prolong labor, so it is usually not started until the cervix has dilated to 4–5 cm. A risk of epidural anesthesia is placental hypotension, which will appear as severe, repetitive fetal heart rate decelerations. This can be treated with maternal IV hydration.
- The most commonly used systemic anesthetics are **narcotics**. These are more easily administered than epidurals, but they can prolong the latent phase if given too early and can cause fetal respiratory depression if given too late. Fetal side effects can be reversed with naloxone (Narcan).
- The most common inhaled analgesic is **nitrous oxide**, although this is not frequently used in the United States. The efficacy of analgesia is not as good as with an epidural, but there is less risk of fetal respiratory depression than with systemic narcotics.

Induction of Labor

Artificially initiating labor is indicated only when continuation of the pregnancy threatens the well-being of the fetus or mother. Augmentation refers to enhancing a labor that has already begun. Common indications for induction include preeclampsia, some concurrent medical diseases, post-dates pregnancy, some fetal abnormalities, Rh isoimmunization, premature rupture of membranes, and chorioamnionitis.

Prior uterine surgery with complete transection of the uterine wall is the most common contraindication to inducing or augmenting labor, although this does not include a prior lower transverse incision as used in cesarean section. A contracted pelvis, an immature fetus, and acute fetal distress are other contraindications.

A Bishop Score determines the readiness of the cervix for delivery, based on effacement, dilation, and station of the fetal head. A low score reflects a lower likelihood of successful induction. Fetal pulmonary maturity must be assessed before induction is begun, and maturation can be hastened by administration of glucocorticoids 24 hours before delivery. For induction, oxytocin is given and adjusted as needed. If the induction is unsuccessful after 3 days, amniotomy may be tried, but a cesarean section is usually necessary.

Forceps Delivery

Obstetric forceps aid in fetal descent by providing traction and rotation. The most common indication is a prolonged second stage of labor, due to either failure of head rotation, inadequate uterine contractions, or cephalopelvic disproportion. Vacuum extraction may also be used when the uterus alone is not providing sufficient power for delivery.

There are several prerequisites for a forceps delivery. Delivery must be mechanically feasible, the head must be engaged, and the presentation must be appropriate, with the

Table 7-2. Relative indications for cesarean section

Fetal issues	Maternal issues	Fetal/maternal issues
Distress	Classic cesarean section	Placenta previa
Malpresentation	Prior uterine rupture	Placental abruption
Cord prolapse	Eclampsia	Cephalopelvic disproportion
	Failed induction of labor	
	Severe preeclampsia	
	Diabetes mellitus	
	Cardiac disease	

position of the fetal head known. The mother must have uterine contractions, ruptured membranes, a fully dilated cervix, an empty bladder, and proper analgesia.

Fetal complications include serious face, scalp, or head injuries and brain damage. Maternal complications include soft-tissue trauma and subsequent heavy bleeding.

Indications for Cesarean Section

The decision to perform a cesarean section is only rarely obvious. A history of previous "classic" cesarean section, in which a vertical incision was made in the uterus, is one absolute indication for repeat cesarean section, because there is a high rate of uterine rupture in vaginal delivery following this procedure. The newer cesarean section technique, in which a low transverse incision into the uterus is made, is not an absolute indication for repeat cesarean section, and a vaginal birth may be attempted following this procedure. The most common reason for cesarean section is dystocia (i.e., difficult labor), or "failure to progress." In general, indications for cesarean section involve a threat to fetal health, maternal health, or both. These decisions are seldom clear-cut, but a list of relative indications is given in Table 7-2.

Abnormal Labor

Preterm Labor

The onset of labor prior to the thirty-seventh week of gestation occurs in about 10% of all pregnancies in the United States. Risk factors include multiple gestation, premature rupture of membranes, uterine anomalies, previous preterm labor or delivery, polyhydramnios, infection, and cervical incompetence. Lower socioeconomic status and poor maternal nutrition are associated with a higher incidence of preterm labor.

SIGNS & SYMPTOMS

Patients may complain of contractions, uterine or low-back pain, and vaginal discharge or bleeding.

Regular uterine contractions (at least 6 per hour) and concurrent cervical change occurring prior to the thirty-seventh week of gestation are the criteria for diagnosis. Cultures for *Chlamydia* and group B *Streptococcus* are needed, and ultrasound can rule out fetal or uterine anomalies, verify gestational age, and assess amniotic fluid volume.

Preterm labor is relieved in half of patients simply by prescribing hydration and bed rest. Tocolytic agents should be administered unless chorioamnionitis, maternal compromise, or fetal distress require immediate delivery. The beta-adrenergic agonists ritodrine or terbutaline are used for tocolysis with a high success rate. Magnesium, prostaglandin synthetase inhibitors, and calcium channel blockers are also used to arrest labor. Corticosteroids may be administered to accelerate maturation of the fetal lungs.

Premature Rupture of Membranes

Spontaneous premature rupture of the membranes (PROM) may occur prior to the onset of labor. Vaginal or cervical infections, abnormal membrane physiology, and cervical incompetence may precipitate this event. If it occurs before the thirty-seventh week of gestation, it is referred to as preterm PROM and has a high associated risk of preterm delivery.

Patients note leaking vaginal fluid, which is generally clear but may be tinged with blood or meconium. Some uterine contractions may be present.

Vaginal fluid loss suggests PROM, and the presence of amniotic fluid in the vagina, with a positive nitrazine or ferning test, confirms the diagnosis.

Only one vaginal exam should be performed, in order to minimize the risk of introducing infection. It can confirm rupture, allow cervical assessment, and permit cervical culture and amniotic fluid sampling for lung maturity tests. The lecithin to sphingomyelin (L/S) ratio of amniotic fluid predicts fetal lung maturity. If the L/S ratio suggests lung immaturity, delivery should be delayed, with bed rest and tocolysis if necessary, to provide time for lung maturation. Corticosteroid administration is not necessary, since PROM decreases the risk of the respiratory distress syndrome in neonates. If the patient develops chorioamnionitis, antibiotics should be given as soon as cultures have been taken and labor should quickly be induced.

Prolonged Latent Phase

A prolonged latent phase extends beyond 20 hours in nulliparous women and beyond 14 hours in multiparous women (see Fig. 7-1). It may result from hypertonic uterine contractions, premature or excessive sedation, and, rarely, hypotonic uterine contractions. In addition, the patient may in fact be in false labor, with no progressive cervical dilation at all.

Protracted labor.

True contractions without full cervical effacement and dilation. The patient is observed over time, while monitoring uterine contractions and cervical change.

A hypertonic uterus usually responds well to morphine, while a hypotonic uterus may respond to IV oxytocin. Sedating medications should be minimized. Amniotomy (artificial rupture of membranes) can sometimes accelerate labor, but it also introduces an increased risk of infection.

Prolonged Active Phase

Protraction of the active phase occurs when progression of active labor is extremely slow or arrests entirely (see Fig. 7-1). Cephalopelvic disproportion is the most common cause. Others include abnormal fetal presentation, hypotonic uterine contractions, and excessive sedation.

Protracted labor.

Protracted cervical dilation occurs when dilation is slower than normal or entirely arrested for 2 hours or more. Protracted descent is slower than 1 cm/hour in a nullipara and 2 cm/hour in a multipara.

No immediate intervention is needed if there are no signs of fetal distress. If the pelvic inlet is normal, amniotomy or oxytocin may improve the power of the uterus. Assisted vaginal delivery or cesarean section are frequently necessary.

Cephalopelvic Disproportion

In some deliveries cephalopelvic disproportion (CPD) is evident, in which the fetal head cannot pass through the maternal bony pelvis because of mechanical difficulties in size or shape. Contraction of the midpelvis is the most common cause. Disproportion at the pelvic inlet prevents descent and engagement of the fetal head.

Protracted or arrested labor. A decreased cervical dilation rate may be noted prior to arrest of descent.

Progression of labor and manual evaluation of the bony pelvis establish the diagnosis. X-ray pelvimetry is controversial but can confirm CPD.

Depending on the stage at which descent is blocked, a mid-forceps delivery or an abdominal delivery is necessary.

Fetal Malpresentations

Breech Presentation

Breech presentation involves the presentation of the fetal lower extremities or buttocks into the maternal pelvis. It is the most common malpresentation. While one-fourth of fetuses are in a breech presentation before 28 weeks' gestational age, few fetuses remain breech by 34 weeks.

Prematurity is a major risk factor for breech presentation, and breech babies often have low birth weight. Fetal anomalies such as hydrocephalus and anencephaly also predispose to breech, in addition to multiple gestation, uterine anomalies, polyhydramnios, and a contracted maternal pelvis.

There are three types of breech presentation (Fig. 7-4). In **frank breech**, both lower extremities are extended at the knee, and both thighs are flexed. The majority of breech infants are in this position. In **complete breech**, one or both knees are flexed, and in **incomplete (footling) breech**, one or both feet are below the buttocks with the thigh extended.

Abdominal palpation shows the fetal head in the fundal region. Vaginal exam permits palpation of the presenting part. Ultrasound confirms the presentation and can sometimes identify the cause.

External version after 37 weeks of gestation is successful in rotating the fetus in most patients, but placental abruption and cord compression are associated risks. Cesarean section is often indicated. Vaginal deliveries of breech infants increase the risk of cord prolapse, head entrapment, asphyxia, and birth injury.

Face Presentation

Face presentation is much less common than breech presentation. Advanced maternal age, high parity, prematurity, and CPD are risk factors, and anencephaly must be excluded. Abdominal and vaginal exam suggest the position, which is confirmed by ultrasound. Normal spontaneous vaginal delivery or low forceps delivery may be possible, and the fetus should be carefully monitored throughout. Cesarean section is indicated for arrested labor.

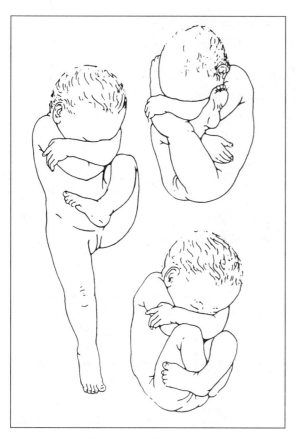

Fig. 7-4. Types of breech presentation. (Adapted from RC Benson. *Handbook of Obstetrics & Gynecology*, Eighth Edition. Norwalk, CT: Lange, 1983.)

Brow Presentation

Brow presentation is a rare condition involving the presentation of a wider diameter than for breech or face presentations. Again, prematurity, grand multiparity, and CPD are associated. Many brow presentations convert to face or vertex and deliver vaginally. The remainder will not fit through the bony pelvis and the baby must be delivered by cesarean section.

The Puerperium

Immediate Care of the Newborn

The following procedures are performed after the birth of a normal infant:

- **Clearing the airway.** Suction with a pump or catheter clears any fluid and prevents aspiration, which is a particular danger if meconium is present in the amniotic fluid.
- **Drying the baby.** This stimulates respiration and prevents heat loss.

- **Clamping the cord.** Delayed clamping results in significantly increased blood volume, increasing the risk of neonatal jaundice and tachypnea. Failure to clamp also prevents an accurate cord gas measurement.
- **Verifying onset of respiration.** Delay of onset for up to 1 minute is acceptable.
- **Apgar scoring.** Assess heart rate, respiratory effort, muscle tone, reflex irritability, and color 1 and 5 minutes after birth. Each factor is scored on a two-point scale. A score of at least 7 at 1 minute and 9 or 10 at 5 minutes is normal.

Physiology of the Normal Puerperium

The puerperium is the period following delivery until about 6 weeks postpartum. During this time, the maternal physiology returns to its prepregnant state.

Pelvic Changes

The lochia (normal uterine discharge) is bloody during the first days postpartum. It grows paler after a few days due to increasing amounts of mucus, and by the tenth day it is white or yellowish-white in appearance and consists primarily of microbes and cellular debris. The uterus decreases in weight, from 1 kg at delivery to 50 g within 3 weeks. The muscles of the pelvic floor gradually regain most of their prepregnancy tone.

Cardiovascular Changes

Immediately after delivery, the maternal peripheral vascular resistance increases sharply because the low pressure uteroplacental component is gone. Some weight loss occurs in the first week as the plasma volume and extracellular fluid levels return to normal. Cardiac functioning returns to its prepregnant state within 3 weeks.

Menstrual Cycle Changes

Nursing mothers generally do not ovulate for several months, but this is variable and is no guarantee of contraception. Women who opt not to nurse typically regain their menstrual flow by 6–8 weeks postpartum.

Lactation and Breast-Feeding

During the first half of pregnancy, the ductal elements of the breast proliferate due to the influence of estrogen. The epithelial cells then develop their secretory ability. High prolactin levels promote milk production, but this is inhibited by estrogen and other hormones. Following delivery, the drop in placentally derived estrogen permits lactation to occur. The baby's suckling evokes release of both prolactin, for production of milk, and oxytocin, which induces contraction of myoepithelial cells in the milk ducts and causes ejection of fluid. Colostrum is initially secreted. It contains protein, fat, secretory IgA, and minerals. Mature milk is present within a week, containing protein, fat, lactose, and water.

The advantages of breast-feeding are many, including complete and inexpensive nutrition for the infant, transmission of immunoglobulins for improved immunity, reduced incidence of allergies and asthma later in life, mother-child bonding, and weight loss for the mother. Mothers often worry during the first days that their milk production is insufficient. They should be reassured that early milk is thin and that it is normal for infants to lose weight in the first week. Breast engorgement in the first few days may cause pain, which is relieved by breast-feeding and by applying hot compresses. There are very few contraindications to breast-feeding; these include HIV infection, active hepatitis infection, and the use of certain medications—particularly tetracycline, chloramphenicol, and warfarin.

Nipple Fissures

Nipple fissures may arise from breast-feeding. They are common and painful. Fissures can serve as sites for bacterial entry and infection, leading to cellulitis, mastitis, or even abscess. A protective cream can facilitate the healing of cracked nipples. During the healing period, breast-feeding should be replaced with manual expression of milk.

Breast-Feeding–Related Mastitis

Breast-feeding–related mastitis, a cellulitis of the periglandular tissue, is most often caused by *Staphylococcus aureus*.

SIGNS & SYMPTOMS

Onset is usually 2–4 weeks after breast-feeding begins. Fever and chills occur with painful erythema and induration of the breast.

DIAGNOSIS

Clinical presentation and breast milk culture.

TREATMENT

Begin a penicillinase-resistant penicillin immediately, prior to culture results. Breast-feeding is not contraindicated.

Postpartum Hemorrhage

Postpartum hemorrhage is defined as blood loss exceeding 500 ml during vaginal delivery or 1,000 ml during cesarean section. It is the second leading cause of maternal mortality. Uterine atony is responsible for the majority of cases and often follows an overdistended uterus (e.g., multiple gestation), grand multiparity, prolonged or augmented labor, and chorioamnionitis. Trauma to the vaginal tract, commonly due to macrosomia or an instrumented vaginal delivery, can also cause hemorrhage. Most serious bleeding occurs early, but delayed postpartum hemorrhage may be due to retained placental tissue.

SIGNS & SYMPTOMS

Excessive blood from the uterus or vaginal tract.

Careful exam will determine the cause. Uterine atony is palpated through the abdominal wall. Vaginal and cervical inspection identify any lacerations. Manual exploration of the uterine cavity can diagnose uterine lacerations, retained products of conception, or partial inversion of the uterus.

Uterine massage and oxytocin help maintain uterine tone. Any lacerations must be sutured. The delivered placenta should be checked to ensure that it is complete. In refractory hemorrhage, blood replacement is indicated. If the uterus remains atonic, hypogastric artery ligation or hysterectomy will save the patient's life.

Postpartum Sepsis

Infection in the postpartum period usually occurs in the uterus, vagina, or urinary tract. It follows cesarean section more often than vaginal delivery. Other risk factors include anemia, preeclampsia, premature and prolonged rupture of membranes, extended labor, multiple vaginal exams during labor, traumatic delivery, and postpartum hemorrhage. Anaerobic organisms cause most postpartum infections, particularly anaerobic streptococci and *Bacteroides fragilis. Escherichia coli* is the most common aerobic pathogen.

A fever and uterine tenderness are key, often accompanied by tachycardia, pallor, chills, and leukocytosis. Reduced lochia is associated with a more severe sepsis. Parametritis (inflammation of connective tissue around the uterus) is characterized by a fixed, painful uterus and high fever. Pelvic thrombophlebitis is a complication of postpartum sepsis that presents as a persistent, spiking fever that is not responsive to antibiotics.

Temperature of 38°C or higher, lasting 2 days and starting between the second and tenth day postpartum. Other sources of fever, particularly mastitis, must be excluded. Blood, cervical, and urine cultures establish the infecting organism.

Antibiotics with broad anaerobic coverage should be given early and continued for 2 days after the fever has resolved. A commonly used regimen of "triple therapy" includes ampicillin, gentamicin, and clindamycin. Heparin therapy is indicated if pelvic thrombophlebitis is suspected.

Postpartum "Blues" and Postpartum Depression

Postpartum "blues" are a common complication of the puerperium, usually occurring 3–10 days after delivery and resolving spontaneously. Unlike postpartum blues, postpartum depression will not resolve in the puerperium. It occurs most often in primipara patients with a history of depression and in patients who do not have good social support. Depressive symptoms may be associated with apathy toward the infant, hallucinations, psychotic behavior, and homicidal or suicidal ideation. Antidepressant medication is helpful.

Postpartum Psychosis

Postpartum psychosis is less common, more severe, and longer lasting than postpartum depression, and the psychotic aspects are pronounced. Hospitalization and antipsychotic medications may be necessary to stabilize the patient.

Contraception

Behavioral Methods

- **Abstinence** involves never having sex. Effective, but dull.
- The **rhythm method** involves monitoring monthly cycles and basal body temperature to estimate the date of ovulation each month. Sexual intercourse is avoided for several days surrounding this date. This method is safe, free, and acceptable to most religions. However, effectiveness rates vary widely, and this method is ineffective if cycles are irregular.
- **Coitus interruptus** (withdrawal of the penis from the vagina just prior to ejaculation) is only about 75% effective, in part because sperm-containing fluid may leak from the penis before ejaculation occurs. It is also associated with decreased pleasure and may be ineffective if withdrawal is not timed properly.

Barrier Methods

- **Diaphragms** and **cervical caps**, used with spermicide, provide barriers that block sperm from entering the cervix. These barriers must be inserted just prior to intercourse and must remain in the vagina for 6–8 hours after intercourse. If used correctly, effectiveness is more than 98%; however, in practice, effectiveness rates are closer to 80% due to inconvenience and accompanying lack of compliance.
- **Condoms** are sheaths that cover the penis during intercourse, preventing sperm from entering the vagina. Made of either latex or lambskin, they are often used in conjunction with spermicidal cream or foam. Under perfect conditions, condoms are 95% effective in preventing pregnancy; however, in practice, effectiveness rates are less than 85% due to improper use and lack of compliance. Condoms made of latex are the most effective method of protection against STDs, including HIV.
- **Intrauterine devices** (IUDs) are placed into the uterus, where they irritate the endometrial lining and inhibit embryonic implantation. These objects are inserted by clinicians and can remain in the uterine cavity for many years. Newer IUDs contain progesterone for further inhibition of implantation. IUDs are associated with increased risks of infertility, spontaneous abortion, uterine perforation, and ectopic pregnancy. They are generally recommended for women who have completed their childbearing.

Hormonal Methods

- **Birth control pills** (BCPs), consisting of low doses of estrogen and progesterone, work by preventing ovulation and by changing the quality of the endometrial lining to interfere with implantation. BCPs are available by prescription only and must be taken daily to be effective. Theoretically, effectiveness rates approach 100%; however, in practice, rates range from 90% to 95%. Side effects include nausea, headache, hypertension, and weight gain. The risk of thromboembolic disease is also increased, and smokers over the age of 40 should not be given BCPs due to high rates of clots. Progestin-only pills ("mini-pills") are associated with fewer side effects but are slightly less effective than estrogen-containing pills.
- **Depo-Provera** is a progestin analogue that prevents pregnancy by suppressing endometrial development. It is administered via injection every 3 months. Side effects are similar to those of BCPs and include weight gain, headache, nausea, and irregular spotting.
- **Norplant** is a set of progestin capsules placed subcutaneously that provides long-term pregnancy prevention. Typically, five capsules are implanted, and protection lasts for 5 years. Side effects are similar to those of Depo-Provera and include weight gain and menstrual irregularities. Patients who wish to become pregnant may have the capsules removed and are usually able to ovulate within 3 months.

Sterilization

Permanent sterilization can be achieved in the male with a vasectomy, in which the vas deferens is cut and sealed. Follow-up semen analysis can verify results. This surgery is simple and effective, and the success of reversal, if desired, is approximately 60%. Tubal ligation in the female can be done at the time of cesarean section or with laparoscopy at any other time. Efficacy is generally excellent, but ectopic pregnancy cannot be excluded in a woman with a prior tubal ligation if she presents with the classic symptoms. Reversal is often effective but places the woman at a particularly high risk for ectopic pregnancies.

Perinatal and Congenital Issues

Common Complications of the Neonatal Period

Intracranial Hemorrhage

Bleeding in or around the brain may occur in three locations:

1. Premature infants are particularly at risk for **intraventricular hemorrhage**, which is caused by hypoxia and by mechanical pressure on the infant's head at birth. Up to 40% of premature infants have these intraventricular hemorrhages, which are often bilateral and occur in the germinal matrix (developing periventricular tissue that is seen in the fetus and is still present in premature babies). Neonates may be asymptomatic but can have apnea and cyanosis. The prognosis varies with the extent of bleeding, but severe neurologic sequelae may result.
2. **Subarachnoid hemorrhages** are more often seen in full-term infants. They may be related to birth trauma or to germinal matrix bleeding. Seizures are common and are typically brief. Patients usually do well, with no long-term sequelae.
3. **Subdural hemorrhages** result from traumatic tears in the bridging veins, which cause bleeding in the subdural space, and are often seen after difficult deliveries or in large infants. Seizures, irritability, and a rapidly enlarging head are seen. The majority of infants survive without any sequelae.

The cerebrospinal fluid (CSF) may contain RBCs or gross blood, particularly with a subarachnoid hemorrhage. Metabolic studies should be performed to rule out other sources of neurologic disturbances.

Ultrasound and CT scan will show blood.

Supportive care. Small subdural taps may be helpful to treat subdural hemorrhages.

Meconium Aspiration Syndrome

Meconium is the neonate's first stool, consisting mostly of sloughed cells, mucus, and bile pigments. When an unborn infant aspirates meconium from the amniotic sac, mechanical obstruction and a chemical pneumonia may result. Obstruction is particularly severe in postterm infants, who have thicker meconium and a smaller volume of amniotic fluid. Complete blockage of the bronchi causes atelectasis, whereas partial obstruction causes air trapping, with associated pneumomediastinum or pneumothorax. Fetal distress secondary to placental insufficiency often precedes meconium aspiration, and persistent pulmonary hypertension is a frequent, treatable complication.

Respiratory distress, barrel-chested appearance, meconium staining of the umbilical cord and nails are all characteristic signs.

Chest x-ray demonstrates patchy atelectasis with areas of hyperinflation.

Immediate aspiration of nose and mouth at delivery helps prevent meconium aspiration. Intubate compromised infants, suction the trachea, and administer humidified air or oxygen.

Transient Tachypnea of the Newborn

Transient tachypnea of the newborn (TTN), a disorder of respiratory distress, results from the delayed resorption of fetal lung fluid. Fluid is normally absorbed across the lung epithelium and expelled when the thorax is compressed during vaginal delivery. Most infants with TTN are full-term but have had cesarean section deliveries with some amount of fetal distress.

Tachypnea, grunting, retractions, and sometimes cyanosis.

Chest x-ray shows that the lungs are hyperinflated with dark perihilar markings and a clear periphery.

With oxygen administration, recovery is complete within 2–3 days.

Hyperbilirubinemia

Jaundice in the newborn may reflect increased production or decreased excretion of bilirubin. Common causes are listed in Table 8-1. The most common type of hyperbilirubinemia is "physiologic" jaundice, in which levels of unconjugated bilirubin are elevated due to high RBC turnover occurring before the liver is mature enough to conjugate the bile. About 50% of full-term infants and even more preemies experience this mild increase in bilirubin, which resolves in 1–2 weeks. With causes other than physiologic jaundice, the main complication is **kernicterus**, a syndrome that occurs when unconjugated bilirubin is

Table 8-1. Causes of hyperbilirubinemia

Overproduction from increased hemolysis
    Fetal-maternal blood group incompatibility (Rh, ABO)
    RBC abnormalities (hereditary spherocytosis, elliptocytosis)
    Enzyme abnormalities (G6PD deficiency, pyruvate kinase deficiency)
Overproduction without hemolysis
    Extravascular hemorrhage (hematoma, intraventricular hemorrhage)
    Polycythemia (maternal-fetal transfusion, delayed cord clamping)
    Increased enterohepatic circulation (GI obstruction, ileus)
Undersecretion
    Physiologic jaundice
    Familial jaundice (Crigler-Najjar)
    Gilbert's syndrome
    Biliary atresia
Mixed
    Intrauterine infection
    Sepsis
    Respiratory distress syndrome

deposited in the basal ganglia and hippocampus, causing nerve cell death and brain damage. Any disorder causing hemolysis may result in hyperbilirubinemia.

SIGNS & SYMPTOMS

Jaundice develops from the head downward. Signs of kernicterus are lethargy, poor feeding, high-pitched cry, hypertonicity, seizures, apnea, and death. Developmental manifestations, including mental retardation, sensorineural hearing loss, athetoid cerebral palsy, and paralysis of upward gaze, are irreversible.

DIAGNOSIS

In physiologic jaundice, the increased bilirubin does not rise above normal levels until the second day of life, never exceeding 14–15 mg/dl. Although no specific level for risk of kernicterus has been established, unconjugated hyperbilirubinemia above 15 mg/dl must be investigated further. Useful tests in diagnosis include blood typing, Coombs' test, and hematocrit.

TREATMENT

Phototherapy is generally used for infants with lower levels of hyperbilirubinemia. The blue or white light converts unconjugated bilirubin into a water-soluble form, which the infant can then excrete in the urine. For more dangerous elevations, exchange transfusions are necessary. The underlying disorder must also be addressed.

Common Perinatal Infections

Neonatal Conjunctivitis

Neonatal conjunctivitis is a common eye infection with several etiologies. Chemical injury, the most common cause, results from silver nitrate drops used for prophylaxis against gonorrheal infection. Chlamydial conjunctivitis is acquired during delivery in one-third of infants born to infected mothers. Other bacteria, particularly *Streptococcus pneumoniae, Haemophilus influenzae,* and *Neisseria gonorrhoeae,* and viruses, such as herpes simplex virus (HSV), are also common agents.

Purulent discharge, eyelid edema.

Culture and Gram's stain of discharge.

Chemical conjunctivitis resolves completely within 1–2 days. Chlamydial disease is treated with oral erythromycin, because systemic antibiotic treatment will prevent chlamydial pneumonia, a later complication of intrapartum chlamydial infection. Gonorrheal disease requires hospitalization and ceftriaxone. Other infections are treated with topical preparations.

Silver nitrate drops applied at birth protect against gonorrheal disease. Topical erythromycin protects against other bacteria as well.

Neonatal Sepsis

Neonatal sepsis is defined as any systemic bacterial infection within the first 4 weeks of life. This is more frequent in low-birth-weight infants, in males, and in infants with respiratory depression. Early-onset sepsis, apparent in 6–72 hours, is due to infection acquired in utero or during delivery, and its risk increases with many complications of labor and delivery. Late-onset sepsis is often nosocomial, usually presenting after about 4 days. Common organisms are group B beta-hemolytic streptococci and gram-negative enteric bacteria, in addition to *Staphylococcus aureus, Staphylococcus epidermidis, Listeria monocytogenes,* and *Enterococcus.*

Symptoms are often subtle and nonspecific, with decreased activity, poor feeding, temperature instability (hyperthermia or hypothermia), apnea, and bradycardia.

Blood, CSF, and urine cultures. The white blood cell (WBC) count is considered abnormal and indicative of possible sepsis if less than 4,000/µl or greater than 25,000/µl. The clinician must always have a high index of suspicion.

Broad-spectrum antibiotics.

Neonatal Pneumonia

The respiratory system may be infected in utero or during delivery. Infection is especially common if prolonged rupture of the membranes has led to amnionitis. Group B streptococci are the most frequent causative organisms, although other bacteria and some viruses are also associated. Chlamydial pneumonia has a later onset (2–6 weeks postpartum) and is often preceded by conjunctivitis.

Tachypnea, retractions, and cyanosis. Severe cases may involve respiratory failure and septic shock.

Chest x-rays frequently show patchy infiltrates, but pneumonia is generally indistinguishable from respiratory distress syndrome, transient tachypnea of the newborn, meconium aspiration, and persistent pulmonary hypertension. Cultures of blood, tracheal aspirate, and CSF are diagnostic.

Broad-spectrum antibiotics.

Neonatal Meningitis

Neonatal meningitis, a bacterial infection of the meninges occurring within 4 weeks of birth, is more common in males and low-birth-weight infants. Meningitis accompanies 25% of neonatal sepsis cases, usually resulting from bacteremia. Infections are commonly due to group B *Streptococcus*, *Escherichia coli*, and *Listeria*. One-third of survivors have significant neurologic sequelae.

Sepsis is usually more apparent than meningitis, but infants may have some central nervous system signs such as lethargy, focal seizures, and vomiting. A full fontanelle and nuchal rigidity are apparent in only a minority of patients.

Blood cultures are positive in 70% of cases. CSF examination provides a definitive diagnosis.

Even with broad-spectrum antibiotics, mortality is about 25%. Antibiotics should be tailored to the specific organism.

Neonatal Listeriosis

Neonatal listeriosis is acquired transplacentally and disseminates, causing granuloma formation in multiple organs. Perinatal infection can also occur, when contaminated amniotic fluid or vaginal secretions are swallowed or aspirated. Poor outcomes of pregnancy, including spontaneous abortion, prematurity, and stillbirth, are common.

Sepsis, respiratory compromise, and circulatory insufficiency. Onset may be delayed several weeks.

Culture from cord blood, peripheral blood, CSF, gastric aspirate, meconium, or the mother's lochia can establish the infecting organism.

Ampicillin and an aminoglycoside.

Congenital Rubella

Transplacental rubella infection occurs in utero, with rates of transmission up to 80% during the first trimester. During these early weeks, the fetus is also at the greatest risk of developing abnormalities. Infected women may be asymptomatic or may experience upper respiratory symptoms, arthritis, and a tell-tale rash.

Fetal effects vary from isolated hearing loss, which is asymptomatic at birth, to death in utero. Multiple anomalies can occur, including intrauterine growth retardation, cataracts, retinopathy, cardiac defects, encephalitis, hepatosplenomegaly, and purpura. Bone radiolucencies are demonstrated on x-ray. Mental retardation and hearing loss may be evident later.

Antibody serology and cultures.

No effective treatment exists.

Prophylaxis is crucial, with immunization or verification of antibody titer level of all girls and women prior to their pregnancies. Immunization is contraindicated during the pregnancy. If an unimmunized woman is exposed to rubella, immunoglobulin can be administered, and termination of the pregnancy may be considered.

Neonatal Herpes Simplex Virus

About 80% HSV-2, neonatal herpes simplex virus infection is usually transmitted by delivery through an infected vaginal tract. Transplacental and nosocomial spread also occur. Mothers may be unaware of their HSV infection, and the risk of transmission is higher during a primary maternal infection.

Within 1–4 weeks, skin vesicles appear in about half of infected infants. Some have only localized disease, with skin, mouth, and eye involvement. However, disseminated infection also occurs, including temperature instability, lethargy, respiratory difficulty, seizures, pneumonitis, hepatitis, and disseminated intravascular coagulation (DIC). Another form of localized disease, encephalitis, tends to occur in infants who do not develop skin lesions. Neurologic involvement results in severe neurologic sequelae in at least 95% of these survivors; 30% of all infected infants also have later neurologic impairment.

Culture of CSF or scrapings from lesions.

Vidarabine or acyclovir decreases mortality by 50% and decreases the sequelae of both localized and disseminated disease.

Neonatal Hepatitis B Infection

Neonatal hepatitis B infection is generally acquired during delivery, so the risk of transmission increases with maternal infection later in the pregnancy. Transplacental transmission is rare. The main risk to the infant is becoming a chronic hepatitis B virus (HBV) carrier, with chronic hepatitis and an increased risk of hepatocellular carcinoma as a result.

Most infants develop chronic hepatitis, which is generally subclinical. Some infants develop acute hepatitis that is self-limited and typically mild.

Hepatitis B virus surface antigen (HBsAg) serology.

Acute hepatitis is treated symptomatically.

Infants of known infected women should receive hepatitis B immunoglobulin and vaccine as soon as possible after delivery. Two subsequent doses of the vaccine are necessary for full immunization.

Cytomegalovirus

Cytomegalovirus (CMV) is the virus most commonly transmitted in utero. The mother is generally asymptomatic, with higher rates of transmission from primary rather than reactivated infection. The infant's infection may be congenital, which is acquired from transplacental infection, or perinatal, acquired from contact with infected maternal secretions during delivery or breast-feeding.

The majority of infected infants are asymptomatic at birth. Only 10% of congenitally infected infants have acute symptoms, which may include prematurity, intrauterine growth retardation (IUGR), microcephaly, hepatosplenomegaly, jaundice, petechiae, periventricular calcifications, chorioretinitis, and pneumonitis. The combination of jaundice and petechiae causes the infant to have a "blueberry corn muffin" appearance. Symptomatic CMV has a 20% mortality rate, and 90% of survivors have sequelae of mental retardation, seizures, hearing loss, and visual defects. Among asymptomatic infected infants, 10% will have neurologic sequelae, most often involving hearing loss. Perinatally acquired infections are generally mild or asymptomatic and without sequelae.

Culture from blood, CSF, urine, amniotic fluid, or the placenta.

None available. Ganciclovir may have some use, although this is unproven.

Congenital Syphilis

Risk of congenital syphilis, a transplacentally acquired infection, depends on the mother's stage of disease during the pregnancy. Interestingly, primary and secondary syphilis are usually transmitted, whereas latent and tertiary syphilis are not.

Mostly asymptomatic at birth. Bullous lesions and a macular rash on the palms and soles are characteristic. Lymphadenopathy, hepatosplenomegaly, and jaundice may be present. Later, the infant may exhibit failure to thrive. "Snuffles" (discharge due to nasal bone necrosis) in a young infant may be the presenting sign. Within 3 months, bone changes may result in bone inflammation or pseudoparalysis. Most infected infants remain in the latent stage throughout their lives, although some have late manifestations.

Dark-field microscopy from lesion scrapings, or RPR and VDRL. Long bone x-rays will show characteristic radiologic abnormalities.

Penicillin is given to infected infants, with a good prognosis.

This disease is entirely preventable with adequate diagnosis and treatment of pregnant women.

Congenital Toxoplasmosis

Congenital toxoplasmosis, a transplacentally acquired infection by *Toxoplasma gondii*, occurs after maternal exposure to cat feces or raw meat.

Manifestations include IUGR, microcephaly, seizures, hepatosplenomegaly, jaundice, pneumonia, and chorioretinitis. Many infants are asymptomatic at birth, but some have later sequelae that include mental retardation, seizures, blindness, and deafness.

IgM and IgG serologies.

Little effective treatment is available for infants.

Teaching pregnant women to avoid cat litter, and treatment of infected women may be helpful.

Congenital Varicella

Varicella infection has only a 5% transmission rate across the placenta. Perinatal varicella, however, may have particularly severe consequences.

Transplacental exposure results in limb hypoplasia, microcephaly, cortical atrophy, chorioretinitis, and cutaneous scars. Perinatal exposure can result in fatal infection.

Increased maternal IgG titers, neonatal IgM, or viral culture.

Pregnant women exposed to varicella should receive varicella immunoglobulin. Women with the disease can be treated with acyclovir.

Tetanus Neonatorum

Although tetanus neonatorum is very rare in the United States, it remains widely prevalent throughout much of the world and is the leading cause of infant mortality in many developing countries. In the United States, its incidence is increasing among illegal immigrants, who may deliver their infants at home without appropriate sanitation. The disease results from infection of the umbilical cord by *Clostridium tetani* spores, and its incidence can be greatly decreased with better hygienic treatment of the cord.

Infection becomes evident between 3 days and 2 weeks of age. Poor feeding is the first sign, followed by muscle stiffness, spasms, convulsions, and death.

Typical clinical syndrome in a previously healthy infant.

Tetanus antitoxin, muscle relaxants, and IV feeds may be somewhat helpful for a minority of patients; however, 85% of infected infants die within a few days.

Prevention is critical, with two doses of tetanus toxoid immunization for all pregnant women who have not been previously immunized, and with improved umbilical cord care. Maternal tetanus immunization is completely protective, as the antibodies are passed to the fetus.

Substance-Exposed Infants

Fetal Alcohol Syndrome

Fetal alcohol syndrome (FAS), an all-too-common result of alcohol ingestion during pregnancy, involves a wide spectrum of defects. While the amount of alcohol ingestion causing FAS is unknown, the fetal effects are dose-related. Infants have intrauterine growth retardation and dysmorphic features, including microcephaly, short palpebral fissures, cardiac anomalies, and joint defects. Later manifestations include mental retardation and hyperactivity. In fact, FAS is the leading known cause of mental retardation.

Narcotic Exposure

Infants exposed to heroin, methadone, and other narcotics in utero are at risk for a withdrawal syndrome after birth. Withdrawal symptoms include irritability, tremors, hypertonicity, high-pitched cry, sweating, and stuffy nose. More severe withdrawal symptoms may involve vomiting, diarrhea, and seizures. The symptoms from methadone exposure are generally more severe and prolonged than those from heroin. Urine toxicology confirms the diagnosis only if the drug has been used within a few days of delivery. Swaddling the infant in a quiet environment is usually sufficient treatment. Otherwise, phenobarbital or tincture of opium may be administered and tapered slowly. These infants are at an increased risk of sudden infant death syndrome (SIDS).

Cocaine Exposure

Cocaine use during pregnancy leads to an increased risk of complications of labor, as well as to a range of fetal effects. Vascular disruption secondary to cocaine use may have early effects on the fetus, causing limb reduction malformations and intestinal atresias. Low birth weight and low Apgar scores are two well-documented outcomes, and cerebral infarcts may be associated. Signs of withdrawal include irritability, jitteriness, sweating, vomiting, tremors, and diarrhea, which are treated by swaddling the infant and providing a quiet, low-stimulation environment.

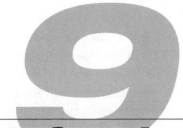

Infectious Disease

Socioeconomic and Social Impact

The occurrence of infectious disease is associated with a number of public health and environmental factors. To cause illness, an infectious agent must come into contact with a susceptible host. Good nutrition, personal hygiene, and public sanitation have a much larger impact on preventing infectious disease worldwide than do vaccines and medical care. People of lower socioeconomic status may live in areas with poor sanitation and little health education and may have poor nutritional status, making them more susceptible to infectious disease than other socioeconomic groups. As illness may require absence from work or school, susceptible people also suffer from the results of increased absenteeism, including lost wages.

Surveillance and Reporting

The monitoring of infectious disease is facilitated by national mandatory reporting of certain diseases to the Centers for Disease Control and Prevention (CDC). This organization can provide information on seasonal and temporal trends, as well as help in the detection and investigation of epidemics. Some of the diseases that must be reported to local health departments are listed in Table 9-1.

Measures to Prevent Transmission

The most effective way to decrease transmission of communicable disease is to address issues of public education, surveillance, containment, and contact tracing. As a community, containment may require the quarantine of individuals with a specific disease. Contact tracing is usually conducted by public health departments and pertains most often to sexually transmitted diseases, although tuberculosis contacts are traced and treated as well.

Individual measures to prevent disease vary with the mode of disease transmission, but include condoms (to prevent the transmission of HIV and other sexually transmitted diseases), hand washing (to prevent the spread of many gastrointestinal and upper respiratory organisms), and face masks (to protect against diseases such as tuberculosis that are spread by respiratory droplets). Even basic actions such as covering one's mouth when coughing can decrease the spread of respiratory diseases.

Isolation Procedures in Hospitalized Patients

Different types of isolation procedures are used in hospitals, depending on the risk posed. The most important types of isolation are described below:

- **Contact isolation** is used to prevent the spread of highly transmissible organisms that are spread through direct contact, such as antibiotic-resistant strains of *Staphylococcus aureus*. Gowns, masks, and gloves are generally required of all individuals who interact with an infected patient.

Table 9-1. Reportable diseases

Sexually transmitted diseases	Immunization-preventable illnesses	Diseases with outbreak potential
Gonorrhea	Measles	Tuberculosis
Non-gonococcal urethritis	Mumps	Hepatitis
Syphilis	Rubella	Meningitis
Chancroid	Polio	Salmonella
Pelvic inflammatory disease	Hepatitis B	Shigella
HIV/AIDS*	Tetanus	

*May vary from state to state.

- **Respiratory isolation** helps prevent the spread of organisms transmitted by coughing, sneezing, or breathing. It involves private rooms for patients and masks for visitors and staff. Pertussis is one infection that requires respiratory isolation. TB requires more stringent isolation and is described below.
- **Strict isolation** is used for organisms that can be transmitted either by direct contact or by airborne spread. Strict isolation includes putting patients in private rooms and requiring visitors to wear gowns, masks, and gloves when entering the room and to wash their hands on exiting. Special ventilation may also be necessary for diseases such as chickenpox.
- **Tuberculosis isolation** is used for all known or suspected cases of TB. It requires private rooms with separate ventilation systems and masks for visitors and staff.
- **Protective isolation** (reverse isolation) is designed to protect immunosuppressed patients from exposure to outside organisms. Protective measures include private rooms with closed doors; gowns, masks, and gloves on entering; and hand washing both when entering and leaving the room. Other measures include separate ventilation systems and sterilized food.

The CDC have recommended the use of "**universal precautions**" for all patients to prevent exposure to HIV, hepatitis B virus, and other bloodborne infections. This entails protection against blood and body fluids, particularly enteric secretions. Precautions include the use of gloves (with double-gloving in high-risk procedures), gowns, and masks when there is a risk of being splashed with blood and body fluids. Hand washing and reporting any needlestick injuries is also suggested.

Immune Defenses

Normal physiology provides some innate resistance that includes general defenses against infection. The most important immune defense is intact skin, although some organisms, such as human papillomavirus (HPV), may invade through skin. The respiratory defenses include mucous membranes and ciliary action in the bronchi. Fever is also an important nonspecific defense. Specific defenses for the major classes of organisms are described below:

- To fight **bacteria**, the humoral (B cell–mediated antibody) and the cellular (T cell–mediated) immune systems work together. First, the bacteria is covered by IgG antibodies (opsonization). Then neutrophils phagocytose the bacteria. Finally, within the neutrophil, lysosomal granules release oxygen radicals to kill the bacteria. Macrophages also engulf and kill bacteria in a similar cycle in order to help the B cells produce antibody directed specifically at the organism.

- **Viruses** must invade a cell in order to grow and replicate. Once the virus enters the host cell, antibodies are an ineffective defense. Macrophages can phagocytose infected cells, and cytotoxic ("killer") T cells are able to recognize and destroy infected cells as well. Interferon is a nonspecific defense against viral diseases. It works by blocking production of viral proteins.
- **Fungal** infections are generally fought by cell-mediated immunity, which can result in the formation of granulomas. Cell-mediated immunity is also involved in both immediate and delayed hypersensitivity reactions to fungi.
- The mainstays of the immune response against **parasites** are eosinophils and IgE antibodies. Parasitic infections are fairly unusual in the United States.

Fever

Fever is defined as an elevation of body temperature above 37.8°C, or 100°F. It is caused by the presence of pyrogens, which are chemicals that act on the hypothalamic temperature regulatory center. Both exogenous (e.g., endotoxin of gram-negative bacteria) and endogenous pyrogens (e.g., interleukin-2) may induce fever. Fever can arise as a response to any type of inflammation, including that of neoplastic and autoimmune diseases. The most common cause of immediate postoperative fever is atelectasis (localized lung tissue collapse), but surgical patients are also at risk for wound infection, which usually causes fever after 3–5 days. A fever in a postoperative patient after more than 2 weeks suggests thrombophlebitis or pulmonary embolism.

SIGNS & SYMPTOMS

A rising temperature may be accompanied by peripheral vasoconstriction, shivering, and chills. Diaphoresis and peripheral vasodilation occur during the reduction of temperature.

DIAGNOSIS

After using a thermometer, it is important to search for the source of inflammation. Specific characteristics of the fever may provide a clue to the source (e.g., cyclic waxing and waning fever suggests malaria).

TREATMENT

Debate still rages over whether or not a fever should be treated. Although fevers are theoretically beneficial (by increasing immune response and metabolism to fight infection), this theory has little concrete clinical support. Antipyretics (medications that reduce fever by inhibiting the production of prostaglandins) must be given to children at risk for febrile seizure. Adults who will suffer if oxygen demands are increased, such as patients with cardiac or respiratory disease, should also receive antipyretics, since fever greatly elevates the body's consumption of oxygen. Other patients may be given antipyretics for symptomatic relief. Typical antipyretics include aspirin, acetaminophen, and a variety of newer nonsteroidal anti-inflammatory drugs (NSAIDs), such as ibuprofen and naproxen.

Fever of Unknown Origin

Fever of unknown origin (FUO) is defined as a fever of greater than 100°F for a period of at least 3 weeks, without known cause despite active investigation for at least 1 week.

Fever of at least 100°F lasting at least 3 weeks.

Complete blood count (CBC) and white blood cell differentials may indicate a specific class of infections (e.g., fungal, bacterial). Multiple blood cultures should be drawn. Antibody titers may be helpful for diagnosing viral infections and autoimmune diseases. Imaging studies may locate neoplasms.

Broad-spectrum antibiotics are usually given while the source of the fever is aggressively sought. Infections are the most common cause of FUO in children, whereas adults are likely to have an infectious, autoimmune, or neoplastic cause.

Inflammation

Inflammation is a reaction against foreign material, such as bacteria and transplanted tissue, or tissue mistaken as foreign, such as in autoimmune diseases. The classic symptoms of inflammation are "rubor, tumor, calor, and dolor" or redness, swelling, warmth, and pain. These symptoms result from increased blood flow to areas of inflammation and increased capillary permeability. Various chemical mediators, such as histamine, play a role in these changes. Elevation of certain blood cell lines may suggest the type of infectious agent present. For example, T cell proliferation often reflects the presence of a viral illness.

Acquired Immunity

Acquired immunity refers to directed protection against specific organisms. **Active acquired immunity** is developed when the individual is exposed directly to the organism in question. Either an infection or a vaccination can introduce antigens that promote active acquired immunity. **Passive acquired immunity** is the temporary protection against an organism that is obtained from administration of serum antibodies produced by another animal that has been exposed to the organism. Examples include antibodies transferred through breast milk and immunoglobulin given in cases of acute illness.

Antibiotic Resistance

Organisms may acquire resistance to some antibiotics by a variety of mechanisms. Those mechanisms of major concern are addressed in Table 9-2.

Table 9-2. Antibiotic resistance

Antibiotic	Mode of action	Basis of resistance
Penicillins, cephalosporins	Inhibition of cell wall synthesis	Beta-lactamases cleave drug
Aminoglycosides	Inhibition of protein synthesis via 30S subunit	Plasmid-encoded enzymes inactivate drug Mutation of 30S unit chromosome
Tetracyclines	Inhibition of protein synthesis via 30S subunit	Plasmid-encoded enzymes reduce drug uptake
Chloramphenicol	Inhibition of protein synthesis via 50S subunit	Plasmid-encoded enzymes inactivate drug
Erythromycin	Inhibition of protein synthesis via 50S subunit	Plasmid-encoded enzymes block drug binding
Sulfonamides	Inhibition of nucleic acid synthesis	Plasmid-encoded increased excretion of drug Target enzyme gene mutation
Rifampin, isoniazid	Inhibition of mRNA synthesis	Chromosomal mutations

Bacteremia and Septicemia

Bacteremia is the term used to describe bacteria in the bloodstream, regardless of whether the patient is symptomatic. **Septicemia** means that bacteria are in the bloodstream of a patient who has signs and symptoms of systemic infection.

SIGNS & SYMPTOMS

Fever, chills, and malaise are typical. Intermittent temperature spiking may occur. Nausea, vomiting, and other GI complaints may also be present.

DIAGNOSIS

Possible sources of infections, such as sites of recent surgery, wounds, urine catheters, and drainage tubes, should be cultured. Serial blood cultures should be drawn at 1-hour intervals. Sputum culture is important if respiratory illness is suspected. Intravenous drug users often have *Staphylococcus* bacteremia due to introduction of bacteria through the skin.

TREATMENT

Broad-spectrum antibiotics are started after the first blood cultures have been drawn. If no improvement is seen, check for possible abscesses that may serve as a source of infection.

Septic Shock

Septic shock is the multiple organ failure and circulatory collapse that occur as a result of infection. "High-output" septic shock refers to the early stages of shock, during which cardiac output is normal or increased. "Low-output" septic shock refers to the later stages, characterized by decreased cardiac output. Septic shock is seen primarily in immunocompromised people. About 70% of infections are due to nosocomial gram-negative bacilli, and the remaining 30% consist of gram-positive cocci and fungal infections.

The initial stages of septic shock involve fever, chills, and altered mental status. Low blood pressure is accompanied by paradoxically warm, dry skin and extremities. Increased heart and respiratory rates are common. Late-stage shock is characterized by cool, pale extremities, oliguria, and disseminated intravascular coagulation (DIC).

White blood cell counts, especially neutrophils and platelets, may be quite low at the onset of septic shock. These values rise significantly after a few hours. Increased blood urea nitrogen (BUN) and creatinine are signs of impending renal failure. Increased lactic acid production can cause metabolic acidosis; this is partially compensated by a respiratory alkalosis as the patient hyperventilates and blows off CO_2.

The above symptoms combined with a likely infectious source should raise suspicion for septic shock.

Septic shock has a high fatality rate, so intensive care treatment is a must. Respiratory support, including intubation, is provided if necessary. Fluid status must be monitored. Blood cultures should be drawn and IV antibiotics given. Dopamine is often necessary to preserve renal blood perfusion.

Infectious Disease in Infants

Neonates and infants are at high risk for infection because of the immaturity of their immune systems. Although newborns have circulating antibodies that they received in utero, the protective effect from these antibodies subsides by about 6 months of age. Additional protection from secretory immunoglobulins is obtained from breast milk. Premature babies are especially at risk of acquiring infection due to the general immaturity of all their organ system defenses.

Infections in neonates must be treated carefully because their metabolic and excretory functions are immature. For example, babies treated with chloramphenicol may develop **gray baby syndrome** because of the high blood levels of chloramphenicol that accumulate due to immature liver metabolism. This syndrome causes cardiovascular collapse and may be fatal.

The most common nosocomial infection that neonates acquire in hospital nurseries is *S. aureus*. This infection causes **scalded skin syndrome**, an exfoliative rash. Most other infections, such as meningitis and viral infections, are acquired perinatally and are discussed in more detail in Chap. 8.

Infectious Disease in the Elderly

Due to the frequent presence of multiple chronic diseases, many elderly persons have decreased resistance to infection. Elderly patients are also more likely to develop dehydration and mental status changes in association with infection. Infectious diseases that

Table 9-3. Organisms commonly seen in immunosuppressed patients

Conditions	Organisms
Nosocomial	*Pseudomonas*
	Proteus
	Candida
Burn	*Pseudomonas*
	Serratia
	Staphylococci
Catheter	Gram-negative organisms
	Staphylococci
	Candida
Cancer or steroid therapy	*S. pneumoniae*
	Haemophilus influenza
	Aspergillus
	Candida

are more common or more debilitating to the elderly include pneumonia, influenza, TB (especially disseminated disease), and herpes zoster. Appropriate preventive measures include pneumococcal vaccine (given once after the age of 65) and annual influenza vaccination.

Infectious Disease in the Immunocompromised

Patients with compromised immune systems are at greater risk for infection with standard pathogens or for opportunistic infections, which are caused by organisms that are not pathogenic in healthy people. Hospital-acquired bacteria and normal flora that have grown out of control (e.g., *Candida*) are often the infectious agents.

Conditions that predispose to opportunistic infections include extremes of age (infants or elderly), chronic disease, extensive burns, prolonged steroid therapy, prolonged chemotherapy, and procedures that have breached normal barriers, such as surgery and foreign body placement (e.g., catheters and tracheal tubes). Common organisms are discussed in Table 9-3. AIDS is discussed in more detail in Chap. 10.

Superinfection is the colonization of an area (e.g., the GI tract) with antibiotic-resistant organisms during treatment with an antibiotic. Factors associated with superinfection include use of broad-spectrum antibiotics and large doses of certain antibiotics. Superinfections usually become symptomatic after 4 or 5 days of antibiotic treatment. Typical organisms include gram-negative enteric organisms, antibiotic-resistant staphylococci, and fungi. One example of superinfection is **pseudomembranous colitis,** a GI infection (see Chap. 1).

Empiric antibiotic treatment should be started as soon as possible. Further treatment will, of course, be tailored to the causative organisms. Since many organisms are antibiotic-resistant, sensitivities should be ascertained by culturing and testing the organism. Chronic immunosuppressive therapies such as steroids should be reduced, if possible, during treatment of the infection.

Antibiotic prophylaxis before procedures, active immunization (e.g., pneumococcus and hepatitis B vaccines), and passive immunization (e.g., immunoglobulin) may help prevent infection. Strict aseptic technique and hand washing should be enforced.

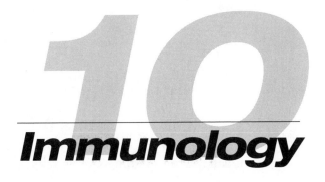

Immunology

Immunizations

Infants and Children

Vaccination schedules for normal, healthy children are shown in Table 10-1.

General Notes

- Vaccinations may be started at 6 weeks of age.
- Vaccinations need not be delayed when the child has a minor illness or is taking antibiotics.
- Vaccinations need not be delayed in premature infants.
- If vaccination status is unknown, assume that no vaccinations have been given. There is generally no harm in extra doses.

Hepatitis B

Infants of mothers who test positive for the hepatitis B virus surface antigen (HBsAG) should receive hepatitis B immunoglobulin (HBIG) and the first dose of hepatitis B vaccine at birth. The second dose should be given at 1 month and the third dose at 6 months.

Diphtheria-Pertussis-Tetanus

The diphtheria-pertussis-tetanus vaccine (DPT) may cause brief, generalized seizures in febrile children. Children with a family or personal history of seizures are at increased risk, but this is not a contraindication to vaccination. Acetaminophen may be given to decrease risk of fever and seizures. True contraindications to DPT are (1) a progressive neurologic disorder and (2) a history of encephalopathy within 7 days of a previous DPT dose. Pertussis vaccine is not indicated in children above age 7 or in those who have had pertussis.

Haemophilus Influenzae Type B

Haemophilus influenzae type B vaccine is not indicated in children above age 5.

Table 10-1. Immunization schedule

Vaccine	Birth	2 mos	4 mos	6 mos	12 mos	15 mos	18 mos	4–6 yrs
Hepatitis B	#1							
		#2		#3				
DPT		#1	#2	#3	#4			#5
H. influenzae		#1	#2	#3	#4			
Polio (OPV)		#1	#2	#3				#4
MMR					#1			#2

(shading indicates acceptable time range for immunization)

Polio

Inactivated poliovirus vaccine (IPV) should be given to patients who are immunocompromised or who have an immunocompromised household contact because there is a risk of causing vaccine-induced paralysis with the live oral polio vaccine (OPV).

Measles-Mumps-Rubella

- The measles-mumps-rubella vaccine (MMR) is not as effective if given before age 1 because maternal antibodies interfere with the development of immunity. Furthermore, the vaccine should not be given until 3 months after a blood transfusion or immunoglobulin because of passively acquired antibodies.
- MMR should not be given to immunocompromised children or pregnant women, but it is safe for those with the human immunodeficiency virus (HIV).
- MMR suppresses tuberculin reactivity. A tuberculin skin test (PPD) should either be given on the same day as the MMR or should be delayed 4–6 weeks.

Adult Immunization

Required immunizations for healthy adults will depend the individual's immunization history. The following recommendations should be noted:

- If they have been properly immunized as children, all adults require **tetanus** booster injections every 10 years. Adults with no history of tetanus immunization should receive two doses of dT (diphtheria and tetanus toxoid) 1–2 months apart, followed by a booster injection at 6–12 months. Tetanus vaccinations are extremely safe and associated with few ill effects other than localized soreness.
- All adults born before 1957 are considered immune to **measles**; persons born between 1957 and 1980 who have not had measles should receive one measles injection as adults. Those born since 1980 should have been fully immunized in childhood. Side effects include fever, rash, and localized swelling. Pregnant women and those allergic to egg albumin should not receive this vaccine.
- The primary purpose of **rubella** immunization is to prevent infection in pregnant women. All women of childbearing (or prechildbearing) age should receive vaccination, as should health care workers. Vaccination of pregnant women is not recommended, although there is no documentation of fetal harm in women who inadvertently receive the vaccine during pregnancy. This vaccine should not be given to immunosuppressed patients, except those with HIV. Adverse effects, which are generally mild, include joint pain.
- **Mumps** injections should be given to all persons born after 1957 who do not have a history of vaccination or disease. The vaccine is associated with very few ill effects, but it should not be given to immunosuppressed patients, except those with HIV.
- A series of three **hepatitis B** injections is recommended for all adults at risk of sexual or bloodborne transmission of hepatitis B, including health care workers, male homosexuals, and IV drug users.

Immunization of Elderly and Immunocompromised Patients

- Annual **influenza** vaccinations are recommended for patients with chronic respiratory and metabolic diseases, nursing home residents, and all adults over age 65. Local reactions of redness and swelling are common; systemic reactions are rare. Influenza vaccination may be associated with false-positive HIV test results.
- One dose of the **pneumococcal** vaccine confers life-long immunity and is recommended for all adults over age 65 as well as asplenic patients and patients with sickle cell disease. It is also recommended for patients who are immunocompromised, although the efficacy of the vaccine in these patients has been questioned.
- The rule of thumb is to avoid giving live vaccines to immunocompromised patients. Current recommendations are provided in Table 10-2.

Foreign Travel Immunizations

Immunization requirements vary from country to country, and they may change depending on the season and the status of endemic illnesses. A listing of required immunizations is available from the World Health Organization. The following is a list of the most common vaccination and chemoprophylaxis indications:

- The killed **cholera** vaccination is fairly ineffective, providing protection for only about half of recipients for a period of 3–6 months; however, it is still required by some nations for entry. It is not recommended for children under 6 months of age.
- The **yellow fever** vaccine is a live virus vaccine that is required in most parts of Africa and South America. It is effective for 10 years. It is not recommended for children under 9 months of age or for pregnant women.

Table 10-2. Immunizations in immunocompromised patients

Not recommended
    Measles*
    Mumps*
    Rubella*
    Yellow fever
Acceptable
    Tetanus
    Influenza
    Pneumococcal pneumonia
    Hepatitis B
    Cholera
    Polio (inactivated form)
    Typhoid (inactivated form)
    Meningitis

* This does not include patients with HIV disease.

- **Tetanus** immunization, usually combined with diphtheria and/or pertussis as a DPT or dT injection, is required every 10 years.
- **Poliomyelitis** is still endemic in many parts of the world. Patients with an uncertain history of polio immunization should receive the injected, killed vaccine (IPV) due to the increased risk of postvaccination polio with the live, attenuated oral vaccine (OPV). Patients with a recorded history of full polio immunization should receive a booster dose of the oral vaccine.
- **Measles** vaccination is recommended for all persons traveling abroad. If the patient received primary injections before 1980 or before 15 months of age, he or she will require reimmunization. Pregnant women and immunocompromised patients (except those with HIV) should not receive the measles vaccine.
- Immunization against **typhoid fever** is recommended for persons traveling to areas of poor sanitation. Both an inactivated, injectable vaccine and a new oral capsular vaccine are available. Patients should not take typhoid vaccine capsules concurrently with antimalarials such as chloroquine.
- **Meningococcal** vaccination is required for travel to parts of Asia and South America. One dose is effective for 3 years, but it is not recommended for children less than 2 years of age.
- A series of three **hepatitis B** injections over a 6-month time period is recommended only for persons planning extended stays in developing countries.
- Passive immunization with **immunoglobulin** (gamma globulin) is recommended for all persons spending more than 1 month abroad. It is effective against a variety of illnesses, including hepatitis A. The injection is effective for 6 months and should be given more than 4 weeks following other active immunizations to prevent interference with immunity development.
- Chemoprophylaxis of travelers to areas endemic for **malaria** includes chloroquine or mefloquine, despite resistance seen to both medications. Chemoprophylaxis should be taken during exposure and for 6 weeks following exposure.

Routine vaccination for **plague**, **typhus**, **rabies**, and **encephalitis** are not required but may be recommended for travel to endemic areas. **Smallpox** has been successfully eradicated from the globe and vaccination is no longer required.

Human Immunodeficiency Virus Disease

Epidemiology

The AIDS epidemic in the United States was first identified among homosexual men in the early 1980s. It has since spread to other groups, and the fastest-growing group of infected individuals currently is heterosexual women. In addition to homosexual and bisexual men, IV drug users, hemophiliacs, infants born of infected mothers, and heterosexual partners of infected people are at high risk for becoming infected. In Africa, the epidemic has very different characteristics, and the virus is spread primarily via heterosexual contact.

HIV transmission requires contact with body fluids, including blood, semen, vaginal secretions, and breast milk. The presence of sexually transmitted diseases (STDs) makes viral transmission during intercourse more likely, presumably due to breaks in the mucosal tissue. The blood supply in the United States is now screened for HIV and is generally quite safe, but a small risk of becoming infected via blood transfusion still exists due to the possibility of an individual giving blood in the "window period" after infection and before seroconversion. Occupational needlestick injuries are a potential source of infection, but it is important to keep the risk in perspective. HIV is transmitted by needlesticks much less readily than is hepatitis B; the risk is estimated to be approximately 1 in 200 needlesticks, but this rate depends on how much blood is involved. Mothers with HIV are advised not to breast-feed their infants because a few cases of HIV transmission by this route have been reported.

The Virus

HIV is an RNA retrovirus. After it infects a cell, it uses an enzyme, reverse transcriptase, to make a DNA copy of itself, which is then integrated into the cellular DNA. HIV infects T-helper cells, which are marked with a membrane glycoprotein called CD4. The progressive loss of these cells, which are integral in the immune system, is the most significant prognosticator of HIV infection.

Initial Infection

The initial infection with HIV is usually completely asymptomatic but is occasionally accompanied by several weeks of a flu-like illness with symptoms including malaise, fever, tender lymphadenopathy, and a skin rash. Viremia is high during this time, but antibody tests are negative because seroconversion has not occurred (Fig. 10-1).

Diagnosis

One to six months after the initial infection, antibodies to HIV can be detected in the blood. The standard test to detect antibodies is the enzyme-linked immunosorbent assay (ELISA). This test is very sensitive (i.e., anyone with anti-HIV antibodies will have a positive test) but not very specific (i.e., many people without the infection will test positive as well). When an ELISA test is positive, the result should be confirmed with a second ELISA test. If it is positive a second time, the more specific Western blot should be used to confirm the diagnosis.

Natural History of HIV and Diagnosis of AIDS

Among adults who contract HIV through sexual intercourse or IV drug use, approximately half become ill with AIDS after 10 years. Progression to disease occurs much faster in children and in adults who receive blood transfusions, presumably due to the higher concentration of virus received.

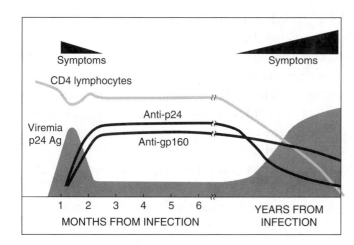

Fig. 10-1. Natural history of HIV infection. Viremia denotes cell-free infectious virus in plasma, p24 Ag denotes circulating viral p24 antigen in plasma, and anti-p24 and anti-gp 160 correspond to antibodies to viral core and envelope proteins.

The Centers for Disease Control and Prevention (CDC) issues a definition of AIDS, primarily to standardize diagnosis across the country. The definition includes a variety of clinical conditions which, if present, confer a diagnosis of AIDS. These include *Pneumocystis carinii* pneumonia, Kaposi's sarcoma, and toxoplasmosis of the brain. A CD4 cell count of less than 200 cells/mm³ is also diagnostic.

Primary HIV Treatment

Treatment for HIV continues to evolve as experience with the disease grows. Zidovudine (AZT) is usually given to patients with CD4 counts less than 500 cells/mm³, although a recent study raises questions about the efficacy of this treatment. Dideoxyinosine (ddI) and dideoxycytidine (ddC) may be useful in combined drug therapy with AZT. Side effects include bone marrow suppression, neuropathy, and pancreatitis. AZT during pregnancy has been shown to dramatically reduce the transmission of HIV from mother to infant.

AIDS-Related Illnesses

As a result of immunodeficiency, HIV patients may experience a number of unusual infections or more severe forms of common infections. The most frequently seen infections are described briefly below:

Cytomegalovirus (CMV), commonly seen in AIDS patients, may be manifested in a number of ways, including pneumonia, retinitis, and gastritis. Treatment with ganciclovir or foscarnet is recommended. HIV-positive patients should receive routine ophthalmologic exams to aid in the early diagnosis of CMV retinitis.

Related viruses, such as **herpes simplex virus, varicella-zoster,** and **Epstein-Barr virus,** are also associated with disseminated infection in HIV-positive patients. Manifestations include respiratory infections, encephalitis, meningitis, and cutaneous lesions. Acyclovir is helpful in symptomatic cases.

In addition to viral pneumonia, AIDS patients are at greater risk of developing **bacterial pneumonia,** usually due to *Streptococcus pneumoniae, Haemophilus influenzae,* or group

B *Streptococcus.* These are typically lobar pneumonias. Diffuse interstitial pneumonia is characteristic of **Pneumocystis carinii.** Trimethoprim-sulfamethoxazole (TMP-SMZ) is used to treat *Pneumocystis.* TMP-SMZ, dapsone, or pentamidine is given prophylactically to AIDS patients to prevent *Pneumocystis* pneumonia.

Mycobacterial infections, such as tuberculosis and *Mycobacterium avium-intracellulare* are seen commonly in AIDS patients, often as gastrointestinal, respiratory, or disseminated disease. Multidrug therapy with antitubercular drugs, such as ethambutol and rifampin, may be helpful but are generally not curative.

Persistent **candidiasis** of the mouth, esophagus, and genital tract is common, and increased frequency of infection may be a sign of declining immune function. Other **fungal infections** include *Cryptococcus neoformans*, *Coccidioides immitis*, and *Histoplasma*, which may cause central nervous system, respiratory, or disseminated infection. Antifungals such as amphotericin B and fluconazole are often used for treatment and as prophylaxis. Other than *Pneumocystis*, common **protozoal infections** include *Toxoplasma gondii*, which causes encephalopathy, and *Cryptosporidium*, which causes GI infection. Antibiotics are helpful, but recurrences are common.

Neoplastic disorders that are seen more commonly in AIDS patients include Kaposi's sarcoma (seen cutaneously as well as internally), non-Hodgkin's lymphoma, and CNS lymphomas.

Prevention in AIDS

Tuberculosis testing (PPD with controls) should be performed annually; if the patient is anergic, a chest x-ray should be performed. Recommended immunizations include MMR, IPV, and pneumococcal vaccine. Hepatitis B series should be given to patients without hepatitis immunity, and influenza vaccination should be given annually.

Cell-Mediated Immunity Deficiency

DiGeorge's Syndrome (Thymic Aplasia)

DiGeorge's syndrome involves a congenital defect of the thymus and parathyroid glands. As a result, these patients suffer from a severe lack of T cells and develop recurrent viral and fungal infections. Associated findings include congenital heart disease and craniofacial abnormalities. These patients present with tetany due to hypocalcemia within the first few days of life. Treatment consists of thymus or bone marrow transplantation.

Chronic Mucocutaneous Candidiasis

Individuals with chronic mucocutaneous candidiasis have a T cell deficiency that is specific to *Candida albicans*. As a result, these patients develop candidiasis on the scalp, skin, nails, and mucous membranes. Treatment consists of antifungal medications.

Ataxia-Telangiectasia

Ataxia-telangiectasia is an autosomal recessive disorder that consists of lymphopenia and IgA deficiency and is associated with ataxia (gait abnormalities), telangiectasia (localized blood vessel dilatation), and endocrine abnormalities. Recurrent infections are common. Treatment consists of immunoglobulin and antibiotics.

Wiskcott-Aldrich Syndrome

Individuals with Wiskcott-Aldrich syndrome, an X-linked disorder, are unable to mount antibody responses against polysaccharide-encapsulated bacteria, such as pneumococci. Associated signs include bleeding (due to decreased platelets), eczema, and recurrent bacterial infections. Treatment consists of splenectomy (to alleviate platelet destruction), antibiotics, immunoglobulin, and bone marrow transplantation.

Chronic Granulomatous Disease

Chronic granulomatous disease is an autosomal recessive disorder that involves decreased bactericidal abilities against certain organisms due to a defect in phagocytic enzymes. Patients experience recurrent bacterial and fungal infections, especially *Staphylococcus aureus, E. coli, Pseudomonas*, and *Aspergillus*, which form granulomas. Treatment consists of antibiotics and bone marrow transplantation.

Chediak-Higashi Syndrome

Chediak-Higashi syndrome is an autosomal recessive disorder that results in ineffective neutrophilic enzymes, leading to recurrent streptococcal and staphylococcal infections. Treatment consists of antibiotic therapy.

Severe Combined Immunodeficiency

Severe combined immunodeficiency (SCID) is a group of recessive disorders that involves deficits of both B cell and T cell function and is usually fatal within the first few years of life. Patients experience recurrent infections from bacteria, viruses, fungi, and protozoa. Immunoglobulin, antibiotics, and bone marrow transplantation may be helpful in some cases.

Humoral Immunity Deficiency

Common Variable Immunodeficiency

Common variable immunodeficiency, a disorder of unknown etiology, consists of decreases of B cell and T cell function, although these cells are present in normal quantities. Onset typically occurs between the ages of 15 and 40, at which time patients experience recurrent bacterial infections. Immunoglobulin and antibiotics are the mainstays of treatment.

X-Linked Agammaglobulinemia (Bruton's Disease)

In X-linked agammaglobulinemia, B cell precursors do not develop into B cells, resulting in low or absent B cells and antibody levels. Infants begin to experience recurrent bacterial infections after about 6 months of age (after maternal antibodies have been depleted). Treatment consists of immunoglobulin injections.

IgA Deficiency

Individuals with IgA deficiency may be asymptomatic or may experience recurrent infections, particularly of the respiratory and GI tract. Patients typically do not receive any treatment, and the administration of immunoglobulin is contraindicated in these patients because they may develop antibodies against them, thereby depleting already low levels.

Hypersensitivity Reactions

Anaphylactic Shock

Anaphylactic shock, an IgE-mediated reaction, occurs when a person who has been previously sensitized to an allergen is re-exposed. Almost any substance can act as an allergen and cause an anaphylactic reaction. Medications (especially penicillin), bee stings, nuts, and seafood are common causes of anaphylaxis.

Within a few minutes of exposure, patients become agitated and flushed. Common complaints include palpitations, dyspnea, chest tightness, coughing, and pruritus. Angioedema causes swelling of soft tissues and may lead to airway obstruction. Less common symptoms include nausea, vomiting, and diarrhea. On exam, wheezing and urticaria (hives) may be noted. In severe reactions, patients may become hypotensive, incontinent, and unresponsive. Convulsions and death may follow.

The above symptoms provide the diagnosis.

Immediate epinephrine administration is essential. In milder cases, this may be followed by antihistamines. More severe reactions require IV fluids to maintain blood pressure and methylxanthines, such as aminophylline, to control bronchospasm. Intubation may be necessary.

Patients experiencing such reactions should be warned to avoid reactive substances whenever possible. They should also carry epinephrine auto-injectors and antihistamine tablets. Desensitization therapy may be helpful, but this requires several years of injections to maintain adequate effects.

Transplant Rejection

Transplants can be classified by the type and origin of the transplanted tissue. **Autografts** consist of transplantation of one's own tissue to another location in the body, such as the use of a saphenous vein for coronary artery bypass grafting in the same individual. An **isograft** is tissue transplanted to an identical twin, while an **allograft** is tissue transplanted to another person. Finally, a **xenograft** consists of animal tissue transplanted for use in humans, such as the use of pig valves in heart valve replacement surgery.

Rejection of transplanted tissue may occur by both cell-mediated and antibody-mediated responses to tissue antigens. The most important of these antigens are the HLA groups and the ABO blood group antigens. T cell–mediated rejection (**host vs. graft reaction**) is the principal mechanism of acute transplant rejection, while later graft rejection generally occurs as a result of **antibody-mediated** damage. If the host has been presensitized against particular antigens (e.g., through a previous blood transfusion), **hyperacute graft rejection** occurs, in which the transplanted tissue is destroyed within minutes. In addition, a **graft vs. host reaction** can occur when blood cells in the transplanted organ attack an immunocompromised host. Methods that are used to control transplant rejection include immunosuppressive drugs, antilymphocyte globulin, and irradiation of the graft and local recipient tissue.

11

Hematology

Basic Principles of Management

Blood Loss

Blood loss may occur due to injury, bleeding disorders, cardiovascular disease, ulcers, complications of pregnancy, and many other conditions. Hemorrhage can occur externally or internally, as large amounts of blood can collect in the abdomen, pelvis, or pleural space. Fractures of the pelvis and long bones generally result in significant blood loss. Rapid hemorrhage can be fatal in minutes.

SIGNS & SYMPTOMS

While many hemorrhages are visible and obvious, internal blood loss is not always evident. Signs of hypovolemia include rapid heart rate and low blood pressure, especially orthostatic hypotension. Abdominal bleeding is suggested by bluish discoloration in the flank or abdomen and by peritoneal signs, such as guarding and rebound tenderness. Hemothorax causes difficulty breathing, dullness to percussion, and decreased breath sounds.

DIAGNOSIS

Presentation and typical vital signs are usually diagnostic of blood loss. Hemoglobin and hematocrit are not good indicators of acute blood loss, since these measures remain normal for several hours before hemodilution occurs.

TREATMENT

If the source of blood loss can be identified, it should be addressed immediately. For stabilization, patients are given crystalloid infusion through a large-bore IV needle while blood is sent for chemistries, clotting parameters, counts, and crossmatch. O-negative blood may be given in an emergency if the patient's blood type is unknown. Transfusions are required for a patient in clinical shock or for patients whose vital signs do not stabilize after crystalloid infusion. The final stabilized hematocrit should be between 25–30%.

Blood Transfusions

Transfusions are generally given to raise hematocrit or blood volume in patients with inadequate blood volume or blood cells. There are four major replacement products used:

- **Fresh whole blood** has RBCs, plasma, and platelets. It is often used during surgery or for hemorrhage.
- **Packed RBCs** will raise the hematocrit about 4% per unit given. If need is anticipated—for example, prior to surgery—the patient may opt to store his or her own blood for autologous transfusion.
- **Leukopoor blood** is given if patients have history of severe leukoagglutinin reactions (described later in this chapter).
- **Frozen blood** is used mostly for rare blood types and has no white blood cells or plasma.

Blood for transfusions is currently screened for a number of viruses, including the hepatitis B virus (HBV) and the human immunodeficiency virus (HIV). The risk of getting blood contaminated with HIV in the United States is now 1 in 100,000 units. There is a higher risk of getting the hepatitis C virus, which currently infects about 1% of blood supplies.

Table 11-1 ABO blood type frequencies

Blood type	Percentage of the caucasian population	Antibodies present
O	45	Anti-A, anti-B
A	42	Anti-B
B	10	Anti-A
AB	3	—

Compatibility testing of the donor blood is crucial. If the incorrect blood is given, patients can suffer severe intravascular hemolysis and death. The most important factor to match is the ABO blood type (Table 11-1). The Rh type should then be considered. If possible, the patient should have an antibody screen and crossmatch performed to assure that cross-reactions will be minimized. In an emergency, when type is not known, give type O-negative packed cells.

Care should be taken with female patients who may later bear children to ensure that they do not receive Rh-positive blood if they are Rh-negative. However, in an emergency, type-specific Rh positive blood is not life-threatening.

Fresh frozen plasma (FFP) is given to patients with coagulation factor deficiencies. It is also given to patients with thrombotic thrombocytopenia purpura (TTP). FFP contains normal levels of the coagulation factors found in blood. **Cryoprecipitate** contains fibrinogen, factor VIII, and von Willebrand's factor (vWF). It is given to patients with factor VIII deficiency, vWF disease, fibrinogen deficiency, and disseminated intravascular coagulation (DIC).

Transfusion Reactions

Transfusion reactions are usually due to clerical errors, so it is vital that all identification labels are checked and confirmed. Immediate reactions to incorrect blood transfusion occur within the first 2 hours, and symptoms include fever, chills, back pain, chest pain, headache, pulmonary edema, urticaria, and hematuria. If a reaction is suspected, the transfusion must be discontinued immediately, and antihistamines and epinephrine should be administered. Delayed reactions can also occur over days to weeks following the transfusion and include hemolysis, thrombocytopenia, rash, fever, and gastrointestinal complaints.

Leukoagglutinin Reactions

Leukoagglutinin reactions occur when the patient reacts to antigens on the donor WBCs or platelets. These reactions are usually seen in patients who have had previous transfusions. Symptoms include fever and chills, shortness of breath, and pulmonary edema, which can become life-threatening. Treatment includes antihistamines, acetaminophen, and steroids. The patient may require leukopoor blood for future transfusions.

Platelet Transfusions

Platelet transfusions are given to patients with thrombocytopenia, as platelet levels below 20,000/mm^3 can result in spontaneous bleeding. One unit of platelets elevates platelet count by approximately 10,000/mm^3. Platelet transfusions are not useful if the thrombocytopenia is caused by autoimmune destruction, since the transfused platelets will quickly be destroyed as well. Transfused platelets may also have poor survival if human leukocyte antigen (HLA) types are very dissimilar. Platelet concentrate is also available; it contains 6 units of platelets and will raise the platelet level about 60,000/mm^3.

Anemia

Anemia is defined as any condition with less than normal amounts of hemoglobin, hematocrit, or number of RBCs. Anemia is typically classified according to whether RBCs are microcytic (mean corpuscular volume [MCV] <80 μm^3), normocytic (MCV 80–100 μm^3), or macrocytic (MCV >100 μm^3). Specific etiologies and diagnoses are described below.

Iron-Deficiency Anemia

Iron-deficiency anemia (IDA) is the most common type of anemia. The reduction in heme production from lack of iron is usually due to blood loss through the GI system (e.g., ulcers or chronic rectal bleeding) or menstruation. Dietary iron deficiency can contribute as well. Pregnancy is a common cause of IDA due to expanding maternal blood volume and additional fetal iron requirements.

SIGNS & SYMPTOMS

Fatigue and pallor. In severe cases, angular cheilosis (irritation at the corners of the mouth and lips), koilonychia (spooning of the nails), and pica (the craving to eat unusual things such as dirt) may occur.

LABS

Hematocrit, hemoglobin, and RBC count are decreased. RBCs are usually microcytic (MCV <80 μm^3) but can be normocytic (MCV 80–100 μm^3) in early stages. Peripheral blood smear typically shows microcytic cells with increased central pallor (hypochromia). Ghost and pencil cells may be present. Reticulocyte count may be low or normal, depending on the severity of the iron deficiency.

DIAGNOSIS

The single best test for diagnosing iron deficiency is measurement of the level of serum ferritin, an iron storage protein. Ferritin levels are proportional to iron stores and will therefore be low (<12 ng/ml) in IDA. Less reliable tests include low serum iron, high total iron-binding capacity (TIBC or transferrin), and low transferrin saturation (serum iron to TIBC ratio). Bone marrow biopsy reveals low or absent iron stores but is usually not indicated in simple IDA.

TREATMENT

Oral iron supplements. IDA should be fully corrected in 6–8 weeks, but an additional 4–6 months of treatment are required to replenish iron stores. Common side effects of oral iron treatment are nausea and constipation.

Anemia of Chronic Disease

Anemia of chronic disease is the most common anemia in hospital patients. It is seen in patients with bacterial infections, malignancies, chronic inflammatory diseases, and diabetes. The anemia is caused by the production of lactoferrin, a storage protein with a greater affinity for iron than transferrin.

The classic symptoms of anemia are present, including fatigue, shortness of breath on exertion, and pallor.

Hematocrit levels are reduced but generally do not fall below 25%. MCV may be normal or low. RBC morphology and reticulocyte count are usually normal.

Laboratory analysis shows decreased serum iron and decreased transferrin. Ferritin levels are generally high (>100 ng/ml), since ferritin is an acute-phase reactant and these patients have some type of inflammatory condition. Bone marrow biopsy shows a normal or increased amount of iron stores.

Treat the primary disorder, if possible. Do not give these patients iron supplementation or transfusions; they may experience iron overload.

Megaloblastic Anemias

Megaloblastic anemia is most often due to vitamin B_{12} or folate deficiency, but it can also result from drugs that inhibit DNA synthesis. It is seen in liver disease, particularly in alcoholics, and in hyperthyroidism. Features include macrocytes (MCV >100 μm^3), macro-ovalocytes (large, elliptically shaped RBCs), and hypersegmented neutrophils (nuclei containing five or more lobes).

Vitamin B_{12} is important for DNA synthesis and myelin formation. It is found in meat, eggs, and milk. Once ingested, vitamin B_{12} binds to **intrinsic factor (IF)**, which is produced in the gastric parietal cells, and the complex is absorbed in the terminal ileum.

Folic acid is also used in DNA synthesis. It is found in green, leafy vegetables and citrus fruits and is absorbed throughout the small intestine.

Vitamin B_{12} Deficiency Anemia

Vitamin B_{12} (cobalamin) deficiency is usually caused by inadequate absorption due to pernicious anemia (lack of IF caused by autoimmune destruction of parietal cells), resection of the terminal ileum, intestinal overgrowth of bacteria, or presence of fish tapeworm. Vitamin B_{12} deficiency due to diet is rare and seen only in strict vegans.

In addition to general signs and symptoms of anemia, vitamin B_{12} deficiency can cause severe neurologic disturbances. These may occur with or without the presence of anemia and include symmetric paresthesias, loss of proprioception, and ataxia. Psychosis and irreversible dementia may develop.

Hematocrit, hemoglobin, and RBC count are decreased and MCV is high (>100 μm^3). Peripheral blood smear reveals macro-ovalocytes and hypersegmented neutrophils. Bone marrow biopsy shows unusually large erythroblasts—hence the name megaloblastic anemia. The serum vitamin B_{12} level is decreased (<140 pg/ml), but serum folate measurements should be normal.

The definitive diagnosis of pernicious anemia is made with the Schilling test, which involves administering an oral dose of radioactively labeled vitamin B_{12} and measuring its urinary excretion. Decreased excretion indicates a lack of appropriate B_{12} absorption. The test is repeated with the addition of intrinsic factor. If absorption is normal with exogenous IF, the patient has pernicious anemia. If absorption is still low, an intestinal cause of B_{12} malabsorption is likely.

Intramuscular injections of B_{12} are given for as long as the need persists, which may be lifelong. Some neurologic symptoms may be irreversible.

Folate Deficiency Anemia

Folic acid deficiency is the most common cause of megaloblastic anemia, since folic acid stores last only 2–3 months. Inadequate dietary sources, from either decreased intake (seen in alcoholics, elderly, and the poor) or increased demand (in pregnancy), are usually the cause. Some drugs, such as sulfasalazine and phenytoin, may reduce the availability of folic acid.

In addition to general symptoms of anemia, signs of impaired epithelial cell proliferation (sore, beefy tongue; diarrhea) result from inadequate DNA synthesis.

Serum folate and/or RBC folate levels are low, and the vitamin B_{12} level is normal. Serum folate levels correct quickly on a hospital diet, whereas the RBC folate level reflects long-term stores.

Daily oral folate supplement.

Aplastic Anemia

Aplastic anemia is pancytopenia (lack of all three blood cell lines: RBCs, WBCs, and platelets) resulting from bone marrow failure. It is associated with an almost complete lack of progenitor cells in the bone marrow. The most common cause of pancytopenia is a drug reaction, often with chloramphenicol, phenylbutazone, gold salts, sulfonamides, and phenytoin. Less common causes include chemotherapy, radiation therapy, and toxins.

Symptoms result from the lack of blood cells and include anemia (fatigue, pallor), neutropenia (recurrent or persistent nonhealing infections), and thrombocytopenia (abnormal or uncontrolled bleeding).

The numbers of RBCs, WBCs, and platelets are decreased, and bone marrow biopsy shows hypocellularity.

Withdrawal of causative factors. Further treatment includes immunosuppressive drugs, transfusions, and bone marrow transplant.

Drug-Induced Anemia

There are three mechanisms by which certain drugs provoke hemolytic anemia. First, some drugs can act as haptens, bind to the RBC membrane, and induce the synthesis of antidrug antibodies. One common drug in this category is penicillin. Hemolysis occurs about 7–10 days after starting the drug. During hemolysis, the direct Coombs' test is positive with IgG reagent, showing that antibody is present on the RBC.

Some drugs form immune complexes with immunoglobulins and start fixing complement, which leads to hemolysis. Quinidine is one example. During hemolysis, the direct Coombs' test is positive with anticomplement reagents.

The third type of drug-induced anemia is induction of synthesis of anti-Rh antibodies, which cause hemolysis. This may involve loss of suppressor cell activity. L-Dopa and alpha-methyldopa are examples of drugs that can cause this reaction, which may continue even after the drug is discontinued.

Hemolytic Disease

Hemolytic Anemia

Hemolysis of RBCs takes place naturally after 120 days. Hemolytic anemia occurs when the normal RBC life span is shortened and marrow production can no longer compensate for the increased destruction. Specific etiologies are generally grouped into three categories: defects external to the RBC (immune hemolysis, mechanical hemolysis, hemolytic disease of the newborn), defects of the RBC membrane (hereditary spherocytosis), and defects of the RBC interior (glucose-6-phosphate dehydrogenase deficiency). These etiologies are described in greater detail below.

Mild cases are asymptomatic. Patients with severe cases have palpitations, dyspnea, pallor, hepatosplenomegaly, chills, fever, abdominal and back pain, and shock. Jaundice occurs when hemoglobin from destroyed RBCs cannot be converted to conjugated bilirubin fast enough to be excreted and unconjugated bilirubin builds up in the tissues. Hemoglobin may be excreted in the urine, causing brownish discoloration.

Reticulocyte count increases as the bone marrow tries to replenish the RBC supply. Unconjugated (indirect) bilirubin may be increased. Increased serum lactate dehydrogenase (LDH), released from RBCs, is also seen.

Immune Hemolysis

Immune hemolysis is usually caused by anti-RBC IgG antibodies that attach most effectively above 31°C (warm-reacting antibodies). Antibody-coated RBCs are removed from circulation by the spleen, resulting in anemia. Thirty percent of cases are idiopathic. An additional 30% are drug-induced (penicillin, quinidine, methyldopa), and the rest are associated with underlying disease, including systemic lupus erythematosus (SLE), lymphoma, and chronic lymphocytic leukemia (CLL).

Peripheral blood smear shows spherocytes, which arise from partial consumption of RBCs by the reticuloendothelial system. The direct Coombs' test, which detects the presence of antibody or complement on the RBC, is positive.

Discontinue the offending drug immediately. Give corticosteroids to suppress the immune response. Splenectomy may be necessary to control hemolysis.

Cold-reacting antibodies form RBC complexes only below 31°C. These IgM antibodies can cause either hemolysis or agglutination of RBCs, leading to infarction of tissues in colder areas of the body (fingers and toes). This form of hemolytic anemia occurs in patients with certain infections (*Mycoplasma*, malaria, Epstein-Barr) and with lymphoproliferative diseases. Avoiding exposure to cold is the primary treatment.

Mechanical Hemolysis

Mechanical hemolysis occurs when RBCs are fragmented by shear forces or by turbulence. Injury to cells can arise in the heart (aortic stenosis, prosthetic heart valve), in the arterioles (malignant hypertension), or in other vessels (thrombotic thrombocytopenic purpura, disseminated intravascular coagulation).

Peripheral blood smear shows odd-shaped RBCs, including schistocytes (helmet cells).

Directed at the underlying process.

Hemolytic Disease of the Newborn (Erythroblastosis Fetalis)

If Rh-positive fetal cells enter the circulation of an Rh-negative mother, the mother may develop anti-Rh antibodies. This can occur during delivery, during a therapeutic abortion, or, less commonly, during third-trimester bleeding. Maternal anti-Rh antibodies can then cross the placenta and cause massive hemolysis and death to any future Rh-positive fetuses that the mother may carry. This is hemolytic disease of the newborn. About 15% of caucasians are Rh-negative. The rate is lower for Asians and African-Americans.

Treatment consists of passive immunization with Rh-immunoglobulin (RhoGAM) given within 72 hours of the delivery or abortion. RhoGAM acts by binding to all fetal Rh-positive cells in the mother's blood, preventing the mother from synthesizing the antibodies. Women who are exposed to bleeding during pregnancy can be given Rh-immunoglobulin in the twenty-eighth week of pregnancy. RhoGAM does not pose any danger to the fetus, since the immunoglobulin antibodies are too large to pass through the placenta.

Hereditary Spherocytosis

Hereditary spherocytosis is a dominantly inherited defect in RBC membrane proteins that results in damaged cells being trapped in the spleen and destroyed.

Splenomegaly is the major finding. Hepatomegaly and cholelithiasis are also common. Aplastic crises can occur during infections.

Spherical RBCs and reticulocytosis are seen on peripheral blood smear. The cells are spherical because surface area is reduced more than volume. Spherical cells are identified as abnormal and trapped by the spleen. Coombs' test is negative, as no antibodies are involved.

Splenectomy will stop hemolysis, although the underlying defect is unchanged.

Glucose-6-Phosphate Dehydrogenase Deficiency

Glucose-6-phosphate dehydrogenase (G6PD) is an enzyme required by the RBC to cope with oxidative damage. Its deficiency is an X-linked disease. Without G6PD, hemoglobin is damaged and accumulates in the RBCs as small densities called Heinz bodies. These cells are then taken out of circulation by the spleen. This oxidation and subsequent hemolysis occur when the patient ingests oxidative drugs (antimalarials, sulfa drugs, aspirin) or fava beans, as well as during febrile illnesses or acidosis. A mild form of the disease is found in 10% of African-American men, and a more severe form occurs in Mediterranean and Middle Eastern men.

Symptoms of acute hemolysis include palpitations, breathlessness, and dizziness, usually occurring 1–3 days after ingestion of an oxidant. Jaundice and splenomegaly are common.

Heinz bodies and "bite cells," cells in which the Heinz body has been "bitten" out during a pass through the spleen, are visible on peripheral blood smear before the onset of hemolysis.

Assay of G6PD levels.

Discontinue the oxidative drug and avoid future oxidants. Transfusion may be necessary.

White Blood Cell Disorders

Agranulocytosis (Neutropenia)

Agranulocytosis is a deficit of neutrophils. Since neutrophil half-life is only 6–7 hours, this disorder can develop rapidly. Causes include inadequate granulopoiesis, as seen in aplastic anemia and leukemia, or accelerated destruction of neutrophils, which is usually caused by drugs such as chloramphenicol, sulfonamides, chlorpromazine, thiouracil, and phenylbutazone.

Constitutional symptoms include fever, chills, weakness, and fatigue. Infections, including ulcerating and necrotizing surface lesions, are common.

The above symptoms, along with laboratory evidence of decreased neutrophils, should suggest the diagnosis. Bone marrow biopsy is helpful in discerning the exact cause.

Antibiotics, steroids, and neutrophil transfusions may be useful.

Eosinophilia

Eosinophilia is characteristic of allergic disorders, asthma, and parasitic diseases. The most common source of eosinophilia in hospitalized patients is an allergic drug reaction. It is also seen in Loffler's syndrome (endocardial fibrosis), pulmonary infiltrates with eosinophilia (PIE), and Addison's disease. A mnemonic for the most common causes of eosinophilia is NAACP: *n*eoplasm, *a*llergy/asthma, *A*ddison's disease, *c*ollagen vascular disease, and *p*arasites.

Asymptomatic, except as related to the underlying disorder.

Increased eosinophil count on complete blood count (CBC).

Remove any allergic stimuli as soon as possible. Otherwise, treat the underlying disorder.

Hemoglobin Abnormalities

Thalassemia

In thalassemia, diminished or absent production of a particular globin chain causes unbalanced amounts of alpha and beta chains. Sufficient normal hemoglobin cannot be produced. Unpaired chains become tetramers and precipitate, damaging the RBC membrane and causing hemolysis.

Two types of thalassemia are commonly seen:

- **Alpha-thalassemia** refers to a group of structural deletions of the alpha chain of hemoglobin. It is seen more frequently in Asians. Depending on the number of deletions, patients may be asymptomatic, may suffer from a mild anemia, or may have more severe manifestations. In one of the more severe forms, **hemoglobin H disease**, alpha-globin is completely absent. Infants with this disorder are often stillborn. Some may survive for a short time due to the presence of fetal hemoglobin, but they will have very severe anemia and splenomegaly.

- **Beta-thalassemia** is characterized by defective expression of the beta chain of hemoglobin. It is generally seen in Mediterranean and African populations. If heterozygous, patients are referred to as having "beta-thalassemia minor" and may be asymptomatic. Homozygotes have "beta-thalassemia major," with severe anemia, delayed growth and development, and shortened life expectancy.

MCV is severely decreased (typically out of proportion to the reduction in hematocrit), reticulocytes are increased, and peripheral blood smear shows abnormal RBC morphology. Alpha-thalassemia is characterized by target cells and acanthocytes (cells with rounded projections). Peripheral blood smear in beta-thalassemia shows basophilic stippling, nucleated RBCs, anisocytosis (variations in size), and poikilocytosis (variations in shape). Definitive diagnosis is performed with hemoglobin electrophoresis.

Transfusions are important for symptomatic disease, with iron chelation therapy to prevent iron overload. Supplemental iron should never be given to thalassemic patients. Bone marrow transplant has been used with some success, and genetic counseling is important to help prevent the most severe forms of both alpha- and beta-thalassemia.

Sickle Cell Anemia

In sickle cell anemia, a recessively inherited disease, the beta-hemoglobin chain is altered, resulting in the production of hemoglobin S (HbS) instead of the normal hemoglobin A. When exposed to a low-oxygen environment, HbS molecules join together to form long crystalline structures that distort the RBC into the classic sickle shape. Acidosis and dehydration also promote sickling. The HbS gene is more common in African-American populations. While 1 in 400 births of African-American infants results in a child with sickle cell anemia, approximately 8% of African-Americans are carriers of the gene. Carriers are referred to as having sickle cell trait, and they are asymptomatic except under extreme conditions. These carriers have a beneficial increased resistance to malaria.

Patients are rarely symptomatic until 6 months of age because of the presence of HbF (fetal hemoglobin). Chronic anemia arises from constant destruction of sickled cells. Most other problems are due to vascular sludging and thrombosis, which result in damage to multiple organs as well as acute, painful crises. Common manifestations include stroke, osteonecrosis, pulmonary hypertension, and acute chest syndrome (characterized by fever, pain, dyspnea, and a pneumonia-like infiltrate on x-ray). Multiple infarcts of the spleen result in autosplenectomy, and patients are susceptible to *Streptococcus pneumoniae* sepsis and *Salmonella* osteomyelitis. Aplastic crises may be triggered by infection of any kind.

Peripheral blood smear may not show sickled cells unless the blood sample is deoxygenated first (sickle cell preparation). Hematocrit is low (20–30%), and the reticulocyte count is high (10–25%), except during an aplastic crisis. Neutrophilia is chronic but may become extreme during a painful crisis, even in the absence of infection.

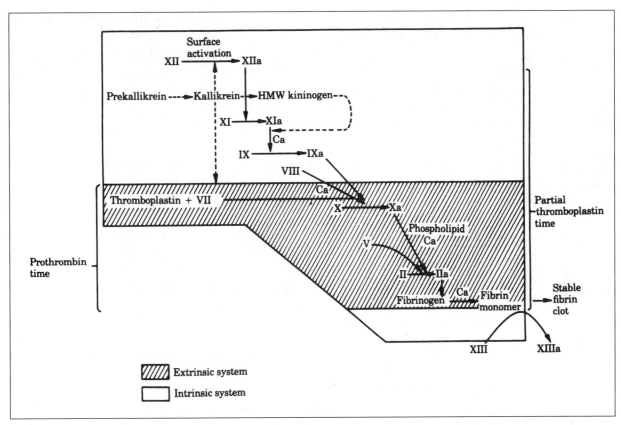

Fig. 11-1. Coagulation cascade. (From HH Friedman. *Problem-Oriented Medical Diagnosis*, Fifth Edition. Boston: Little, Brown, 1991.)

Solubility tests (Sickledex) may be used, but hemoglobin electrophoresis showing HbS without HbA is the gold standard.

Preventive care includes avoidance of dehydration or low-oxygen environments. Prophylactic penicillin should be given to decrease risk of pneumococcal sepsis, and pneumococcal vaccine should be administered as soon as the child's system can respond to it (at 2 years of age). Treatment of crises includes oxygen, hydration, and narcotic analgesics. Blood transfusions may be required in aplastic crises, but iron overload is a concern.

Clotting Disorders

Hemophilia

Hemophilia A is an X-linked recessive disorder caused by reduced quantity or activity of factor VIII of the coagulation cascade (Fig. 11-1). It is often asymptomatic but can become severe when factor VIII activity drops to less than 1% of normal. Incidence is about 1 in 10,000. **Hemophilia B** (Christmas' disease) is also an X-linked recessive disease, which is similar to hemophilia A but is much less common, with an incidence of 1 in 100,000. Hemophilia B is related to factor IX deficiency.

Uncontrolled bleeding can arise spontaneously or following minor trauma. Bleeding occurs most often in the joints (hemarthroses) and soft tissues, but also in the GI tract, genitourinary tract, central nervous system, and elsewhere.

Lab evaluation shows a prolonged partial thromboplastin time (PTT), but definitive diagnosis is made only with factor activity assay. Factor activity assay shows low activity of factor VIII (hemophilia A) or factor IX (hemophilia B).

Infusions of factor concentrates and FFP may be useful. DDAVP, an analogue of antidiuretic hormone (ADH), has been shown to raise factor VIII levels. Most adults with hemophilia are HIV-positive if they received transfusions before widespread blood screening was available.

Von Willebrand's Disease

Von Willebrand's disease, an autosomal dominant disease, involves deficiencies in both factor VIII and von Willebrand's factor (vWF), resulting in a disorder of both coagulation and platelets.

Uncontrolled bleeding from the skin and mucous membranes, including epistaxis, menorrhagia, and bruising. Hemarthroses are rare, even though these patients have factor VIII deficiency.

Prolonged PTT and bleeding time (time taken for bleeding to discontinue after a skin cut) are typical. Ristocetin cofactor assay or vWF immunologic assays shows specific deficiencies and provides the definitive diagnosis.

Cryoprecipitate and FFP.

Vitamin K Deficiency

Vitamin K is a cofactor in the liver's synthesis of clotting factors II, VII, IX, and X. It is supplied by leafy green vegetables, as well as by normal bacteria in the intestine. Thus, poor diet or prolonged antibiotic treatment may lead to a deficiency. The drug warfarin acts by interfering with vitamin K–mediated clotting factor synthesis, and therefore patients using this drug appear to have a vitamin K deficiency.

The primary symptom is spontaneous bleeding or prolonged oozing.

Prothrombin time (PT) and PTT are prolonged, although the PT is generally more affected.

Vitamin K injections.

Platelet Disorders

Qualitative Platelet Disorders

Qualitative platelet disorders involve malfunctioning platelets. The hereditary forms are rare and include abnormalities of platelet membranes, attachment, and storage. Acquired platelet disorders occur with the use of aspirin or other NSAIDs that can irreversibly acetylate cyclooxygenase, resulting in deficits of platelet aggregation. The effect lasts for the life of the platelet (approximately 7–10 days) and is not dose-dependent. Uremia can cause a platelet disorder that is associated with renal failure, although the mechanism by which this occurs is unknown. Symptoms of qualitative platelet disorders include easy bruising, epistaxis, prolonged oozing, and menorrhagia. Treatment with cryoprecipitate and renal dialysis may be helpful. Platelet transfusions are not beneficial.

Quantitative Platelet Disorders

Quantitative platelet disorders involve inadequate numbers of circulating platelets, which can result from a variety of etiologies. The following causes are common:

Decreased production of platelets
- Aplastic anemia
- Bone marrow damage (e.g., secondary to drugs, radiation)
- Myelophthisis (reduction of cell-forming ability of the bone marrow)
- Ineffective thrombopoiesis (e.g., vitamin B_{12} and folate deficiency)

Increased destruction of platelets
- Idiopathic thrombocytopenia purpura (ITP, see below)
- Underlying disease (e.g., SLE, CLL)
- Drug-induced antibodies (e.g., quinine, quinidine, thiazide diuretics, sulfa drugs, heparin)
- Viral infections (e.g., CMV, EBV, HIV)

Increased consumption of platelets
- Disseminated intravascular coagulation (DIC, see below)
- Thrombotic thrombocytopenic purpura (TTP, see below)
- Hemolytic-uremic syndrome (HUS, see below)

Common symptoms of quantitative platelet disorders include petechiae (small hemorrhages in the skin) and purpura (larger skin hemorrhages).

Diagnosis and treatment are discussed with the individual disorders.

Disseminated Intravascular Coagulation

Disseminated intravascular coagulation (DIC) is caused by widespread activation of the coagulation sequence. Formation of microthrombi causes infarcts, while massive consumption of platelets, fibrin, and coagulation factors causes uncontrolled bleeding. Significant damage may occur in the kidneys, lungs, and brain. Common causes include obstetric complications (50%), malignancy (33%), infections, and massive tissue trauma.

Presentation varies widely. Physical manifestations include hemolytic anemia, respiratory difficulty, neurological symptoms, acute renal failure, and shock.

Decreased platelets, fragmentation of RBCs, prolonged PT and PTT, decreased fibrinogen, and increased fibrin degradation products.

Heparin, antithrombin III, and FFP may be useful.

Thrombotic Thrombocytopenic Purpura

Thrombotic thrombocytopenic purpura (TTP) involves the reaction of platelets with endothelial cells, resulting in occlusion of vessels and platelet consumption. The cause of TTP is unknown but is not thought to be autoimmune. Patients are generally between the ages of 20 and 50, and women are affected more often than men.

TTP is characterized by the acute onset of thrombocytopenia, fever, anemia, jaundice, fluctuating neurologic deficits, and renal failure.

Lab evaluation shows low platelet count, decreased hematocrit, and increased reticulocytes. Serum LDH levels are usually markedly elevated.

Corticosteroids, platelet aggregation inhibitors, and plasma exchange transfusions are generally effective. If untreated, TTP is usually fatal within 3 months.

Idiopathic Thrombocytopenia Purpura

Idiopathic thrombocytopenia purpura (ITP) is an autoimmune disease caused by the development of antibodies against the patient's own platelets. Massive phagocytosis of immune complexes then occurs in the spleen. ITP is more common in children and frequently follows a mild viral infection. The childhood form has a better prognosis than the adult form. ITP is also common in AIDS patients.

Patients are generally asymptomatic except for mucosal and skin bleeding due to lack of platelets. Purpura, petechiae, epistaxis, and menorrhagia are common.

Platelet counts are markedly low (<10,000/mm^3). Other blood cell counts are generally normal, and the peripheral blood smear is normal.

ITP is usually self-limited in children, but the condition may require treatment in adults. Medical treatment consists of corticosteroids. Splenectomy may be indicated if phagocytosis is severe and the disorder is unresponsive to steroids. Approximately 40–50% of ITP patients are cured within a short time, while the rest go on to have chronic ITP.

Hemolytic-Uremic Syndrome

In hemolytic-uremic syndrome (HUS), rapid destruction of RBCs causes acute renal failure, in part due to obstruction of small renal arteries. The associated thrombocytopenia (secondary to thrombi formation) can result in severe hemorrhage. This disorder is mainly seen in infants and children, but it can occur in adults, particularly pregnant women or patients with infectious diseases. Toxin-producing *Escherichia coli* is associated with 75% of HUS cases.

Patients present with abdominal pain and diarrhea, usually following a flu-like prodrome. Manifestations are similar to TTP and include thrombocytopenia, anemia, and renal failure. Hypertension may be seen, but unlike TTP, CNS involvement is not common.

The hallmark finding is RBC fragments on peripheral blood smear in association with the above symptoms. Platelet counts are low, and serum LDH is usually markedly elevated.

Conservative management is generally sufficient. FFP and plasmapheresis are sometimes necessary.

Neoplastic Disorders

Acute Lymphocytic Leukemia

Acute lymphocytic leukemia (ALL) is the malignant expansion of the lymphoid line of white cells (B and T cells) (Fig. 11-2). It comprises 80% of all childhood leukemias, with peak ages of incidence from 3 to 7 years. Eighty percent of ALL is of B cell origin.

Symptoms are varied and result mainly from bone marrow infiltration. Pale skin and mucosa and fatigue result from anemia. Infections are common due to leukopenia. Purpura, petechiae, and bleeding occur due to thrombocytopenia. Splenomegaly, hepatomegaly, lymphadenopathy, and bone tenderness may also be present.

Blasts are abundant, although they may be absent in some cases. Total WBC may vary from low to high. Decreased RBC and platelet count occur because the bone marrow has been taken over by lymphocytic cells. Hyperuricemia may be noted.

Bone marrow biopsy reveals many lymphoblasts and few other cells. Hyperdiploidy (51–60 chromosomes) in the nuclei of B cells is associated with a good prognosis. The Philadelphia chromosome, found in about 15% of adult ALL, is associated with a poorer prognosis.

ALL must be differentiated from a leukemoid reaction, in which patients with severe inflammatory diseases have increased numbers of WBCs and blasts.

Chemotherapy alone achieves a cure rate of 60% in children and 40% in adults. Those who are not cured may be candidates for bone marrow transplant.

Acute Myelocytic Leukemia

Acute myelocytic leukemia (AML) neoplastic cell disorders affect the myeloid cells (neutrophils, basophils, eosinophils, erythrocytes, and megakaryocytes) (see Fig. 11-2). In contrast to ALL, AML is more common in adults.

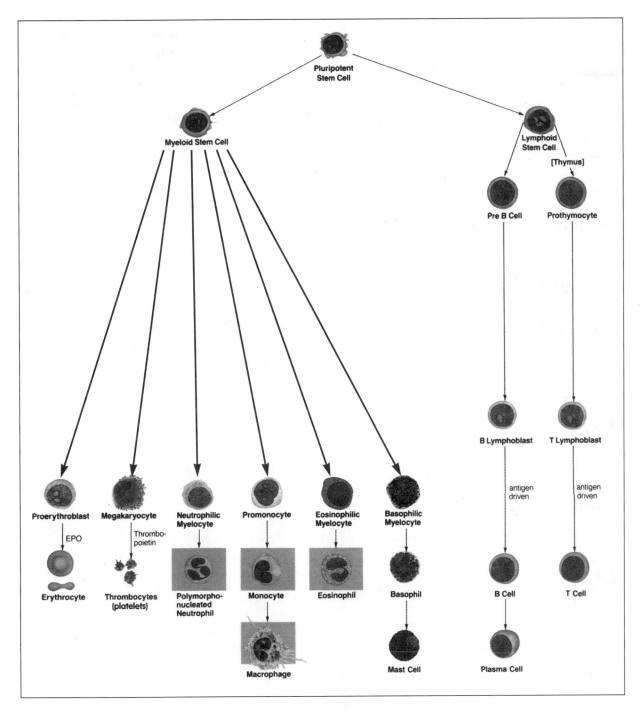

Fig. 11-2. Development of lymphoid and myeloid cell lines. (Adapted from ML Turgeon. *Clinical Hematology: Theory and Procedures*, Second Edition. Boston: Little, Brown, 1993.)

Symptoms are similar to those of ALL and include infections and bleeding. DIC may be seen with AML. Neutropenic patients are at risk for a number of infections with gram-negative bacteria and fungi, such as *Candida* and *Aspergillus*.

Labs vary depending on which cell line has expanded. Examination of the cells may show the presence of Auer rods, red-staining intracellular inclusions that are pathognomonic for AML. Bone marrow histochemistry reveals staining with myeloperoxidase or para-aminosalicylic acid (PAS).

The majority of patients go into remission with chemotherapy, but they tend to relapse within 12–18 months. Bone marrow transplant may be beneficial to those who relapse. Long-term survival is generally only 10–15%.

Chronic Myelocytic Leukemia

Chronic myelocytic leukemia (CML) describes a group of disorders of myeloid cells. Unlike AML, the tumors cells are more mature myeloid forms rather than blasts, and they retain the ability to differentiate. The disease may remain stable for several years before progressing to an acute leukemia. It is usually diagnosed in middle age. Genetically, CML is characterized by the Philadelphia chromosome, an acquired translocation of chromosomes 9 and 22.

Fatigue, nights sweats, chronic low-grade fevers, and splenomegaly.

Leukocytosis is often an incidental finding, with WBC counts greater than 150,000/mm^3. Other lab abnormalities include increased uric acid and increased serum vitamin B$_{12}$, because the B$_{12}$ carrier protein is produced by WBCs. Leukocyte alkaline phosphatase may be low or absent. RBCs are normal in appearance and number.

Treatment with chemotherapy and alpha-interferon is palliative, not curative. As the disease progresses, patients experience a "blast crisis," which signifies rapid worsening of the disease. Survival is typically about 4 years after onset. Bone marrow transplant increases survival time but is rarely curative.

Chronic Lymphocytic Leukemia

Chronic lymphocytic leukemia (CLL) is a neoplastic disorder of mature B cells (T cell types are rare). Typically, these B cells do not differentiate into plasma cells. Some B cells may create auto-antibodies to RBCs and platelets, resulting in hemolytic anemia and thrombocytopenia. CLL strikes men more often than women. Patients are generally over the age of 50, with 65 the median age at diagnosis.

Patients with CLL are often asymptomatic or experience nonspecific symptoms such as fatigue and anorexia. Generalized lymphadenopathy, splenomegaly, and hepatomegaly may be noted on physical exam. Due to a relative lack of plasma cells, many patients have hypogammaglobuline-mia and experience frequent infections as a result.

WBC count is elevated, with an isolated increase in lymphocytes. Peripheral blood smear shows numerous small, mature-appearing lymphocytes. Small amounts of IgM paraprotein may be detected in the patient's serum.

Treatment is primarily symptomatic, with benefit in some patients from chemotherapy. Prognosis varies, but median survival is 6 years. Unlike CML, there is no "blast crisis" transformation to acute leukemia signaling a poorer prognosis.

Hairy Cell Leukemia

Hairy cell leukemia is a neoplastic transformation of B cells that involves tumor cells with fine, hairlike projections. It is predominantly a disease of middle-aged men.

Symptoms are nonspecific, often including generalized fatigue. Unlike CLL, there is usually no lymphadenopathy, and virtually all patients have splenomegaly. Recurrent infections, especially of mycobacteria, are common.

Lab evaluation is notable for pancytopenia, with leukocytosis in only 25% of patients. Peripheral blood smear reveals the "hairy cells." Bone marrow may be inaspirable but may show infiltration. Infiltration of the red pulp of the spleen is also present (as opposed to white pulp infiltration, which is common in lymphomas).

Chemotherapy achieves complete remission in more than 80% of patients. The course of the disease is indolent, with survival of 10 years or more.

Hodgkin's Lymphoma

Hodgkin's lymphoma, a cancer of macrophage origin, has a bimodal distribution, with peak ages of presentation in patients in their 20s or later in their 50s.

Patients present with painless lymphadenopathy, especially in the neck, and generalized symptoms, such as fever, weight loss, night sweats, and pruritus.

Lymph node biopsy shows Reed-Sternberg cells. These large, multinucleated reticular cells are pathognomonic of Hodgkin's disease.

Radiation therapy and chemotherapy. Currently, patients with Hodgkin's disease have a good prognosis, and cure rates approach 80% even for stage III disease.

Non-Hodgkin's Lymphoma

Non-Hodgkin's lymphoma (NHL), a large group of neoplasms of the lymphocytes, has a wide range of severity and prognoses. In general, however, prognosis is poorer for NHL than for Hodgkin's disease.

As in Hodgkin's disease, patients usually present with localized or generalized painless lymphadenopathy, as well as with nonspecific symptoms of fever, night sweats, and weight loss.

Lab evaluation is often normal, although one-third of patients have anemia due to bone marrow infiltration. Peripheral blood smear may be normal or reflect the overgrowth of a particular white cell line. At this point it is often difficult to distinguish NHL from other types of leukemia. Serum LDH is increased if the disease has spread.

Definitive diagnosis is made by lymph node biopsy. The disease is often disseminated by the time of diagnosis, and bone marrow is frequently involved. Bone marrow biopsy shows lymphoid aggregates around the bone trabeculae.

Treatment is primarily palliative, although radiation therapy and chemotherapy are used with variable effectiveness. Survival ranges from months to several years depending upon the aggressiveness of the disease.

One form of NHL is **Burkitt's lymphoma**, which affects B cells. It is endemic in parts of Africa, and it is more common in children and young adults. In the United States, symptoms include abdominal pain and fullness due to a predilection of the disease for the abdomen, whereas jaw involvement is common in Africa. Burkitt's lymphoma has been associated with chromosomal translocation (8;14) and may also be related to the Epstein-Barr virus.

Multiple Myeloma

Multiple myeloma is a neoplastic proliferation of plasma cells and monoclonal immunoglobulin. The disorder strikes men and women equally, and peak incidence occurs between 50–60 years of age. Survival is generally 1–3 years from diagnosis.

Replacement of the bone marrow with plasma cells results in anemia, bone pain, pathologic fractures, and nephrosis. Plasma cell infiltration of the liver, lungs, and nodes also occurs. Because of leukopenia, infections may be frequent, especially with encapsulated organisms such as *S. pneumoniae*.

Diagnosis is made by finding "paraproteins" (abnormal plasma proteins) in the blood via serum protein electrophoresis (SPEP). X-rays may show osteolytic bone lesions.

Chemotherapy and radiation therapy may be effective, depending on the stage of the disease. Bone marrow transplant has also been used with the potential for cure. Palliative care includes treatment of infections and the hypercalcemia that results from bone degradation.

Waldenström's Macroglobulinemia

Waldenström's macroglobulinemia is characterized by malignant transformation of a single B-lymphocyte cell line, resulting in monoclonal IgM overproduction. Peak incidence is in the sixth decade, and survival is about 3–5 years from diagnosis.

Constitutional symptoms of weakness, fatigue, and weight loss. Hyperviscosity may occur, along with bleeding, and visual and neurologic problems. Cellular proliferation in the liver and spleen causes hepatomegaly and splenomegaly.

Decreased hematocrit, usually with normal WBC and platelet counts. Peripheral blood smear reveals RBCs in a "rouleau formation," in which several red blood cells pile on one another, forming a cylinder. Bone marrow biopsy shows increased plasma cells, but no osteolytic lesions are seen on x-ray.

Definitive diagnosis is made by the presence of a monoclonal IgM spike on SPEP.

Plasmapheresis to reduce hyperviscosity and chemotherapy to slow lymphocyte production are commonly used.

Mycosis Fungoides

Mycosis fungoides is a neoplastic tumor involving clonal proliferation of CD4 T cells. It usually infiltrates the dermis and epidermis and may involve nodal and visceral spread. Median survival is usually 8–9 years.

SIGNS & SYMPTOMS

Skin lesions may initially be confused with eczema, psoriasis, or contact dermatitis. They later thicken and become nodular, with an area of central clearing.

DIAGNOSIS

Skin biopsy.

TREATMENT

Topical medications and phototherapy may be used for early lesions. Further progression of the disease requires systemic chemotherapy such as methotrexate and cyclophosphamide. Cure is usually possible in early stages.

Polycythemia Vera

Polycythemia vera is a common acquired disorder of the bone marrow stem cells that results in overproduction of all three blood cell lines, but predominantly RBCs. RBC counts can exceed 1,000,000/mm^3 and hematocrit can rise above 60%. Polycythemia vera is seen in both men and women, with peak incidence around age 60. The disease can last for decades but may progress to leukemia.

SIGNS & SYMPTOMS

Symptoms are due to increased blood viscosity. Headache, dizziness, blurred vision, and fatigue are common. Some patients may experience generalized pruritus, especially after a hot bath, which is attributed to the increased number of basophils. Splenomegaly and hepatomegaly may be present. Major morbidity and mortality are primarily related to thrombotic events, particularly strokes and deep venous thromboses (DVTs).

DIAGNOSIS

Hematocrit and RBC count are increased. Bone marrow biopsy shows hypercellular marrow with absent iron stores. The most important differential diagnosis is spurious polycythemia, in which the hematocrit is artificially elevated due to decreased plasma volume or dehydration, and secondary polycythemia, in which RBC mass is a reaction to decreased oxygenization.

TREATMENT

Phlebotomy is used to maintain hematocrit under 45%. Allopurinol may be given for hyperuricemia, antihistamines for itching, and aspirin to prevent thrombotic events. Iron should not be given despite low or absent iron stores, as it may exacerbate the overproduction.

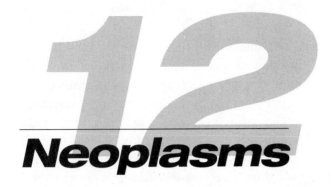

Neoplasms

Note: Cancers of specific organ systems are found in their respective chapters.
This chapter deals with broad concepts of neoplastic disease.

Community Measures to Prevent Cancer

Many cancers are entirely preventable, and the sequelae of those that are not may be prevented if the cancers are detected early. Community prevention measures include anti-smoking or antialcohol campaigns, education about the danger of sun exposure, and efforts to encourage Pap smears and mammograms. Communities may also provide or promote screening programs. To be effective, screening programs must use tests that are both sensitive and specific, must target the population at highest risk (Table 12-1), and must identify a disease for which early intervention is available and useful. The positive predictive value of the test (i.e., the chances of having the disease if the test is positive) and the consequences of a false-positive or false-negative result must also be considered.

Individual Measures to Prevent Cancer

One's lifestyle greatly affects the risk of developing cancer. Such well-known measures as not smoking, eating fruits and vegetables, and staying out of the sun can significantly reduce risk. Regular screening, performed by the individual (e.g., monthly breast exams) or by a clinician (e.g., for cervical, colon, and breast cancer) is also important. The National Cancer Institute provides schedules of screening for different cancers, discussed in Chapter 17.

Surveillance and Reporting

Population-based tumor registries are maintained both internationally and nationally. The International Agency for Research of Cancer (IARC) maintains data on common worldwide cancers. In the United States, the National Cancer Institute maintains the Surveillance, Epidemiology, and End Results (SEER) tumor registry. These data are used to direct research efforts and funds, to plan education campaigns, and to monitor effects that may contribute to the incidence of each cancer.

Epidemiology of Neoplastic Disease

Cancer is the second leading cause of death in the United States, accounting for 22% of deaths each year. (Cardiovascular disease is the number one cause of death.) Age is the most important predictor of cancer incidence, with the incidence of cancer generally rising with increasing age. Overall, the mean age of diagnosis is 65 years old. Gender may also be a predictor for some cancers; for example, men are more likely than women to develop lung cancer, although much of this effect is due to the higher rates of smoking among men. Lung cancer is the leading cause of death in this country, and 90% of cases are attributed to tobacco use. Certain cancers are more prevalent in some racial groups than in others. For example, the rate of prostate cancer is much higher in African-American men than among any other group. Socioeconomic status (SES) may be an inde-

Table 12-1. Risk factors for cancer

Risk factor	Associated cancer
Tobacco	Lung
	Head and neck
	GI
	Kidney and bladder
	Pancreas
Alcohol	Liver
	GI
	Head and neck
Ionizing radiation	Leukemia
	Lymphoma
	Thyroid
	GI
	Bladder
Sun exposure	Basal and squamous cell skin cancer
	Malignant melanoma
Drugs (e.g., DES)	Cervix
	Vagina
Infectious agents	
Epstein-Barr virus	Burkitt's lymphoma
Hepatitis B and C viruses	Liver
Human papillomavirus	Cervix
Schistosomiasis	Bladder
Nutritional factors	
High fat/low fiber	Colon
Aflatoxins (from fungi)	Liver

pendent risk factor for disease. In addition, lower SES may be associated with poor access to medical care, delayed diagnosis, and therefore poorer prognosis.

Leading Causes of Cancer Death and Disability

The most common causes of cancer and cancer death are shown in Tables 12-2 and 12-3.

Cancer Screening Recommendations

Table 12-4 provides a brief review of the American Cancer Society's screening recommendations. Patients with a family history of cancer may require more frequent screening.

Table 12-2. Estimated cancer incidence by site and sex, 1994*

Type	Men (%)	Women (%)
Melanoma of skin	3	3
Oral	3	2
Lung	16	13
Breast	—	32
Pancreas	2	2
Stomach	2	—
Colon and rectum	12	13
Prostate	32	—
Ovary	—	4
Uterus	—	8
Urinary	9	4
Leukemia and lymphomas	7	6
All other	14	13

* Excluding basal and squamous cell skin cancers and carcinoma in situ.
Source: Adapted from *CA Cancer J Clin* 44:7, 1994.

Table 12-3. Estimated cancer deaths by site and sex, 1994

Type	Men (%)	Women (%)
Melanoma of skin	2	1
Oral	2	1
Lung	33	23
Breast	—	18
Pancreas	4	5
Stomach	3	—
Colon and rectum	10	11
Prostate	13	—
Ovary	—	5
Uterus	—	4
Urinary	5	3
Leukemia and lymphomas	8	8
All other	20	21

Source: Adapted from *CA Cancer J Clin* 44:7, 1994.

Table 12-4. Current American Cancer Society screening recommendations*

Organ system	Frequency	After age
Breast		
Breast self-examination	Every month	20
Clinical breast exam	Every 3 years	20–40
	Every year	40+
Mammography	Every 1–2 years	40–50
	Every year	50+
Uterus/cervix		
Pelvic examination	Every 1–3 years	18–40
Pap smear	Annually for 3 years, then every 1–3 years	18
Endometrial biopsy	Once	Menopause
Colon		
Occult stool blood	Every year	50
Sigmoidoscopy	Every 3–5 years	50
Digital rectal exam	Every year	40
Prostate		
Digital rectal exam/PSA	Every year	50

PSA = prostate-specific antigen.
*Note that the American Cancer Society recommendations may suggest different or more frequent tests than those recommended by the United States Preventive Services Task Force (see Chap. 17).

Treatment Strategies

Any cells that can replicate can also undergo malignant transformation. Infection or some insult, such as radiation, can damage cells' DNA and alter normal cellular function. If appropriate regulation of the cell cycle is lost, division and growth continue unchecked, and cancer is the result. In a clinical setting, several treatment strategies exist:

• **Chemotherapy.** Since tumor cells and normal cells are very similar, selective destruction of tumor cells is quite difficult. Most antineoplastic agents target cells that are actively dividing, so they have more of an effect on the rapidly growing tumor than on the body's normal cells. DNA and RNA replication and protein synthesis are crucial for cell division; therefore, interference at this level prevents further division and can destroy the affected cells.

Two major types of chemotherapeutic agents are used. **Cell cycle–specific agents** interfere with DNA synthesis or with mitosis. **Cell cycle–nonspecific agents** damage the cells regardless of whether they are dividing, so these are more effective against slow-growing tumors. Because chemotherapy inflicts damage anywhere that frequent cell division occurs, bone marrow suppression, nausea and vomiting, and hair loss are common side effects. Table 12-5 classifies the major classes of chemotherapeutic agents.

Table 12-5. Drugs used in cancer chemotheraphy

Agent	Mechanism	Tumor types
Nitrogen mustards	Block DNA transcription	Lymphoma
Cyclophosphamide		Ovarian
Chlorambucil		Testicular
Nitrosureas	Block DNA transcription	CNS tumors
		Lymphoma
Cisplatin/carboplatin	Crosslinks DNA	Ovarian
Antimetabolites	Block nucleotide synthesis	Leukemia
Methotrexate		GI tumors
5-Fluorouracil		
Antibiotics	DNA strand breakage	Leukemia
Doxorubicin		Sarcomas
Bleomycin		GI tumors
Vinca alkaloids	Microtubule destruction	Leukemia
Vincristine		Hodgkin's disease

- **Surgery.** Surgical excision of a tumor may be curative, or it may be used to debulk a tumor that is later treated with chemotherapy and/or radiation. If the tumor is detected before it has spread beyond the confines of the organ, surgery is often curative.
- **Radiation.** Radiation therapy offers both curative and palliative effects. Radiation directed against primary tumors halts cell division by targeting DNA synthesis. Cancers that are commonly treated by radiation include lymphomas, prostate cancer, breast cancer, and head and neck tumors.

Basic Staging Classifications

Cancer staging helps determine the extent of disease, the appropriate treatment, and the prognosis. The two basic staging systems are the international system and the American system.

The international system uses the TNM terminology, in which T stands for primary tumor, N for nodal involvement, and M for metastasis. The T ranking ranges from T1 to T4, depending on the size of the primary tumor, while T0 indicates carcinoma in situ. The N ranking ranges from N0, indicating no nodal involvement, to N3, indicating more extensive nodal involvement. The M ranking ranges from M0, indicating no metastases, to M2, generally indicating extensive metastases.

The American system uses a 0–IV ranking system. The meaning of the ranks differs from one tumor type to another. In general, stage 0 represents carcinoma in situ, stage I refers to cancer confined to the primary organ, stages II and III describe progressive involvement of adjacent structures, and stage IV indicates distant metastases.

Paraneoplastic Disorders

Paraneoplastic disorders are syndromes caused by the indirect effects of tumors at distant sites. Most paraneoplastic disorders result from secretion of ectopic hormones from tumor cells. These complications occur in approximately 10% of patients with advanced malignancies. The malignancies most often responsible are small-cell and squamous cell lung cancer, breast cancer, and thyroid cancer. Commonly secreted hormones include insulin, vasoactive intestinal polypeptide (VIP), epinephrine, adrenocorticotropic hormone (ACTH), vasopressin, calcitonin, and parathyroid hormone (PTH).

SIGNS & SYMPTOMS

The effects are determined by the specific hormone secreted. For example, insulinomas cause hypoglycemia; pheochromocytomas, which secrete epinephrine and norepinephrine, lead to hypertension. Cushing's syndrome due to ectopic ACTH secretion and hyperthyroidism due to ectopic TSH secretion are other possible clinical manifestations.

DIAGNOSIS

The constellation of symptoms should suggest the diagnosis in a patient with a known malignancy. Otherwise, the malignancy must be sought.

TREATMENT

Treat the underlying malignancy as much as possible. Control of symptoms may be achieved with medications specific to the hormonal effects.

Management of Acute Problems

Acute complications of malignancies can be severe and even life-threatening, but many can be alleviated by proper care. For example, central nervous system (CNS) edema due to a brain tumor may be temporarily relieved by administration of high-dose corticosteroids, and gastrointestinal perforation or obstruction can be surgically repaired. The common complications of each particular tumor are discussed in the appropriate sections throughout this book.

Chronic Care

Pain management is a critical issue in the chronic care of a cancer patient. Addiction is not a concern for terminally ill patients, so narcotics should not be withheld if needed for pain control. Constant dosing schedules, rather than "as needed" administration, are used to avoid breakthrough episodes of pain.

Infections occur frequently in patients with cancer due to immunosuppressive therapies, the effects of chronic disease, and chemotherapy-induced bone marrow suppression. The decision to give antibiotics should be based on the potential to improve both quantity and quality of life. Although nutrition is also often a concern, enteral or "forced" feedings are generally not recommended. The decreased food intake may be a necessary result of progressing illness, and excess food may cause discomfort and reduce the quality of life.

Psychiatric Elements

Serious illnesses are accompanied by many stressors, both physical and emotional. Depression and social withdrawal are common, and patients should receive supportive and psychological counseling if needed. All treatment decisions should be discussed openly, and the patient's wishes regarding the acceptance or refusal of care must be respected.

Hospice Care

Hospice care is given to patients with terminal illnesses, usually during their last 6 months of life. It is provided in many settings, including private homes, hospitals, nursing homes, and specially designed hospice facilities. Hospice care focuses less on invasive medical treatments for prolonging life and more on physical and emotional comfort. Hospice care does not encourage euthanasia or assisted suicide, but attempts to provide the support that a patient needs to die comfortably and with dignity.

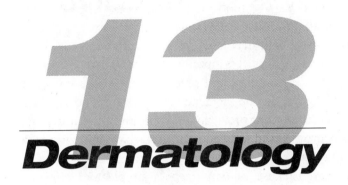

Dermatology

Skin Disorders Secondary to Sun Exposure

Sunburn is an acute reaction to sun overexposure. It may range in severity from mild erythema to severe pain, swelling, and blisters, with constitutional symptoms of fever and even shock.

Effects of chronic sun exposure include wrinkling and precancerous lesions known as actinic keratoses (described later in this chapter). The incidence of squamous and basal cell carcinoma increases in proportion to the amount of previous sun exposure. Melanoma incidence may also increase with sun exposure. Darker-skinned individuals have more melanin, which protects against all types of sun damage, including cancer.

Prevention of these effects through the use of sunscreen is simple and effective. Sunscreens containing para-aminobenzoic acid (PABA) or opaque creams with zinc oxide protect the skin well. Sunscreens are rated on the FDA's sun protection factor (SPF) scale, with a rating of 15 considered adequate protection.

Drug Reactions

Any medication can cause an allergic reaction with cutaneous manifestations. Antibiotics, nonsteroidal anti-inflammatory drugs (NSAIDs), and anticonvulsants are common offenders, but all medications, including nonprescription medicines, must be considered in a careful history. Skin eruptions can vary in severity from a mild maculopapular rash to the potentially lethal **toxic epidermal necrolysis**, in which large areas of epidermis become loosened and detached. The edematous wheals of **urticaria** ("hives") are common, especially with penicillin allergies.

Dermatitis

Contact Dermatitis

There are two types of contact dermatitis. **Primary irritant contact dermatitis** is caused by direct injury to the skin, affects all individuals who contact the irritant, and occurs at the first exposure to the irritant. The vast majority of occupational dermatoses are irritant contact dermatoses, usually resulting from detergents, solvents, and other caustic chemicals. **Allergic contact dermatitis** (ACD) is a type IV delayed hypersensitivity reaction mediated by T cells. It never occurs at first exposure because susceptible individuals must first be sensitized to the agent. Common substances causing ACD are poison oak, poison ivy, ragweed, and nickel.

Effects range from redness to severe swelling and blistering. Itching is common. Distribution of the reaction depends on the area of contact; the extremities and face are commonly affected.

SIGNS & SYMPTOMS

If the history is not diagnostic, patch testing may be useful.

DIAGNOSIS

Remove or avoid the offending substance. An antihistamine for itching and topical or, in severe cases of ACD, systemic corticosteroids may be used.

Seborrheic Dermatitis

Seborrheic dermatitis is a chronic, inflammatory hyperproliferation of the epidermis. It occurs in teens and adults and is generally worse in winter and in times of stress. Mild scalp involvement is called dandruff or, in infants, "cradle cap." Eyelid involvement is called **seborrheic blepharitis.**

Involved skin is erythematous. Greasy yellow scales are typically noted on the scalp, forehead, nasolabial folds, and ears.

Selenium or tar shampoo reduces epidermal turnover, decreasing the severity of the symptoms. Corticosteroid cream may be used on the face. Baby shampoo is usually sufficient to treat cradle cap.

Psoriasis

Psoriasis, a condition of increased proliferation of epidermal tissue, is often familial. Psoriatic arthritis is a condition found in 20% of patients with psoriasis. It is associated with HLA-B27 and a family history of psoriasis. Its symptoms are similar to those of rheumatoid arthritis, but patients are rheumatoid factor (RF)–negative.

Sharply demarcated, salmon-colored papules or plaques covered by silvery scales are typical. Most common locations are the scalp, knees and elbows, intergluteal cleft, and back. Pinpoint bleeding results if scales are removed. Nails are frequently pitted or thickened.

Ultraviolet light, topical corticosteroids, and topical tar may be used to decrease epidermal proliferation. NSAIDs (e.g., indomethacin), phenylbutazone, and methotrexate may be used to control symptoms of psoriatic arthritis.

Decubitus Ulcers

Decubitus ulcers, or pressure sores, result from ischemic damage when tissues are exposed to continuous pressure. They are most commonly seen in patients who do not sense pain and pressure or cannot move to alleviate this pressure (e.g., paralyzed, bedridden, or comatose patients). They may also occur under casts and on the legs of diabetic patients with poor microcirculation. Sores are most frequent over bony prominences, including the sacrum, trochanter, ankles, and heels.

The first sign of pressure sores is redness of the skin. The ulcer may ultimately extend through fat and muscle to bone.

Relieve pressure and keep wounds clean and dry. Severe sores may require surgical debridement and closure.

Change patient's position every 2 hours. Keep skin clean and dry. Water beds, "egg-crate" mattresses, and protective padding at susceptible sites may help. Avoid oversedation and encourage activity. Diabetic patients should be taught how to examine and care for their feet.

Infections

Herpes Simplex

The herpes simplex virus has two types, HSV-1 and HSV-2. These generally cause oral and genital herpes lesions, respectively, though there is considerable overlap. Transmission usually occurs via oral or genital secretions from active and, occasionally, inactive cases. The virus infects its new host, and the viral DNA remains in the neurons of the sensory ganglia, becoming periodically activated by sunlight, illness, or stress. (See Chap. 6 for discussion of genital herpes.)

The most common site of oral herpes lesions is the lower lip. Recurrences are often preceded by a prodrome of local itching or burning. Small, painful vesicles on an erythematous base are characteristic. After a few days, the vesicles crust over and heal.

Microscopic examination of the vesicular fluid using a Tzanck preparation reveals multinucleated giant cells. Viral culture of the fluid is also diagnostic.

Although usually not necessary, acyclovir may shorten the duration of the recurrence.

Chickenpox

Chickenpox is a highly contagious, acute viral illness caused by the varicella-zoster virus. The virus is spread by infectious respiratory droplets and direct contact with skin lesions. Symptoms develop in 2–3 weeks, but communicability begins only 10 days after exposure and continues until skin lesions have crusted over. Epidemics tend to occur in winter.

A prodrome, which becomes more severe with age, includes headache, malaise, and fever and is usually present for 24–36 hours before pruritic skin lesions appear. The typical skin lesion progresses from macule to papule to vesicle before it crusts over. New lesions, which appear in crops as old lesions are crusting over, may continue to appear for 5–6 days. Skin lesions may become secondarily infected. Pneumonia is a complication seen more frequently in adults and immunocompromised patients.

Clinical inspection of the lesions.

In mild cases, symptomatic treatment to control itching is helpful to prevent later scarring. In severe cases or in immunocompromised patients, IV acyclovir may be given.

For exposed newborns and immunocompromised patients, intramuscular varicella-zoster immunoglobulin (VZIG) given within 4 days of exposure may prevent or lessen the severity of disease. A vaccine has recently been approved and may be used more commonly in the future.

Herpes Zoster

Also known as "shingles," this condition is caused by the varicella-zoster virus, which can remain dormant in the sensory nerve root ganglia for years after the patient has chickenpox. Reactivation of the virus characteristically affects only one dermatome. Unlike herpes simplex infections, recurrence is rare. Zoster occurs frequently in the elderly and immunocompromised.

After a 3-day prodrome of fever and malaise, crops of vesicles on an erythematous base appear along one dermatome. The affected area is quite painful. Vesicles begin to scab over after 4–5 days. The most common site of eruption is the thorax; however, herpes zoster ophthalmicus, which results from involvement of the ophthalmic branch of the trigeminal nerve, can have the most serious consequences. In this condition, vesicles on the tip of the nose indicate possible involvement of the cornea and risk to vision. Elderly patients are particularly susceptible to postherpetic neuralgia, which is pain at the site that may last for months or years.

Vesicles in the characteristic distribution are usually diagnostic. Viral culture of the lesion is confirmatory.

Pain medication. Corticosteroids may reduce later postherpetic neuralgia. Acyclovir is used in immunocompromised patients.

Cellulitis

Cellulitis is an acute, spreading infection of the skin and subcutaneous tissues. The most common pathogen is *Streptococcus pyogenes* (group A beta-hemolytic *Streptococcus*). *Staphylococcus aureus* can cause a less extensive cellulitis, usually if an open wound is present. The severe **necrotizing fasciitis** is caused by a mixture of aerobes and anaerobes.

Typically, infection begins on the lower extremities at the site of a break in the skin, though this break may not be evident. The area is erythematous, hot, tender, and edematous. Regional lymphadenopathy may be present. Systemic symptoms, such as fever and chills, tachycardia, and hypotension, may precede cutaneous findings by a few hours. In necrotizing fasciitis, the skin may turn purple, and bullae and dermal gangrene develop.

Leukocytosis.

Diagnosis is based on clinical findings, since culturing the organism is often difficult.

Penicillinase-resistant penicillins (e.g., nafcillin, dicloxacillin) can be used in uncomplicated cases. Necrotizing fasciitis requires broad-spectrum antibiotics and extensive wound debridement. Mortality is 30%.

Carbuncle

A carbuncle is an abscess of the skin and subcutaneous tissue that is created when several follicular infections (called furuncles or boils) coalesce. Carbuncles are most common on the back or nape of the neck. Multiple drainage sites may develop and the patient may be febrile. *S. aureus* is frequently the cause, though gram-negative bacteria may be involved. Treatment is with drainage, culture, and antibiotics if there are systemic signs. Usually, a penicillinase-resistant penicillin or cephalosporin is used.

Abscess

An abscess is a collection of pus, usually from a bacterial infection. Cutaneous abscesses result from implantation of bacteria through breaks in the skin. The most common causative organisms are *S. aureus* and *S. epidermidis*. Perineal abscesses are frequently caused by anaerobic bacteria (e.g., *Peptococcus*, *Bacteroides*). Examination reveals fluctuant soft-tissue swelling surrounded by erythema. Treatment involves incision and drainage, followed by gauze packing. Antibiotics are only necessary if the patient has signs of systemic infection or is immunocompromised or if the abscess is in an area of the face drained by the cavernous sinus. If not properly treated, orbital or central facial abscesses can lead to **cavernous sinus thrombosis**.

Gangrene

Gangrene is tissue necrosis resulting from lack of circulation. The skin is blackened and wrinkled in "dry" gangrene. When bacterial superinfection occurs, "wet" gangrene results, and the tissue oozes fluid.

Gas gangrene results from a wound contaminated with gas-producing anaerobes, usually of the *Clostridium* species. Infection develops hours to days following a severe crushing or penetrating injury. The patient has severe pain, fever, and shock. Crepitus (a crackling sound or sensation) is noted in the subcutaneous tissues, and the wound may have a foul-smelling discharge. X-ray will show gas in the fascial planes. Treatment requires immediate wound debridement and antibiotics.

Dermatophytoses

Dermatophytes are fungi that cause dermatophytoses, also known as tinea or ringworm. These fungi invade dead tissue, including the epidermis, nails, and hair. Common causative organisms include *Microsporum, Trichophyton,* and *Epidermophyton.* Certain types of fungal infections are more common in warm weather and in warm, moist areas of the body, such as between toes and in skin folds. Scalp infections are contagious and primarily affect children.

Tinea corporis (ringworm of the body) and **tinea cruris** ("jock itch") have characteristic round lesions with raised borders that expand peripherally and clear centrally. **Tinea pedis** ("athlete's foot") occurs between the toes and on the sole of the foot. The skin may be scaly or macerated (soft and pulpy). **Tinea unguium** (infected toe nails) are thickened and discolored. **Tinea capitis** (ringworm of the scalp) causes patchy hair loss, with or without scalp inflammation.

KOH preparation showing hyphae and fungal culture are diagnostic.

Topical antifungals (miconazole, clotrimazole) or oral antifungals (griseofulvin) may be used.

Pilonidal Cysts

In pilonidal cysts, a congenital tract exists in the skin of the sacrococcygeal area. This tract is lined with hair and ends in a cavity. Infection of the cavity results in a tender, erythematous pilonidal cyst. Treatment is by incision and drainage, followed by excision of the tract.

Viral Warts

There are 35 different types of human papillomavirus (HPV), all of which can cause epithelial tumors, or viral warts. Some HPV types are associated with malignancies, such as cervical cancer. Warts are contagious and frequently occur at the site of local irritation or trauma. Common warts (**verrucae vulgaris**) are sharply demarcated, rough tumors up to 1 cm in diameter. Color may vary. Plantar warts are common warts on the sole of the foot. They are flat, surrounded by cornified epithelium, and frequently tender. Warts occasionally disappear spontaneously, but chemical or cryotherapy may be used to destroy them.

Neoplasms

Actinic Keratosis

Actinic keratosis is a precancerous lesion that develops on sun-exposed skin and may lead to squamous cell carcinoma. Atypical keratinocytes grow to form a firm, well-marginated, reddish papule with rough, yellow-brown scales. Diagnosis is made by biopsy. Cryotherapy is frequently used to destroy the lesion.

Squamous Cell Carcinoma

A squamous cell carcinoma tumor may arise from normal tissue or from a preexisting actinic keratosis. It occurs on sun-exposed areas of the body and is more common in outdoor workers and frequent sunbathers. Light-skinned individuals are more susceptible.

SIGNS & SYMPTOMS

The tumor is initially a red papule with a crusted surface but later can become nodular, ulcerate, and invade the underlying tissue. Metastasis occurs infrequently.

DIAGNOSIS

Biopsy.

TREATMENT

Excision.

Basal Cell Carcinoma

Basal cell carcinoma is the most common cancer found in humans. Like squamous cell carcinoma, it is found in light-skinned patients on sun-exposed areas.

SIGNS & SYMPTOMS

The typical lesion is a pearly papule with dilated blood vessels (telangiectasia) and a central depression or ulceration. Lesions grow but rarely metastasize.

Biopsy.

Treatment is usually with excision, but radiation, electrocautery, or cryotherapy may be used for better cosmetic results.

Nevi

Pigmented nevi (benign moles) vary widely in size, color, and texture, but they are generally uniform in appearance. Most appear on sun-exposed areas in childhood or adolescence. Half of malignant melanomas arise from melanocytes in moles, so a biopsy should be performed on any mole that enlarges suddenly, changes color, ulcerates, bleeds, or begins to itch or hurt.

Dysplastic nevi are generally larger (5–12 mm in diameter) and more irregular than simple moles. They occur more frequently on unexposed areas of the body and continue to appear into adulthood. The syndrome of **multiple dysplastic nevi** runs in families and is associated with a high risk of melanoma. Dysplastic nevi should be carefully monitored, and the threshold for biopsy should be low. People with dysplastic nevi should avoid sun exposure, as they are at risk for melanoma.

Melanoma

Melanoma is a malignant tumor of melanocytes that may occur in the skin, mucous membranes, eye, or central nervous system. Although four types have been described, the superficial spreading type accounts for 70% of cases. Lesions may arise from preexisting nevi or from normal skin in sun-exposed areas. The prognosis is much worse than for other skin cancers and is correlated with the amount of vertical extension of the tumor. Metastasis occurs to the skin or internal organs with increasing frequency as the lesion invades deeper than 0.76 mm.

The patient may report that a mole has increased in size. The lesion has irregular borders and color. Initially brown or black, later stages may show spots of red, white, or blue. Plaques and nodules may itch, ulcerate, and bleed.

Biopsy, preferably excisional.

Wide excision is the treatment for local disease. Chemotherapy is added if metastasis has occurred.

Hemangiomas

Hemangiomas are benign tumors of hyperplastic blood vessels and are present in one-third of newborns. They are either congenital or occur shortly after birth. There are three types of hemangiomas. A **nevus flammeus** (port wine stain—think Mikhail Gorbachev) is a flat purple lesion that usually does not fade with time. Laser treatment is used with some success. **Capillary hemangiomas** (strawberry marks) are raised, bright-red lesions that usually regress spontaneously by age 5. Treatment with prednisone is indicated only when the lesion is obstructing the eye, urethra, or anus. **Cavernous hemangiomas** are raised red or purple lesions created by enlarged vascular spaces. Prednisone or surgical excision are treatment options.

14

Musculoskeletal and Connective Tissue Disorders

Health Maintenance

Exercise, Fitness, and Physical Conditioning

With regular exercise, a "training effect" occurs, in which the body adapts to new physical and metabolic demands placed on it by increasing its capacity to meet these demands. The particular type of physical conditioning that occurs depends on the type of exercise performed (e.g., weight-lifting increases strength, whereas running increases endurance). Moderate-intensity exercise has demonstrated benefits for patients with coronary heart disease, adult-onset diabetes, osteoporosis, and other medical conditions. Many individuals who exercise say that the most beneficial aspect of regular physical activity is an improved psychological status, including less anxiety, less depression, and more self-confidence.

Weight Reduction

To lose weight, a patient must take in fewer calories than he or she burns. People who include exercise in their weight loss programs are more likely to maintain their optimal weight successfully. Calories are burned during exercise, but the metabolic rate remains higher even after exercise has stopped. As a result, people who exercise burn more calories than sedentary people both while they exercise and while at rest. (See Obesity in Chap. 1.)

Inherited, Congenital, and Developmental Disorders

Congenital Hip Dislocation

Congenital hip dislocation occurs when the femoral head is partially or completely displaced from the acetabulum. Dislocations may be unilateral or bilateral. Since dislocations may be difficult to detect at birth, periodic exams should be performed throughout the first year of life.

The thigh cannot be completely abducted to the surface of the exam table when the hip and knee are flexed. This maneuver causes a palpable "clunk" as the femoral head pops into the acetabulum. ("Clicks" are more common, less significant, and usually disappear within a few months.) If the dislocation is unilateral, the skin folds of the thighs may be asymmetric.

X-rays are difficult to interpret and are only helpful if they confirm the clinical suspicion.

The hip must be held in an abducted, laterally rotated position. A large, padded diaper may be sufficient for this purpose, though other more effective devices exist. This position encourages the acetabulum to form normally. If treatment is delayed, permanent deformity can result.

Phocomelia

Phocomelia is a developmental anomaly characterized by the absence of the proximal portion of the arms or legs, so that the hands or feet are attached to the trunk by a small, irregularly shaped bone. The sedative thalidomide, which was prescribed in Europe in the 1950s and early 1960s, caused an epidemic of babies with this condition. This is an FDA success story, as thalidomide was never approved for use in the United States.

Osteochondritis

Osteochondritis is the inflammation of both bone and cartilage. Osteochondritis can vary greatly in location and etiology; however, a common presentation in active adolescents is **Osgood-Schlatter disease**, an osteochondritis of the tibial tubercle. It is thought to be due to continuous traction on the immature epiphyseal insertion by the patellar tendon.

In Osgood-Schlatter disease, pain, swelling, and tenderness occur at the site of the patellar tendon insertion.

X-ray may show fragmentation of the tibial tubercle.

Patients should avoid excessive activity, particularly deep knee bends, until the condition resolves. The course is usually several weeks to months. Immobilization and surgery are necessary only in extreme cases.

Slipped Capital Femoral Epiphysis

In slipped capital femoral epiphysis, the femoral head literally slips with respect to the femoral shaft. The condition is most common in overweight teen-agers.

The onset of symptoms is gradual. Hip stiffness leads to limping, which is followed by hip pain that radiates down the anteromedial thigh to the knee. The leg is externally rotated.

X-ray shows widening of the epiphyseal line or posterior and inferior displacement of the femoral head. Early diagnosis is crucial because avascular necrosis may develop if the blood supply to the femoral head is disrupted.

Surgical correction.

Infections

Osteomyelitis

Osteomyelitis is an infection of the bone that may develop locally, by extension from a nearby infection site, or via hematogenous spread. Local spread is usually initiated by a fracture, surgery, bite, or other trauma. Hematogenously spread osteomyelitis generally occurs in bones with rich blood supplies, such as long bones and vertebral bodies. Before puberty, infection usually occurs in the metaphysis (shaft) of long bones because the epiphysis is protected by the epiphyseal plate. Common infecting organisms are *Staphylococcus aureus* and *Pseudomonas*. In patients with sickle cell anemia, *Salmonella* osteomyelitis is most common.

Pain, tenderness, redness, and swelling are present over the involved bone. Fever and chills may be present in acute presentations. Subacute and chronic osteomyelitis are subtle and may escape detection until a sinus draining to the skin develops.

Leukocytosis and elevated erythrocyte sedimentation rate (ESR).

X-rays are not helpful in diagnosing early disease. Radionuclide bone scans will show the lesion within 72 hours of clinical onset. Needle biopsy followed by culture and Gram's stain are necessary to select appropriate antibiotics.

Drainage of pus and debridement of dead tissue are required, followed by a long course (4–6 weeks) of organism-specific antibiotics.

Septic Arthritis

Septic arthritis, an infectious monoarthritis, is usually caused by hematogenous spread of microorganisms. *S. aureus* is the most common causative organism, except in sexually active young people, in whom *Neisseria gonorrhoeae* is more frequent. Gram-negative organisms account for only 10% of cases and usually occur in patients with diabetes, cancer, or other underlying illnesses. Joints with preexisting arthritis are particularly susceptible to infection.

The affected joint is warm, red, tender, and swollen. Movement causes intense pain. Fever is common, but the patient may or may not appear acutely ill.

Synovial fluid has markedly elevated leukocyte counts, and the organism may be cultured from this fluid. Blood cultures and Gram's stains of synovial fluid sometimes reveal the organism but cannot be relied on.

Use ceftriaxone if gonococcal arthritis is suspected. Otherwise, a penicillinase-resistant penicillin (e.g., nafcillin) should be used. An aminoglycoside should be added if the patient is susceptible to gram-negative infections.

Lyme Disease

Named after the town in Connecticut where it was first described, Lyme disease is caused by the spirochete *Borrelia burgdorferi*, which is transmitted to humans by the *Ixodes* tick. The disease has a variety of presentations and may affect the joints, heart, or nervous system.

Within a month of being bitten, the patient develops an expanding, erythematous rash with central clearing (**erythema chronicum migrans**). Accompanying symptoms include fever, chills, fatigue, arthralgias, and headache. Several months later, the patient may develop mono- or oligoarticular arthritis, usually in the larger joints, particularly the knees. Meningoencephalitis and myocarditis are other potential late complications of untreated disease.

In early stages, diagnosis relies on clinical presentation, although blood cultures are occasionally positive. Later, immunologic assays, such as the enzyme-linked immunosorbent assay (ELISA), will detect antispirochete antibodies. Synovial fluid culture is not helpful in diagnosis.

Choice and duration of antibiotic depends on clinical presentation, but doxycycline, tetracycline, or amoxicillin are typically used.

Metabolic and Nutritional Disorders

Osteoporosis

Osteoporosis is a progressive decrease in the mass of otherwise normal bone. This condition is most common in postmenopausal white and Asian women. Smoking, excessive alcohol intake, sedentary lifestyle, and low estrogen levels all predispose to disease.

Secondary causes of osteoporosis include long-term corticosteroid therapy, Cushing's syndrome, hyperparathyroidism, and hyperthyroidism. It is estimated that 1–2 million fractures in the United States each year are due to osteoporosis.

The disease is usually asymptomatic until a fracture occurs. Hip and wrist (Colles') fractures are common. Vertebral compression fractures cause back pain, loss of height, and kyphosis.

Quantitative CT and photon absorptiometry studies show decreased bone density. Serum calcium and phosphorus are usually normal.

Sufficient dietary calcium, weight-bearing exercise, and estrogen all help slow bone loss. Etidronate inhibits osteoclast activity and is used in men and in women who cannot take estrogen.

Bone density is built up until roughly age 35. Thereafter, bone is lost with age. Prevention of osteoporosis involves maximizing total bone density and slowing bone loss. These goals are achieved with high dietary calcium, weight-bearing exercise, and, if necessary, exogenous estrogen.

Gout

Gout is a peripheral arthritis that results from the deposition of sodium urate crystals in the joints. Primary gout is usually idiopathic, although patients with renal disease are predisposed due to decreased urate clearance. The vast majority of patients are middle-aged men.

The typical presentation is the sudden nocturnal onset of excruciating pain and swelling in a single joint, most commonly the metatarsal joint of the big toe (**podagra**). The joint is exquisitely tender, and the overlying skin is tense and dark red or purple. The patient may also have fever, chills, or malaise. Initial attacks resolve spontaneously, but later attacks may last for weeks and involve multiple joints. Half of patients with untreated gout will develop chronic tophaceous gout, in which urate crystals are deposited in the joints, ears, or other surfaces. Permanent deformity results.

The diagnosis is suspected in a patient with the typical presentation and a high serum uric acid level. If necessary, the diagnosis is confirmed by analyzing the synovial fluid and finding negatively birefringent needle-shaped crystals within leukocytes. X-rays show tophi as "punched out" radiolucent areas.

Colchicine or NSAIDs are used to treat an acute attack. Preventive measures include limiting alcohol and foods high in purines (liver, sardines, anchovies) and taking colchicine daily. Allopurinol inhibits the formation of uric acid and is used in conditions of high nucleic acid turnover, such as leukemia or psoriasis.

Pseudogout

Pseudogout is a condition caused by inflammation due to calcium pyrophosphate dihydrate crystals in the synovial fluid. Although the overall presentation is similar to that of gout, the knee is most commonly affected, and positively birefringent crystals are found in the synovial fluid. Colchicine can be used for prevention and for acute attacks.

Rickets

Rickets is a metabolic bone disease in children resulting from vitamin D deficiency. (The same deficiency with differing clinical effects is called **osteomalacia** in adults.) Lack of exposure to sunlight and poor dietary intake are necessary for clinical disease to develop in otherwise normal patients. Defects in vitamin D metabolism may also predispose to disease. Clinical disease results when the epiphyseal cartilage of growing bones becomes hypertrophic without calcification.

In young children, walking is delayed, and bowlegs and kyphoscoliosis may occur. In older children and teen-agers, walking causes pain, and bowlegs may develop in extreme cases.

Very low levels of the vitamin D metabolites $25\text{-}(OH)_2D_3$ and $1,25\text{-}(OH)_2D_3$ are detected in the serum. Parathyroid hormone (PTH) is elevated, serum phosphorus is low, and calcium may be low or normal.

Vitamin D, calcium, and phosphorus supplementation.

Degenerative Disorders

Degenerative Joint Disease

Degenerative joint disease, or osteoarthritis, affects all of us lucky enough to reach age 70. Joint cartilage wears away with age and exposes subchondral bone, which then proliferates to form bone spurs, or osteophytes. There is no associated inflammation.

A gradual onset of pain in the affected joint(s) and increasing morning stiffness is the most common presentation. Distal and proximal interphalangeal joints are commonly affected, as are hips, knees, and joints of the cervical and lumbar spine. Deformities of the distal interphalangeal joints (**Heberden's nodes**) and proximal interphalangeal joints (**Bouchard's nodes**) are caused by bony protuberances at the joint.

X-rays show osteophytes, irregular narrowing of the joint space, and increased radiologic density of subchondral bone.

Joint rest, local heat, and analgesics. Weight reduction may be helpful.

Degenerative Disk Disease

The intervertebral disk consists of the nucleus pulposus, which is surrounded by the annulus fibrosus (Fig. 14-1). Degenerative changes allow the nucleus to herniate posteriorly or posterolaterally, through the annulus fibrosus, and impinge on the spinal cord or roots. This occurs most commonly in the lumbosacral region, but it may occur in the cervical region as well. Thoracic herniations are rare.

Pain is felt both locally and along the distribution of the affected nerve root. In lumbosacral herniations, **sciatica** (pain down the leg in the L4–S3 distribution) is characteristic (Fig. 14-2). Pain is aggravated by movement and by the Valsalva maneuver, in which increased pressure of the subarachnoid space is transmitted to the herniated disk during coughing or straining. Passive straight leg lifts increase pain in lumbosacral herniations. There may be muscle weakness and depressed reflexes at the affected nerve level (Table 14-1). The **cauda equina syndrome** is caused by a large midline posterior herniation that compresses the cauda equina. Urinary and bowel incontinence and bilateral leg weakness are classic symptoms.

CT scan or myelography (x-ray of the spinal cord following injection of contrast medium into the subarachnoid space) is useful in demonstrating the disk protrusion. Electromyography (EMG) will help assess nerve damage.

Conservative approaches include bed rest, local heat, NSAIDs, and physical therapy. Surgery may be necessary for unrelenting pain, progressive neurologic impairment, or the cauda equina syndrome.

Inflammatory and Immunologic Disorders

Polymyalgia Rheumatica

Polymyalgia rheumatica is an inflammatory connective tissue disorder that primarily affects older patients, particularly women. There is a strong association with giant cell (temporal) arteritis.

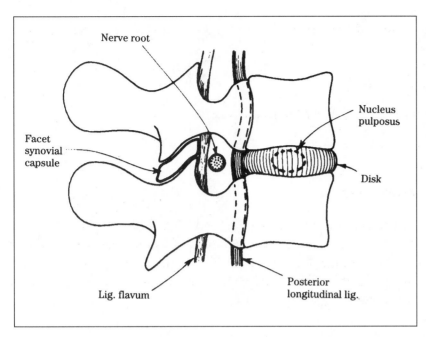

Fig. 14-1. Intervertebral disk and surrounding structures. (From MA Samuels. *Manual of Neurologic Therapeutics*, Fifth Edition. Boston: Little, Brown, 1995.)

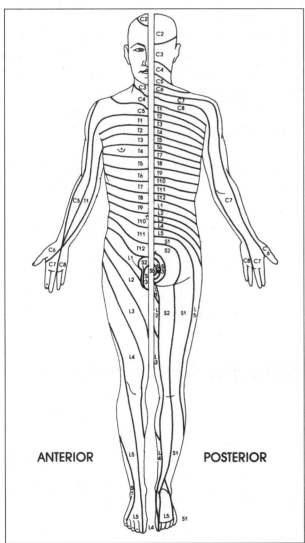

Fig. 14-2. Sensory dermatomes. (From A Guberman. *An Introduction to Clinical Neurology.* Boston: Little, Brown, 1994.)

Table 14-1. Signs and symptoms of nerve root compression

Nerve Root	Location of pain	Muscle weakness	Diminished reflex	Sensory deficit
C5	Shoulder, outer aspect of upper arm	Deltoid	Biceps	Shoulder
C6	Shoulder, scapula, inner aspect of upper arm	Biceps, wrist extension	Brachioradialis	Lateral forearm
C7	Shoulder, scapula, back of upper arm, forearm	Triceps, wrist flexor	Triceps	Middle finger (inconsistent)
C8	Scapula, back of entire arm, medial forearm	Finger flexion	—	Medial forearm, ring and little finger
L4	Hip, front of thigh, knee	Quadriceps, foot inversion	Knee jerk	Medial leg and foot
L5	Outer thigh and leg, dorsal foot	Extension of great toe (patient cannot heel-walk), dorsiflexion of foot	—	Lateral leg and dorsum of foot
S1	Back of thigh and leg, heel	Plantar flexion and eversion of foot, gastrocnemius, gluteus maximus	Ankle jerk	Lateral and plantar surface of foot

Symmetric pain in the neck, shoulder, and/or pelvic girdle muscles. Morning stiffness is so extreme that patients may have difficulty getting out of bed. Swelling may occur in only one or two joints, unlike rheumatoid arthritis. There is no muscle weakness, unlike polymyositis. If temporal arteritis is present, the patient may have headaches, blurred vision, jaw claudication, or blindness.

Anemia is common.

A very elevated ESR is characteristic. Rheumatoid factor (RF) is negative. The pattern of illness, including morning stiffness and prompt response to corticosteroids, confirms the diagnosis. If temporal arteritis is present, biopsy will show giant cell arteritis.

If temporal arteritis is suspected, high-dose corticosteroids must be started immediately to avoid blindness and ophthalmologic consultation is necessary. Improvement is seen within 36 hours. Most patients may be tapered off steroids gradually, but some continue to take small doses for years.

Systemic Lupus Erythematosus

Systemic lupus erythematosus is a multisystem autoimmune disorder in which the body makes antibodies to its own nuclei and to double-stranded DNA. Most manifestations occur because antigen-antibody complexes trigger inflammatory responses in various locations of the body. This disease occurs predominantly in young women and is more common in blacks. The most common causes of death in lupus are infection, nephritis, and central nervous system disease.

Certain drugs, including procainamide, hydralazine, isoniazid, methyldopa, quinidine, and chlorpromazine, can cause lupus-like syndromes, which are reversible after discontinuing the medication.

Presentation varies widely and may involve all body systems. Most patients have constitutional symptoms and cutaneous and musculoskeletal manifestations. Other clinical effects are listed in Table 14-2.

If renal disease is present, there may be proteinuria and elevated blood urea nitrogen (BUN) and creatinine. If anemia is present, check for hemolytic anemia with a Coombs' test.

Clinical presentation and serum antibody tests. Antinuclear antibodies (ANA) are found in more than 95% of lupus patients, but they may be found in other autoimmune diseases as well (i.e., the test is sensitive, but not specific to lupus). Anti-dsDNA antibodies are found in only 50–75% of cases, but they are not found in other disorders (i.e., the test is not as sensitive, but it is very specific to lupus).

Table 14-2. Clinical manifestations of systemic lupus erythematosus

Constitutional	Fatigue, fever, weight loss
Mucocutaneous	"Butterfly rash" (erythematous rash on bridge of nose and cheeks), discoid rash (erythematous patches), cutaneus vasculitis, Raynaud's phenomenon, alopecia, oral ulcers
Musculoskeletal	Arthritis (distribution similar to RA, including symmetric involvement of PIP, MCP, wrists, knees, and feet), morning stiffness, myalgias
Renal	Immune-complex glomerulonephritis, interstitial nephritis
Neurologic	Headaches, psychosis, seizures, strokes, aseptic meningitis
Cardiovascular	Pericarditis, myocarditis, verrucous endocarditis, coronary vasculitis
Pulmonary	Pleuritis, pneumonitis, pulmonary vascular obstruction
Gastrointestinal	Abdominal pain, vomiting
Ocular	Conjunctivitis, episcleritis
Hematologic	Anemia of chronic disease, autoimmune hemolytic anemia, leukopenia, thrombocytopenia, circulating anticoagulant

TREATMENT

Avoidance of sunlight reduces cutaneous effects. Control joint pain with NSAIDs or hydroxychloroquine, an antimalarial medication. Corticosteroids or other immunosuppressants should be used when necessary to control systemic manifestations.

Polymyositis and Dermatomyositis

Polymyositis is a disease involving inflammation of skeletal muscle. One-third of patients also have cutaneous involvement, in which case the disease is called dermatomyositis. One-third develop myocarditis or cardiac conduction defects. A coexisting malignancy is present in 10% of cases.

SIGNS & SYMPTOMS

Symmetric, progressive, proximal muscle weakness develops. Hips and shoulders are affected first, and the typical first complaint is difficulty climbing stairs. Muscle atrophy or tenderness may also be present. Patients with dermatomyositis have a red, scaly rash and may have a violet discoloration of their upper eyelids. This "heliotrope" rash is pathognomonic of the disease.

LABS

Elevation of serum muscle enzymes (CPK, SGOT, SGPT, LDH, aldolase).

DIAGNOSIS

Electromyogram shows spontaneous fibrillations. Muscle biopsy shows inflammatory cells and muscle degeneration.

TREATMENT

High-dose corticosteroids, which can be tapered over many months. Monitor improvement by measuring muscle enzymes. Search for occult malignancy.

Rheumatoid Arthritis

Rheumatoid arthritis (RA) is a chronic inflammatory disorder in which the synovial joints are infiltrated by inflammatory cells, resulting in progressive destruction of the cartilage and bone. Middle-aged women are most often affected.

RA is a symmetric polyarthritis. Diffuse joint pain and swelling are common. Any synovial joint may be affected, but the PIP and MCP joints of the hands and the MTP joints of the feet are often the first to be involved. The DIP joints are seldom affected. Advanced cases will show a typical "swan neck" deformity (flexed DIP and hyperextended PIP) and the "boutonniere" deformity (flexed PIP). Extra-articular manifestations include subcutaneous nodules (common on pressure sites), pleuritis, pericarditis, and scleritis.

Rheumatoid factor (antibodies against the Fc portion of IgG) is present in 70% of patients. ANA is found in half of patients. Elevated ESR and normocytic, normochromic anemia is common. X-rays may show soft-tissue swelling or periarticular osteoporosis, joint space narrowing, and marginal erosions.

A number of diagnostic criteria involving the presentation and lab results must be met for the diagnosis to be made formally.

The first-line drug is aspirin or another NSAID. Second-line drugs are methotrexate, antimalarials, or gold salt. Immunosuppressive agents are third-line drugs. Corticosteroids may be used to control flare-ups but should not be used on a chronic basis.

Ankylosing Spondylitis

Ankylosing spondylitis (AS) is an inflammatory disease of the axial skeleton and large peripheral joints in which involvement of the sacroiliac joint is considered diagnostic. The disease is frequently mild, but it can result in permanent, extreme kyphosis. Most common in white men, AS is strongly associated with HLA-B27.

Insidious onset of back pain, often nocturnal, with morning stiffness is the typical presentation. Patients unconsciously ease back pain by bending over slightly, so some absence of normal lordosis is seen. Some patients have self-limiting episodes of uveitis, an inflammation of the vascular tunic of the eye.

Elevated ESR. Absence of both RF and ANA.

Presence of sacroiliitis on x-ray. The classic "bamboo spine," with vertebral squaring, bony outgrowths, and paraspinal ligament calcification, is a late finding.

Indomethacin or another NSAID controls pain and allows the patient to do maintenance exercises. Strengthening exercises and diligent attention to posture may help prevent permanent deformity.

Bursitis

A bursa is a fluid-filled sac located at sites of friction between tendons, muscles, or bones. Bursitis is the chronic or acute inflammation of the bursa. Bursitis of the shoulder (subdeltoid or subacromial) is most common, though any bursa may be involved. Chronic overuse, infection, inflammatory arthritis, gout, or rheumatoid arthritis may be the cause.

Pain and limitation of movement are common. Swelling and redness are seen if the bursa is superficial or if a bacterial infection is present.

Immobilization and NSAIDs. Use antibiotics if infection is present. Aspiration of the bursa and injection of corticosteroids and anesthetic may help relieve symptoms. Exercises to improve range of motion and strength can be started when symptoms subside.

Tendonitis

Tendonitis is inflammation of the tendon and/or tendon sheath (tenosynovitis). Trauma, strain, or excessive exercise are the most common causes. Incidence is higher in older patients, presumably because of decreased blood flow in the tendons, which makes the tendons more susceptible to microtrauma. In young adults, disseminated gonococcal infection may cause gonococcal tenosynovitis or gonococcal arthritis.

Pain with movement and tenderness along the tendon. The tendon sheath may be visibly swollen due to fluid accumulation. If it is dry, friction rubs may be felt or heard with a stethoscope.

Immobilization, hot or cold compresses (whichever the patient prefers), and NSAIDs relieve discomfort. Injection of corticosteroids into the tendon sheath may also help. Increase exercise as tolerated. Gonococcal infection must be treated with appropriate antibiotics.

Fibromyalgia

Fibromyalgia is a syndrome of unknown etiology that causes pain in muscles and tendons. No histologic abnormality has been identified. The disorder is most commonly seen in middle-aged women.

Diffuse, achy muscle pain, poor sleep, and morning stiffness are common complaints. "Trigger points" are present, which, when palpated, reproduce the pain. Anxiety, depression, and irritable bowel syndrome may be associated.

Once other systemic diseases have been ruled out, diagnosis is made on the basis of the symptoms.

Stretching exercises, heat, massage, and biofeedback may be tried. Trigger points may be injected with anesthetics. Psychotherapy and antidepressants are sometimes useful.

Neoplasms

Osteosarcoma

Osteosarcoma is a tumor most common in rapidly growing teen-age boys. Although it can occur in many bones, the most frequent sites are the distal femur and proximal tibia. Metastases occur in the lung.

Pain, swelling, and limitation of movement of the knee or other involved joint.

X-ray shows bone destruction and a soft-tissue mass.

Biopsy is necessary.

Aggressive chemotherapy and surgery, either "limb-sparing" or amputation.

Bone Metastases

The most common cancers that metastasize to bone are carcinomas of the breast, lung, prostate, kidney, and thyroid. Symptoms of bony metastases may occur before a primary tumor is suspected. While advanced lesions will be visible on x-ray, early bony metastases may be identified only by using whole-body bone scans with radioisotopes. Bone biopsy may help identify the primary tumor, and treatment will depend on this identification.

Pulmonary Osteoarthropathy

Pulmonary osteoarthropathy is a paraneoplastic disorder (i.e., a physiologic disturbance that is unrelated to the primary tumor, metastases, or treatment). This disorder involves inflammation of the periosteum, with subperiosteal formation of new bone. It occurs in patients with lung cancer (except small cell carcinoma), and clubbing of the fingers is also frequently present. Although patients typically complain of joint pain, it is the bones themselves that are affected. The distal long bones of the arms and legs are most commonly involved, and the sites may be tender and swollen. Surgical vagotomy is sometimes effective treatment.

Miscellaneous Disorders

Shoulder-Hand Syndrome

Shoulder-hand syndrome is a rare disorder thought to be caused by sympathetic nervous stimulation. The syndrome is characterized by pain and stiffness in the shoulder, along with pain, swelling, and vasomotor changes in the hands and arms. It develops weeks to months after a myocardial infarction or other acute illness. Treatment is with physical therapy, analgesics, and corticosteroids.

Dupuytren's Contracture

Thickening and contracture of the palmar fascia results in limitation of finger extension in Dupuytren's contracture. This condition typically occurs in middle-aged and older men and is more common in alcoholics, invalids, epileptics, and patients with tuberculosis, diabetes, and liver disease. Diagnosis is by inspection and palpation of the palm. Surgery is required in severe cases.

Carpal Tunnel Syndrome

Neuropathy in carpal tunnel syndrome is caused by compression of the median nerve as it passes through the carpal tunnel. More common in women, this syndrome is associated with occupations that require repetitive hand movements, pregnancy, acromegaly, and myxedema.

Numbness, tingling, and pain occur in the first three digits of the hand. Gentle percussion of the palmar longus tendon of the wrist causes tingling (Tinel's sign). Placing the dorsal surface of the hands together with wrists flexed at 90 degrees for 60 seconds exacerbates symptoms (Phalen test).

History and physical, as described. Decreases in nerve conduction can be measured.

Physical therapy and corticosteroid injection into the tunnel. Surgery may be necessary.

Paget's Disease of Bone

Paget's disease is a skeletal disorder seen in adults. Overactive osteoclasts produce osteolytic lesions, and overactive osteoblasts fill these lesions with improperly formed bone. Because the bone lesions are highly vascular, high-output cardiac failure may develop. Osteosarcoma occurs in rare instances.

The disease is most often asymptomatic. Symptoms may include bone pain, headaches, hearing loss, and increased skull size ("Doc, my hats don't fit anymore!"). The patient may have a visibly enlarged skull with rounded forehead (frontal "bossing"), bowed thighs, and a shortened spine due to vertebral flattening, giving the appearance of long arms.

Serum alkaline phosphatase is elevated. Calcium and phosphorus levels are normal.

The disease is often diagnosed incidentally on x-ray. Early in the course of the disease, x-rays show osteolytic lesions. Later, bone with chaotic architecture or overgrowth may be seen. The skull may have a characteristic "cotton wool" appearance.

No treatment is needed for asymptomatic cases. NSAIDs may reduce pain. Orthopedic appliances or surgery may be needed to improve gait disturbances. Because this is a chronic condition requiring lifelong treatment, chemotherapy to reduce bone cell activity is reserved for extreme exacerbations.

Eosinophilic Granuloma

Eosinophilic granuloma is a disorder of unknown etiology typically occurring between ages 20 and 40. Granuloma formation in the bone involves proliferation of histiocytes, eosinophilic infiltration, and fibrosis. These osteolytic lesions may be painful or asymptomatic. Some patients have lung infiltration as well. Diagnosis is by x-ray and biopsy. Local radiation can be used for treatment, but multiple lesions are associated with a poor prognosis.

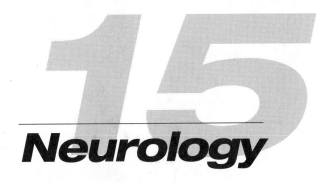

Neurology

(continued)

Blindness

Visual acuity of 20/400 or worse with the best possible correction (e.g., glasses) is the legal definition of blindness. In the United States, prophylaxis of newborns with silver nitrate to prevent gonococcal infection has effectively eliminated a major cause of blindness. Another preventable form of blindness, amblyopia (misalignment of the eyes), can often be corrected early in life with glasses or surgery. Finally, congenital cataracts, which are associated with a number of prenatal infections such as rubella, may be prevented or treated early to maximize useful vision.

In adults, the major causes of blindness are glaucoma, diabetic retinopathy, cataracts, and macular degeneration. These disorders are discussed in more detail below.

Open-Angle Glaucoma

Glaucoma refers to increased intraocular pressure, resulting in varying degrees of visual loss. Open-angle glaucoma is the most prevalent form of the disease. It is characterized by a gradual rise in intraocular pressure, leading to bilateral visual loss. The cause is unknown. Open-angle glaucoma is more common in the elderly, diabetics, and African-Americans. It tends to be familial.

SIGNS & SYMPTOMS

Patients are asymptomatic until late stages of the disorder, when they experience gradual loss of peripheral vision, resulting in "tunnel vision." Eventually, central vision is lost as well. Patients may complain of "halos" around lights if the intraocular pressure is severely increased. On examination, cupping of the optic disc may be noted.

DIAGNOSIS

Tonometry (pressure testing), optic nerve visualization, and visual field testing confirm the diagnosis. One elevated pressure reading does not confirm the presence of glaucoma, since intraocular pressure varies throughout the day.

TREATMENT

Beta-adrenergic antagonists, such as timolol and pilocarpine, must be used daily. These medications decrease the production of aqueous humor, reducing the intraocular pressure. If medication is not effective, widening of the drainage canal by surgical or laser procedures may be necessary.

PREVENTION

All persons over age 40 should undergo tonometry and careful ophthalmoscopic evaluation every 3–5 years. African-Americans and individuals with a family history of glaucoma should begin testing at an earlier age.

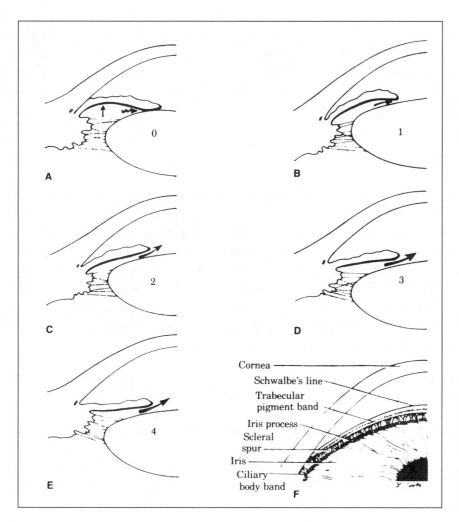

Fig. 15-1. Ocular anatomy in open-angle and closed-angle glaucoma. (Adapted from Anterior Chamber Angle Estimation Card, Allergan Pharmaceutical Co., Irvine, CA.)

Closed-Angle Glaucoma

Closed-angle glaucoma is characterized by the rapid onset of increased intraocular pressure due to a blockage of the aqueous drainage of the eye (Fig. 15-1). Approximately 1% of the population, predominantly Asians, elderly persons, and people with hyperopia (far-sightedness), have preexisting narrowness of the anterior chamber angle; however, the vast majority of these individuals do not develop disease. Angle closure may occur with pupillary dilation (e.g., sitting in a darkened room or receiving a pharmacologic mydriatic during an eye exam).

Severe eye pain, blurred vision, and "halos" around lights are often accompanied by nausea and abdominal pain. The cause of the abdominal manifestations are unclear. On exam, patients have a reddened eye, upper lid edema, a steamy-appearing cornea, and a dilated, nonreactive pupil. Increased pressure also causes the eye to seem "hard" if palpated.

Tonometry reveals a markedly increased intraocular pressure.

Administration of oral glycerin, carbonic anhydrase, or mannitol will rapidly reduce intraocular pressure. Frequent administration of beta-adrenergic antagonists, which produce miosis, is also indicated. Permanent correction involves laser or surgical iridectomy and is usually performed on the unaffected eye as well. Untreated acute-angle glaucoma usually results in permanent loss of vision within days.

Diabetic Retinopathy

The development of diabetic retinopathy is related to the duration of diabetes and is seen frequently in type I diabetes. Hypertension may hasten the onset. Damage to the retinal vasculature, including microaneurysms, ischemic changes, and neovascularization with abnormal vessels, is primarily responsible for the resulting visual loss.

Vision is normal until later stages, when patients complain of decreased visual acuity. Other frequent symptoms include black spots, "cobwebs," and flashing lights. Ophthalmoscopic examination reveals cotton-wool spots (infarctions of the vessel walls), neovascularization (new tortuous blood vessels), and hard, yellow exudates (chronic capillary damage).

The above physical exam findings in a diabetic patient suggest the diagnosis.

Laser photocoagulation or vitrectomy may decrease or eliminate neovascularization and hemorrhage.

Good control of glucose levels and hypertension may delay the onset of diabetic retinopathy but cannot reverse preexisting damage. Diabetic patients should receive annual ophthalmologic exams to monitor and treat asymptomatic development of retinal changes.

Cataracts

Cataracts are a painless clouding of the lens. They are often bilateral. Cataracts may occur congenitally, following trauma, with certain medications, or with increasing age. Age is the most common cause. Cataract development is also associated with smoking and alcohol use.

Patients complain of painless and progressive blurring of vision, often over several months. Gray opacities of the lenses may be seen with ophthalmoscopic or slit-lamp exam. Red reflex may be absent.

The above signs and symptoms suggest the diagnosis.

Glasses may be helpful in early stages, but lens extraction and replacement surgery provide definitive treatment and are performed routinely.

Senile Macular Degeneration

Senile macular degeneration is the primary cause of vision loss in the elderly. It is caused by atrophic degeneration or leakage of the retinal vessels, resulting in scarring and fibrosis of the retina. It is usually bilateral and may be hereditary.

Patients typically experience a gradual loss of visual acuity, especially of central vision, although acute changes occur in some cases. Fundoscopic examination shows hemorrhagic or pigmented areas in the macule.

Fluoroscein angiography may demonstrate the presence of neovascular membranes (Bruch's membrane).

Laser photocoagulation may arrest further loss of vision.

Eye Infection

Conjunctivitis

Acute inflammation of the conjunctiva (the mucosal surface of the eye and eyelid) is typically caused by viruses, bacteria, or allergens. Adenoviruses are the most common cause, followed by staphylococci, streptococci, and *Haemophilus* species. *Neisseria gonorrhoeae* and *Chlamydia trachomatis* may be involved in more severe infections. Conjunctivitis is highly transmissible and can develop after contact with infected hands, towels, and handkerchiefs.

Copious discharge, accompanied by mild discomfort with little or no visual blurring, is the common presentation. On exam, the conjunctiva appears inflamed and injected. Bacterial conjunctivitis is accompanied by purulent discharge.

Gram's stains and culture of the discharge may provide the diagnosis of bacterial conjunctivitis. Most cases are diagnosed by the history and examination findings.

The majority of cases are self-limiting, but sulfonamide ointments may speed recovery of bacterial conjunctivitis. Conjunctivitis caused by allergy may be treated with steroid solutions. The patient should wash his or her hands frequently to prevent the spread of infection.

Uveitis

The uveitis group of disorders is characterized by inflammation of the uveal tract (iris, ciliary body, and choroid layer). Multiple diseases are associated with uveitis, including collagen vascular diseases (e.g., Reiter's syndrome and rheumatoid arthritis), infections (e.g., cytomegalovirus, syphilis, and tuberculosis), gastrointestinal diseases (e.g., Crohn's disease and ulcerative colitis), and diseases of unknown etiology (e.g., sarcoidosis).

Subtle changes in vision, such as haziness or floating spots, are characteristic. Photophobia and redness are seen in cases of iridocyclitis. A "salt and pepper" fundus is characteristic of syphilis.

Slit-lamp examination shows cells with keratin precipitates on the corneal endothelium.

Topical or systemic corticosteroids may be helpful. Patients should also be evaluated for signs of related systemic diseases, such as tuberculosis or rheumatoid arthritis.

Retinal Disorders

Central Retinal Artery Occlusion

Occlusion of the central retinal artery presents as the sudden, painless loss of sight in one eye. Common causes include thromboembolic disease and temporal arteritis. Examination may show a pale fundus with a "cherry-red spot" fovea and the "boxcar" appearance of veins. Emergency referral to an ophthalmologist is essential. Treatment includes oxygen, ocular massage, and fluid removal from the eye.

Central Retinal Vein Occlusion

Occlusion of the central retinal vein typically occurs in elderly patients with atherosclerosis, but it is also associated with diabetes, glaucoma, and hypertension. Unilateral painless loss of sight is also seen with this disorder, but it is more gradual in onset than in arterial occlusion. Examination shows swelling of the optic disk, cotton-wool spots, and tortuous, dilated veins. There is no widely accepted treatment; however, emergent ophthalmologic evaluation is important to distinguish this from any treatable causes of visual loss.

Retinal Detachment

The retina may separate from the pigment layer of the epithelium due to chronic damage (e.g., diabetic retinopathy) or following acute trauma. The accompanying unilateral, painless loss of vision is generally described as a "curtain" coming down over the eye. Fundoscopic exam reveals a gray retina hanging within the vitreous humor. Treatment includes laser photocoagulation and retinal reattachment.

Retinoblastoma

Retinoblastoma is a childhood malignancy of the immature retina that is often hereditary and may be associated with other malignancies, such as osteosarcoma, in later life. On exam, these children have a white reflex, or "cat's eye." Ophthalmologic surgery may be curative if the tumor is caught in its early stages.

Common Symptoms of Eye Disorders

Diplopia

Also known as "double vision," diplopia can occur in a number of contexts. Misalignment, cranial nerve dysfunction, and vascular disturbances may all be involved. Trauma resulting in damage to the muscles or orbit may also cause diplopia. Monocular diplopia (double vision when one eye is covered) is usually caused by lens abnormalities.

Papilledema

Bilateral swelling of the optic disks due to increased intracranial pressure is termed papilledema. Patients are often asymptomatic but may complain of mild changes in vision, such as enlargement of the blind spot. Common causes include cerebral trauma or hemorrhage, meningitis, severe hypertension, and tumors.

Optic Atrophy

Degeneration of the optic nerve is often due to inflammation. The optic disk may be whitish or gray and often has indistinct edges. Loss of vision is generally proportional to the amount of degeneration. The presence of optic atrophy requires further investigation into its origin. In some cases (e.g., tumor removal), sight can be completely restored.

Hearing Loss and Other Auditory Disorders

Hearing loss is divided into two major categories: conductive hearing loss, which is caused by damage to the middle or external ear canal, and sensorineural hearing loss, which results from damage to the inner ear or auditory nerve.

Two commonly used tests of hearing are Rinne's test and Weber's test. With Rinne's test, a vibrating tuning fork is held against the mastoid process and then adjacent to the pinna. Normally, the position in front of the pinna is perceived as louder; if not, the patient may have a conductive hearing loss. In Weber's test, the tuning fork is held against the midline of the forehead. A patient with unilateral conductive hearing loss hears the sound more loudly in the affected ear, while a patient with unilateral sensorineural hearing loss hears the sound more loudly in the unaffected ear. An audiometer can provide more specific information about the extent of hearing loss.

Presbycusis

Presbycusis is the normal loss of hearing that occurs with aging. It is sensorineural in origin, resulting from stiffening and deterioration of the hair cells and basilar membrane. It initially affects high-frequency sounds, and it may be related to noise exposure. Men are more frequently affected than women. Amplification with a hearing aid and lip reading may be helpful.

Otitis Externa

Also known as "swimmer's ear," otitis externa is an infection most frequently caused by gram-negative rods such as *Escherichia coli*, *Pseudomonas*, and *Proteus*, although *Staphylococcus aureus* may cause localized inflammation (a "furuncle"). Predisposing factors include frequent cotton swab use and the presence of irritants such as hair spray.

Patients typically complain of itching, pain, and discharge from the affected ear. More severe cases result in hearing loss due to swelling of the ear canal. On exam, the external auditory canal appears red and swollen, and purulent discharge may be present.

The above symptoms and physical findings suggest the diagnosis.

After removal of superficial debris, topical antibiotics and corticosteroids may be helpful.

Otitis Media

Otitis media, infection of the middle ear, typically occurs in children younger than 3 years of age, due to the short length and horizontal position of the eustachian tube in children of this age group. Common organisms include *Streptococcus pneumoniae*, *Haemophilus influenzae*, *Branhamella catarrhalis*, *Streptococcus pyogenes,* and *S. aureus*. Newborn infants may develop perinatal otitis infection from *E. coli* and *S. aureus*.

Persistent ear pain and fever are typical. Temporary hearing loss may occur. On exam, the tympanic membrane is red and bulging, with loss of tympanic bony landmarks and light reflex. Bloody or purulent discharge may be present in later stages of infection.

Diagnosis is based on the clinical presentation and exam. Pharyngeal cultures are generally not helpful.

Antibiotics, such as amoxicillin, are given for 12–14 days. In resistant cases, a cephalosporin may be used. In adults, decongestants may also be helpful. Serious complications of inadequately treated infections include mastoiditis, meningitis, and permanent hearing loss.

Mastoiditis

Infection of the mastoid process generally occurs several weeks after inadequately treated otitis media. Streptococcal mastoiditis may be associated with perforation of the tympanic membrane.

Redness and swelling of the mastoid process, accompanied by pain, tenderness, and fever is the typical presentation. Hearing loss may also occur.

X-ray reveals destruction of the mastoid air cells and fluid in the air pockets. CT scan may provide a definitive diagnosis.

Intravenous antibiotics are necessary. If complete resolution does not occur, surgical drainage may be required.

Vertigo

Vertigo is an inappropriate sensation of rotational movement that is often associated with disturbances in balance and gait. It occurs in the context of a number of disorders, including Ménière's disease, but it may also be associated with inner ear disorders and lesions of the eighth nerve. Neurologic exam of the cranial nerves and cerebellum is indicated.

Tinnitus

Tinnitus refers to the perception of noise without the presence of an exogenous source of the sound. The most commonly perceived sound is that of ringing, but buzzing, whistling, and roaring noises are also common. Brief episodes of tinnitus may be normal; more prolonged episodes may be associated with a multitude of disorders, including Ménière's disease, ear infection, ototoxic drug use, and excessive noise exposure. Treatment is directed at the underlying cause, and nortriptyline may be helpful in some cases.

Ménière's Disease

Ménière's disease is a disorder of unknown etiology that is characterized by severe vertigo, hearing loss, and tinnitus.

Sudden attacks of vertigo, which may last up to 24 hours, are accompanied by nausea and vomiting. Over several years, significant hearing loss occurs. Tinnitus may be constant and often worsens during a vertiginous attack.

The above symptoms suggest the diagnosis.

Symptomatic relief of the vertigo is achieved through anticholinergics and antihistamines. Diazepam may also be effective. Surgical intervention may be helpful if medical treatment is not sufficient.

Acoustic Neuroma

Also known as vestibular schwannoma, acoustic neuromas are tumors of the eighth cranial nerve that may expand and invade the cerebellum and brainstem.

Hearing loss, dizziness, and tinnitus are common complaints. On examination, the hearing loss appears sensorineural in origin.

Audiography and CT scan confirm the presence of a tumor.

Surgical excision.

Toxic Ear Damage

Toxic ear damage may occur as a result of intense noise or ototoxic drugs. Drugs most commonly associated with ear damage include aminoglycosides (e.g., neomycin, gentamicin), furosemide, salicylates, and quinine. Prevention measures include ear protectors (for excessive noise) and avoidance of ototoxic drugs, especially in pregnancy or in patients with pre-existing hearing loss.

Headache

Migraine

Migraine headaches involve recurrent headaches of characteristic quality. They affect twice as many women as men, usually begin between the ages of 10 and 30, and often disappear spontaneously by age 50. Patients may have a family history of migraine. Precipitating factors include stress, bright lights, menstruation, fatigue, and foods containing tyramine (cheeses), monosodium glutamate, and nitrites (hot dogs).

SIGNS & SYMPTOMS

Patients with classic migraines experience an aura prior to the onset of the headache. The aura often involves visual disturbances such as scintillating scotomas (small areas of visual loss). The headache is dull, throbbing, and frequently unilateral. Nausea and vomiting, sensitivity to noise, and photophobia are common. Without medical intervention, migraines can last for hours or days.

DIAGNOSIS

The clinical presentation is diagnostic in the absence of abnormal neurologic findings.

TREATMENT

Prophylaxis is useful for patients with frequent or severe migraine headaches. Medications for this purpose include ergots, NSAIDs, amitriptyline, propranolol, and calcium channel blockers. Treatment of an acute migraine attack includes NSAIDs, ergots, and sumatriptan.

Cluster Headache

Cluster headaches primarily affect men aged 20–50. Precipitating factors include alcohol and vasodilators.

SIGNS & SYMPTOMS

Cluster headaches are severe, brief, nonthrobbing unilateral headaches that recur or "cluster" around the same time each day for weeks or months at a time. Remissions can last months or years. Horner's syndrome (ptosis, miosis, anhidrosis) and periorbital pain are often associated disorders.

DIAGNOSIS

Diagnosis is by presentation and exclusion of other disorders.

TREATMENT

Treatment for an acute attack includes ergots and lidocaine. Prophylactic therapies against recurrent symptoms include prednisone, ergots, and lithium.

Tension Headache

Chronic headaches that do not resemble migraine or cluster headaches may be "tension headaches." Despite its name, the cause of tension headaches is unknown. Tension headaches are by far the most common type of headache seen in adults.

Patients complain of a bilateral, occipital, constant head pain. Their neck and scalp muscles are usually tightly contracted.

Diagnosis involves ruling out migraine, cluster, or other possible causes of headache.

Acute management involves NSAIDs and ergots. Prophylactic therapies include amitriptyline, propranolol, physical therapy, and relaxation techniques.

Tumor-Associated Headache

Tumor-associated headaches typically present as progressively increasing, dull, nonthrobbing headaches. They are frequently exacerbated by postural changes and exertion, and they often disrupt sleep. These headaches are often associated with nausea and vomiting. CT scan or MRI may be required for definitive diagnosis.

Temporal Arteritis

Also known as giant cell arteritis, temporal arteritis is a chronic inflammatory disease of large blood vessels. It occurs in the elderly and most commonly involves arteries of the carotid distribution. Without treatment, patients are at risk for blindness.

Patients present with a bilateral, diffuse headache, temporal artery tenderness, and jaw claudication. Visual disturbances and polymyalgia rheumatica are also fairly common (see Chap. 14).

The erythrocyte sedimentation rate (ESR) is elevated in 95% of patients. Anemia and altered liver function tests may also be noted.

Suspicion of diagnosis should be verified by a temporal artery biopsy.

To prevent blindness, prednisone should be started in a patient with a suggestive clinical presentation, even before the biopsy results are available.

Trigeminal Neuralgia

Also known as tic douloureux, trigeminal neuralgia is typically seen in older adults. Although its etiology is unknown, some theories suggest microvascular compression as a possible cause.

Excruciating, lightening bolt-like bouts of facial pain in the V1 and V2 distribution are characteristic. Stimulation of trigger zones (e.g., brushing the teeth) can precipitate the neuralgia.

The above symptoms in the absence of other neurologic abnormalities are diagnostic.

Medical approaches include carbamazepine and phenytoin. Patients unresponsive to medical therapy may benefit from surgical decompression of fifth cranial nerve fibers.

Epilepsy and Seizure Disorders

Seizures result from a synchronized discharge of neurons in the central nervous system and can have a variety of causes (Table 15-1). In idiopathic epilepsy, seizures arise from a focus of epileptic tissue within the brain. Electrical discharge of this focus may spread to other brain regions. Other causes of seizures may be due to CNS infections, fever, metabolic defects, or cerebral trauma.

Partial Seizures

Partial seizures arise from a specific focus in the brain and generally begin with localized symptoms.

Simple partial seizures involve a focal symptom, whether sensory (e.g., visual hallucinations), motor (e.g., lip smacking), or psychomotor (e.g., purposeless pattern of movement). Consciousness is retained. The seizure may spread to involve adjacent cortical regions. For instance, in **jacksonian seizures**, focal muscle twitches spread progressively from their initial source across the patient's body as an adjacent motor cortex becomes involved. **Secondary generalization** refers to simple seizures that evolve into grand mal seizures. In these cases, consciousness is lost.

Table 15-1. Causes of seizures among different age groups

Children	Adults	Elderly
Fever	Idiopathic epilepsy	Neoplasms
Infection	Drug intoxication	Stroke
Metabolic defect	Trauma	Trauma
Idiopathic epilepsy		

Complex partial seizures involve stereotyped psychomotor symptoms due to an epileptic focus in the temporal or medial frontal lobes. Seizing patients may show automatism (i.e., coordinated motor activity) and may experience olfactory hallucinations, fear, or déja vu. Patients lose contact with their environment during the seizure and experience postictal confusion afterward.

Electroencephalogram (EEG) during or immediately after the episode shows distinctive changes.

Control of seizures may be achieved with phenytoin, carbamazepine, or valproate.

Generalized Seizures

Generalized seizures involve the entire cerebral cortex, but they may produce only minor symptoms. These seizures are frequently genetic and usually present during childhood.

Absence seizures, also known as petit mal, involve very brief and frequent losses of consciousness without loss of muscle tone. Rapid eye blinking is common during the seizure. Patients experience no aura or postictal confusion. Symptoms may resolve as the patient ages.

Grand mal seizures, also called tonic-clonic seizures, may be preceded by an aura of epigastric discomfort or mood change. In the tonic phase, which lasts up to 30 seconds, the patient falls unconscious to the ground in tonic contraction with an arched back. A 1-minute clonic phase follows, during which the patient undergoes rapid alternation of muscle contraction and relaxation. As long as 30 minutes may pass before the patient regains consciousness. Postictal confusion and headache can last another 10–30 minutes.

Symptoms and EEG are diagnostic.

Ethosuximide is the primary drug used for absence seizures. Phenytoin, carbamazepine, or valproate is effective for control of grand mal seizures.

Status Epilepticus

In status epilepticus, seizures are continuous, not separated by any periods of regained consciousness. Status epilepticus may develop from grand mal seizures, but it can also arise from the rapid withdrawal of anticonvulsant medications.

Uninterrupted seizures may last hours or even days. If untreated, the patient may experience high fever, circulatory collapse, and brain damage.

The clinical presentation is diagnostic. Lab studies, including blood glucose, electrolytes, and toxicology, may suggest an etiology.

Diazepam is given until the seizures are controlled, while airway, breathing, and circulation are maintained. Glucose, thiamine, and naloxone may be given intravenously to treat potential causes. Fever is managed with cooling blankets and curare, if necessary.

Cerebrovascular Disease

Ischemic Disorders

Ischemia of the brain occurs when the blood supply becomes inadequate. Decreased blood flow to the brain can be due to atherosclerosis affecting the carotid or vertebral arteries, intracranial thrombosis, vascular inflammation, and cerebral embolism arising from an atherosclerotic vessel or from a cardiac thrombus. If ischemic conditions persist, infarction of brain tissue results.

Transient Ischemic Attack

Transient ischemic attacks (TIAs) are caused by sudden, brief episodes of impaired blood flow to the brain. They are generally due to emboli or arterial stenosis. Predisposing conditions for TIAs include obesity, smoking, diabetes, and hyperlipidemia. TIAs are frequently recurrent and most commonly seen in elderly or middle-aged patients.

Focal neurologic abnormalities begin suddenly and disappear within an hour. Consciousness is not impaired. Longer lasting symptoms suggest infarction. Carotid artery involvement produces unilateral symptoms, with contralateral hemiparesis and parasthesias and ipsilateral blindness. Aphasia is seen if the dominant hemisphere is involved. Vertebrobasilar system involvement produces symptoms of brainstem dysfunction, including vertigo, confusion, blindness, diplopia, weakness, and parasthesias of the extremities.

The clinical presentation suggests the diagnosis and the location of the impairment. Carotid bruits or thrills suggest extracranial lesions. Ultrasonography or arteriography can identify stenosed arteries.

Anticoagulants and platelet inhibitors are used in patients with obstruction. Aspirin therapy may be used in place of stronger anticoagulants in patients with infrequent TIAs. Patients with carotid TIAs and marked obstruction or ulcerating plaques in the carotid arteries may benefit from surgical endarterectomy.

Stroke

A stroke is caused by prolonged ischemia of the brain, resulting in infarction. Risk factors are the same as those for TIAs.

Neurologic symptoms depend on the site of the infarct (Fig. 15-2).

- The distribution of the middle cerebral artery is most often involved. Contralateral limb weakness, sensory loss, and homonymous hemianopsia are common symptoms. Involvement of the dominant hemisphere leads to aphasia, while involvement of the nondominant hemisphere results in sensory neglect and apraxia (inability to perform learned actions—e.g., dressing). In addition, ipsilateral ocular defects may be present with internal carotid artery involvement.
- Occlusion of the posterior cerebral artery may lead to contralateral homonymous hemianopsia and sensory loss, spontaneous thalamic pain, or a sudden onset of hemiballistic movement disorder.
- Vertebrobasilar artery involvement is frequently fatal. Unilateral occlusion in the vertebrobasilar system produces ipsilateral cranial nerve abnormalities and contralateral body weakness and sensory deficits. Complete occlusion of the artery results in ophthalmoplegia, defects of pupillary constriction, bilateral weakness or paralysis of the extremities, and a decrease in consciousness. Dysphagia and dysarthria may occur as well.

A completed stroke presents with stable neurologic deficits and most often develops within a few minutes. A stroke in evolution presents with a progressive increase in neurologic abnormalities over 1–2 days. Severe brainstem signs, impaired consciousness, mental deterioration, and aphasia indicate a poor prognosis.

The clinical presentation is usually suggestive of stroke. CT or MRI may differentiate ischemic stroke from intracerebral hemorrhage, hematoma, or tumor. Shortly after a stroke, the scan is usually negative.

Anticoagulants are contraindicated in hypertensive patients and are not useful in acute completed strokes. Heparin, however, helps to stabilize an evolving stroke and may also prevent additional cardiac emboli, if this is the source of the stroke. Supportive care is critical. The prognosis is better in younger patients and in patients with limited motor or sensory defects, intact mental function, and a strong support network. Physical and occupational therapy can help the patient to re-establish normal life patterns.

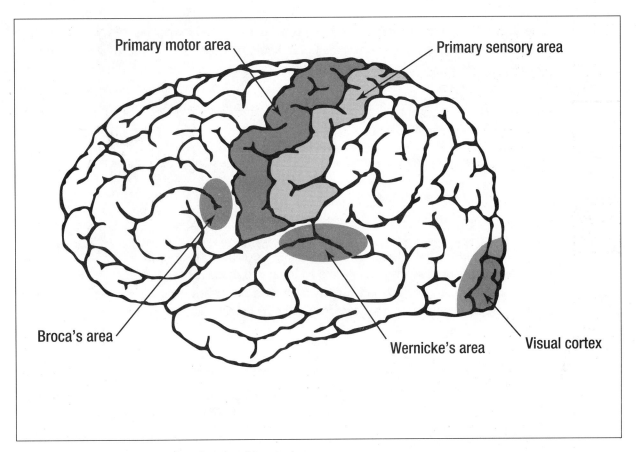

Fig. 15-2. Cortical areas often involved in stroke.

Aneurysm

Aneurysms, localized dilations of blood vessels, are a common cause of subarachnoid hemorrhage. Congenital berry aneurysms, occurring around the circle of Willis, are common and are sometimes associated with polycystic kidney disease and aortic coarctation.

The most dangerous feature of an intracranial aneurysm is its risk of rupture, which results in subarachnoid or intracerebral hemorrhage. Typically, aneurysms are asymptomatic until hemorrhage occurs. Headache, optic abnormalities, syncope, vomiting, and altered level of consciousness are common symptoms of hemorrhage.

Intracerebral Hemorrhage

Bleeding into the tissue of the brain usually results from the rupture of an atherosclerotic vessel. Chronic hypertension or local thrombus formation with secondary ischemia is usually responsible. Hypertensive hemorrhages are often large and frequently fatal.

As the vessel bleeds, pressure from the forming hematoma compresses and displaces adjacent brain regions. A supratentorial hematoma can cause transtentorial herniation, with brainstem compression and midbrain bleeding. Cerebellar hematomas can produce acute hydrocephalus by blocking cerebrospinal fluid (CSF) flow.

The acute onset of headache with progressive neurologic abnormalities is typical. Symptoms may begin during exercise. Small cerebral hemorrhages cause focal neurologic deficits. Supratentorial hemorrhages may produce hemiparesis, while subtentorial hemorrhages produce brainstem or cerebellar defects, including pinpoint pupils or other ocular abnormalities. Loss of consciousness, coma, focal or generalized seizures, nausea, vomiting, and delirium are all common.

CT or MRI is used to show bleeding and structural changes and to rule out ischemic stroke.

Supportive care is the mainstay of treatment. Codeine relieves headaches, and diazepam reduces anxiety. Surgery may be indicated if the hemorrhage is easily accessible. More than half of patients with large hemorrhages die within days of onset of the hemorrhage. While some impairment often remains in survivors, recovery may be complete in some cases.

Subarachnoid Hemorrhage

Subarachnoid hemorrhage refers to bleeding between the pia and arachnoid layers of the meninges. It usually arises from rupture of a cerebral artery aneurysm or an arteriovenous malformation. Hemorrhage leads to a sudden increase in intracranial pressure. Patients are typically in their 50s, and the mortality rate is about 35%.

A sudden, explosive headache is typically characterized as "the worst headache" of the patient's life. Patients may have syncope, with later nuchal rigidity, vomiting, and nonfocal neurologic abnormalities. A decreased level of consciousness, which may be due to increased intracranial pressure, suggests a large hemorrhage.

CT scan shows subarachnoid blood. If negative, lumbar puncture is mandatory.

Management of increased intracranial pressure includes intubation and hyperventilation, osmotic agents, elevation of the patient's head, and fluid limitation. Exertion and anticoagulants are contraindicated. Surgical obliteration or isolation of an aneurysm reduces both the long-term mortality and the probability of a recurrence.

Cavernous Sinus Thrombosis

Cavernous sinus thrombosis is a dangerous condition involving the presence of a septic thrombus in the cavernous sinus. Infection is associated with chronic bacterial sinusitis and may spread from the sphenoid or ethmoid air sinuses.

The patient presents with cranial nerve palsies, as well as fever, exophthalmos, papilledema, headache, decreased consciousness, and occasionally seizures.

CT scan of the cavernous sinus and the air sinuses confirms the diagnosis. Blood and nasal discharges are cultured to identify the infecting organism.

IV antibiotics should be administered immediately. Surgical drainage of the air sinuses may be useful, especially if the patient does not respond to antibiotics.

Traumatic Disorders

Head injury is the leading cause of death in males less than 35 years old. Brain tissue may be damaged at the point of impact (coup) or opposite the point of impact (contrecoup). Skull penetration and fractures can lead to tissue damage and to hematoma formation. Intracranial injury is a blanket term involving subdural and epidural hematomas, cerebral contusion, and cerebral laceration.

Acute Subdural Hematoma

Acute subdural hematoma occurs from rapid bleeding between the dural and arachnoid layers of the meninges, usually due to tearing of the bridging veins. It is a common cause of death in patients with head injury.

Symptoms progress more slowly with this venous bleed than with arterial hemorrhage. Signs of transtentorial herniation develop, including deepening coma with decorticate and then decerebrate posturing, mid-position or dilated fixed pupils, and spastic hemiplegia with increased deep tendon reflexes.

CT or MRI is diagnostic. Lumbar puncture is contraindicated because the procedure may precipitate herniation.

Surgical drainage of the hematoma.

Chronic Subdural Hematoma

Chronic subdural hematoma is the delayed or slowed formation of a subdural clot. Symptoms may develop weeks after a head injury. This condition is particularly common in the elderly and in alcoholics.

Patients present with a progressive, daily headache, fluctuating consciousness, and mild hemiparesis.

MRI or angiogram.

Surgical drainage.

Epidural Hematoma

Epidural hematomas, bleeding between the dura and the skull, are not as common as subdural hematomas. Epidural hematomas typically arise from injury to arteries, most commonly the middle meningeal artery. Because it is an arterial bleed, an epidural hematoma can cause rapid brain compression with permanent neurologic sequelae or death.

Patients typically experience a brief lucid interval after a head injury, followed by progressive headache, decreasing level of consciousness, motor deficits, and pupillary abnormalities. Temporal fracture lines may be noted on exam.

CT, MRI, or angiogram confirms the diagnosis.

The extradural clot must be quickly removed. In the absence of imaging devices, burr holes through the cranium provide both diagnosis and treatment.

Concussion

Concussion refers to injury to the brain due to blunt trauma without evidence of significant lesions or sequelae.

Transient loss of consciousness typically lasts seconds to minutes. Although unconscious, the patient has intact brainstem function without signs of hemiplegia or decerebrate reflexes. Afterward, the patient may experience a post-traumatic confusional syndrome, with transient retrograde and anterograde amnesia, and longer lasting headache, vertigo, and mild cognitive dysfunction.

Clinical presentation.

Careful observation for development of more severe signs is all that is necessary.

Cerebral Contusion and Laceration

Cerebral contusions and lacerations are often associated with skull damage and depressed fragments of bone. They may result in brain edema and transtentorial herniation, leading to coma, decorticate or decerebrate posturing, and death. Signs of brainstem injury suggest a poor prognosis. The clinical presentation usually suggests the diagnosis, which is confirmed by CT or MRI scan. Depressed skull fractures should be repaired, and supportive care is critical.

Toxic Neurologic Disorders

Toxic Vestibulopathies

Many drugs can interact with the peripheral nervous system, resulting in vestibular disorders.
- **Alcohol** can cause positional vertigo within 2 hours of ingestion, and symptoms may last as long as 12 hours. The patient experiences vertigo and nystagmus, especially while lying down and with closed eyes.
- **Aminoglycosides** are ototoxic agents that can produce symptoms of both vestibular and auditory dysfunction. Patients present with vertigo, nausea, vomiting, and ataxia. Romberg's sign may be present. These symptoms last 1–2 weeks and then gradually improve. Extended or repeated therapy can produce progressive vestibular dysfunction.
- **Salicylates** used chronically or in high doses can cause reversible vertigo, tinnitus, and sensorineural hearing loss. Headache, nausea, vomiting, hyperventilation, and thirst may also be present.
- **Quinine** and **quinidine** can both cause cinchonism, an idiosyncratic drug effect involving color vision defects, tinnitus, hearing loss, vertigo, flushed skin, nausea, vomiting, abdominal pain, and sweating.
- **Cisplatin** is an antineoplastic drug that causes ototoxicity in about half of patients. Reversible vertigo, tinnitus, and hearing loss occur, in addition to a sensory neuropathy.

Toxic Neuropathies

Many chemical exposures may result in neurologic effects.
- **Lead** can produce a multiple motor mononeuropathy. It can also cause an acute encephalopathy in children.

- **Dapsone**, used in leprosy and HIV, can produce a reversible motor polyneuropathy.
- **Organophosphates** can cause delayed motor neuropathies, in addition to cholinergic crisis.
- **Alcohol** frequently causes a bilateral, distal sensorimotor neuropathy. Chronic use is also associated with Wernicke's encephalopathy and Korsakoff's amnestic syndrome.
- **Arsenic** can cause acute-onset, symmetrical sensorimotor polyneuropathy.
- **Thallium** can produce a sudden-onset, symmetrical sensorimotor polyneuropathy.
- **Isoniazid**, used in the treatment of tuberculosis, produces a reversible sensory polyneuropathy that is prevented by concurrent pyridoxine administration.
- **Gold**, used in the treatment of rheumatoid arthritis, may produce a symmetrical polyneuropathy.
- ***N*-hexane**, used in solvents and glue, produces a sensory polyneuropathy.

Infections

Bacterial Meningitis

Bacterial meningitis, an infection of the meninges of the spinal cord or brain, is most common in the first month of life. Group B streptococci and *E. coli* predominate at this time. *Haemophilus influenzae* is responsible for most meningitis in children older than 1 month, and *S. pneumoniae* causes the majority of cases in adults. *Neisseria meningitidis*, harbored in the nasopharynx of 5% of the population, causes disease in people of all ages.

Bacteria reach the meninges from the blood, from nearby infected structures (such as the sinuses), and from contamination of the CSF. The bacteria then attract neutrophils. The resulting exudate may cause hydrocephalus, ischemia, and cranial nerve damage.

A sore throat may precede symptoms of fever, confusion, headache, vomiting, and neck stiffness. Stupor or coma may be present, in addition to cranial neuropathies and seizures. A petechial rash is found in more than half of patients with meningitis caused by *N. meningitides*. Brain infarction or systemic complications can cause death within hours. Signs of meningeal irritation include a positive Brudzinski's sign, in which neck flexion in the supine patient causes involuntary hip and knee flexion, and a positive Kernig's sign, in which extension of the knee in a patient with a flexed hip is painful.

CSF analysis, including WBC count, Gram's stain, and culture, confirms that meningitis is present. A low glucose level, a high neutrophil count, and a high protein concentration suggest bacterial meningitis (Table 15-2).

Administration of antibiotics should begin immediately after CSF has been taken for culture. Empiric therapy typically includes a third-generation cephalosporin in adults and in children older than 3 months, and ampicillin and cefotaxime in infants and neonates. Once the culture results are available, an antibiotic specific to the infecting organism should be used.

Table 15-2. CSF findings in different neurologic conditions

	Pressure	Glucose	Protein	White blood cell count
Bacterial meningitis	High	Low	High	High neutrophils
Aseptic meningitis	Normal	Normal	Normal	High lymphocytes
Fungal/TB meningitis	High	Low	High	High lymphocytes
Guillain-Barré	Normal	Normal	High	Normal

Aseptic Meningitis

Aseptic meningitis is nonbacterial meningeal inflammation. Viruses, other organisms, and host responses to exogenous chemicals may be responsible. Viral meningitis is often associated with community epidemics.

SIGNS & SYMPTOMS

Aseptic meningitis has basically the same clinical presentation as bacterial meningitis, including fever, headache, vomiting, neck stiffness, and an altered level of consciousness. The symptoms may be more mild than with bacterial infection.

DIAGNOSIS

CSF analysis shows high lymphocytes, normal glucose, mild protein increases, and a negative Gram's stain and bacterial culture.

TREATMENT

Supportive treatment is usually sufficient, and the patients generally recover fully.

Subacute and Chronic Meningitis

Subacute and chronic meningitis involve the slow but progressive onset of meningeal infection. Subacute meningitis develops over 2 weeks in the absence of treatment. Chronic meningitis lasts longer than 1 month without antibiotic intervention.

Subacute or chronic meningitis can develop in patients with HIV/AIDS, cytomegalovirus, Lyme disease, syphilis, tuberculosis, sarcoidosis, or neoplasms. Immunosuppressive therapy and AIDS have increased the frequency of fungal meningitis, particularly *Cryptococcus*.

SIGNS & SYMPTOMS

Symptoms of meningitis appear slowly over a period of several weeks.

DIAGNOSIS

CSF analysis confirms meningeal inflammation, showing a high lymphocyte count, low glucose (normal in syphilis), and sometimes high protein. Fungi may be seen in the CSF. Tuberculosis can often be identified by acid-fast stain of the CSF, and blood VDRL is positive in syphilis. Because of the many treatment possibilities, the causative agent must be identified.

Treatment varies with etiology. Amphotericin B is used in fungal infections.

HIV Infection and AIDS Meningitis

HIV infection can cause a transient meningitis, usually around the time of seroconversion. It may last up to 1 month before spontaneously resolving. Symptoms, signs, and diagnosis are those of meningitis. In addition, blood lymphocytosis is evident, and the patient may be in a state of acute confusion.

Encephalitis

Encephalitis, acute inflammation of the brain tissue, may be caused by direct viral invasion or by host hypersensitivity to a virus. Primary encephalitis may be sporadic, caused by endemic viruses such as varicella-zoster virus, herpes simplex virus, and mumps, or it may be epidemic, caused by Coxsackie, polio-, echo-, or arboviruses. Secondary encephalitis arises from an immunologic response to viral infection, most commonly chickenpox, measles, and rubella.

Signs of cerebral dysfunction may include seizures, paresis, cranial nerve defects, and altered level of consciousness. Symptoms and signs of meningitis may be present.

A viral etiology is suggested by CSF lymphocytosis, normal glucose, and a negative bacterial culture.

Acyclovir is started immediately and continued for 10 days. Permanent cerebral damage is more common in infants than in adults.

Reye's Syndrome

Reye's syndrome follows a viral infection and involves an acute encephalopathy with fatty infiltration of various organs. It is seen primarily in children with influenza or chickenpox infection who are given aspirin products. For this reason, salicylates are contraindicated in children.

Symptoms of a viral infection (typically an upper respiratory infection) are followed by severe nausea, vomiting, and an acute change in mental status. Signs of hepatic dysfunction occur in about half of patients. Seizures, loss of muscle tone, fixed and dilated pupils, coma, respiratory arrest, and death may all result.

The sudden onset of encephalopathy, severe vomiting, and liver dysfunction suggests Reye's syndrome. CSF pressure is increased. Liver biopsy showing fatty infiltration provides the definitive diagnosis.

No treatment is available, but early and intensive supportive care is useful.

Cytomegalovirus

Immunosuppressed patients with reactivated or primary cytomegalovirus (CMV) infections may develop CNS, pulmonary, renal, or gastrointestinal involvement. This risk is particularly high in transplant patients and in AIDS patients. Detecting CMV antibodies or isolating the virus from body fluids is not useful for diagnosis of an acute illness since CMV is a common infection and many people have antibodies or subclinical infection. Ganciclovir is used to treat CMV infection.

Lyme Disease

Lyme disease is a tick-borne infectious disease caused by the spirochete *Borrelia burgdorferi* (see Chap. 14). A minority of patients with Lyme disease develop neurologic defects within weeks to months. These abnormalities may last several months before resolving completely. The most common neurologic conditions arising in Lyme disease are aseptic meningitis, meningoencephalitis, sensory or motor radiculopathies, and cranial neuritis. Bell's palsy is a particularly common cranial neuritis, and it is often bilateral in Lyme disease.

Brain Abscess

A brain abscess is a collection of pus in the brain usually resulting from bacterial infection. It may be caused by extension from cranial infections (mastoiditis, sinusitis), by direct inoculation after a head wound, or by hematogenous spread from a bacterial source elsewhere in the body. Anaerobic bacteria are usually responsible.

Following an infection or injury, patients develop progressive headache, nausea, vomiting, lethargy, papilledema, and focal neurologic abnormalities. Seizures and personality changes may be present. Brain abscesses are fatal if left untreated.

CT or MRI is diagnostic. Because of the risk of transtentorial herniation, LP is contraindicated.

Antibiotics should be geared to the likely organism. The patient's response to antibiotics may be evaluated by serial CT scans. Surgical excision or aspiration is necessary in patients who are likely to herniate.

Neurosyphilis

Late or tertiary syphilis can cause CNS infection and symptoms. Symptomatic neurosyphilis develops in only 5% of patients with untreated syphilis infection.

Patients with meningovascular neurosyphilis present with headache, dizziness, decreased concentration, diplopia, and neck stiffness. A characteristic sign is the Argyll Robertson pupil, an irregular, small pupil that reacts to accommodation but not to light. The spinal cord may also be involved, leading to bulbar symptoms and weakness and atrophy of the arms. Other symptoms include paralysis, memory loss, dementia, insomnia, lethargy, and irritability. Psychiatric disorders, such as delusions of grandeur, may develop. Patients with bilateral lesions of the posterior columns may also develop tabes dorsalis (i.e., irregular, intense, stabbing leg pain; ataxia; sensory deficits; and loss of tendon reflexes).

The serum VDRL is positive and the CSF shows elevated WBCs, increased protein, and a positive rapid plasma reagin (RPR). With tabes dorsalis, however, the reagin test may be negative.

Procaine penicillin G is given for 21 days. Analgesics may be used to control pain from tabes dorsalis, but this manifestation may progress despite appropriate therapy. The CSF should be examined every 3–6 months until it has been normal for 2 years.

Rabies

Rabies is an acute viral disease that is transmitted by a bite from an infected animal. Rabid dogs provide the greatest risk to humans worldwide, but wild animals are the primary source of infections in the United States. The rabies virus travels from the site of inoculation through peripheral nerves to the spinal cord and brain. It proliferates in the brain and then spreads by efferent nerves to the salivary glands.

The incubation period after being bitten ranges from 30–50 days. Patients experience malaise, fever, and restlessness initially, and symptoms rapidly progress to extreme excitement and painful laryngeal and pharyngeal spasms. Death is from asphyxia, exhaustion, or paralysis and usually occurs within 2 weeks of initial symptoms.

Any animal that bites a human should be isolated. If the animal appears normal after 10 days of observation, it was probably not infectious at the time of the bite. If it becomes rabid, its brain must be analyzed for the virus, and the patient must begin prophylactic therapy. Viral testing of patients once symptoms begin confirms the diagnosis.

Thorough cleaning of the wound reduces the likelihood of contracting rabies. In patients bitten by a rabid animal or by an animal not available for observation, prophylaxis involves passive immunization with rabies immunoglobulin and active immunization with vaccine. Aggressive symptomatic treatment of patients who develop rabies may help; without treatment, mortality is 100%.

Poliomyelitis

Poliovirus is transmitted through fecal-oral contact and may spread to the brain and motor neurons.

Most polio infections, especially in infants and young children, are mild and do not involve the CNS. If the illness progresses, it usually presents with signs of aseptic meningitis, including headache, fever, stiff neck, and muscle pain. Focal or extensive paralysis then occurs. Sensation is not compromised.

Asymmetric paralysis during a febrile illness suggests polio. For diagnosis, the virus must be isolated from the throat or feces, or an increase in polio-specific antibody must be shown.

Therapy is palliative. Artificial respiration is necessary in cases of respiratory failure. More than half of patients with paralytic poliomyelitis recover completely.

Prophylaxis is by active immunization using the oral polio vaccine (OPV) or, in immunocompromised patients, the inactivated polio vaccine (IPV).

Neoplasms

Primary Neoplasms

Brain tumors present most commonly in young and middle-aged adults. Local growth causes most of the symptoms and complications. A common effect is increased intracranial pressure, due to mass effect, cerebral edema, hydrocephalus, obstructed venous sinuses, or obstructed CSF resorption. **Glioblastoma multiforme**, a malignant glioma, is the most common brain tumor in adults, and it has a very high mortality rate. **Meningioma** is the most common benign tumor of adults. Meningiomas may grow very large before they create symptoms. The most common primary childhood tumors include **cerebellar astrocytomas** and **medulloblastomas**.

Headache and vomiting are prominent early symptoms. Patients may present with lethargy, stupor, personality changes, and mental deterioration. Convulsive seizures are more frequent with lesions of the cerebrum, particularly meningiomas and slow-growing astrocytomas. Focal manifestations due to local mass effects are also commonly seen.

CT, MRI, and biopsy are used in diagnosis.

Treatment involves resection when possible, as well as radiation and chemotherapy. Prognosis varies depending on the tumor type.

Metastatic Neoplasms

Metastatic brain tumors in adults most frequently originate from bronchogenic carcinoma, breast adenocarcinoma, and malignant melanoma. They account for more than 20% of adult brain tumors, but they are uncommon in children.

Headache, focal deficits, and seizures are typical.

CT or MRI scan.

Resection and irradiation can be used to treat metastasis. The underlying cancer should be treated as much as possible. Prognosis is typically poor.

Degenerative Disorders

Alzheimer's Disease

Alzheimer's disease is a slowly progressive dementia of unknown cause. It is the most common cause of dementia, affecting the elderly (typical onset after age 80), those with trisomy 21, and those with the autosomal dominant familial Alzheimer's disease (typical onset after age 60).

Progressive memory loss is the first symptom, followed by disorientation, depression, agitation, and other symptoms of dementia. Later stages tend to show psychiatric abnormalities, such as paranoia, delusions, and psychosis. Eventually the patient becomes bed-ridden and incontinent. Death occurs within 5–10 years of onset of symptoms.

No definitive premortem diagnostic test exists, so the diagnosis is made primarily on clinical grounds. CT shows cortical atrophy.

No treatment exists. Well-established routines, tools for orientation, and supportive care may help the symptomatic progression somewhat. Support for caregivers is essential.

Huntington's Disease

Huntington's disease is a progressive and hereditary disorder involving abnormalities in movement and mental function. It is an autosomal dominant disorder that does not become symptomatic until patients are between the ages of 30 and 50 years old.

Patients initially show subtle features of dementia, including irritability and antisocial behavior. Initial movement disturbances may also be subtle, but they eventually develop into chorea (sudden involuntary movements of the face and extremities). The chorea and dementia progress slowly, leading to death about 15 years after onset.

A positive family history is very useful in diagnosis. CT or MRI shows atrophy of the caudate nucleus and cerebral cortex.

No treatment exists for the disease itself. Chorea can be partially controlled with a D2-receptor antagonist, such as haloperidol. Genetic counseling for the patient and family is important.

Parkinsonism

Parkinsonism is a syndrome characterized by a resting tremor, decreased movement, muscular rigidity, and postural instability. The most common cause is idiopathic Parkinson's disease, in which the loss of dopaminergic cells in the substantia nigra leads to an imbalance of cholinergic input into the striatum. Other etiologies include therapeutic drugs, such as phenothiazines, and illicit drugs, such as MPTP.

Most patients develop a resting tremor that is initially confined to one limb (a "pill-rolling" tremor). Voluntary movement and automatic movement decrease, and the patient develops masklike facies, infrequent blinking, and a lack of arm-swinging while walking. The characteristic rigidity of the parkinsonian patient is caused by increased tone affecting both agonist and antagonist muscles, and cogwheel rigidity is common. Patients have difficulty initiating movement. They walk with small, shuffling steps, in some cases with increasing speed (festinating gait), and they often have difficulty stopping.

Clinical presentation.

Dopaminergic agonists and cholinergic antagonists are useful in the treatment of Parkinson's disease. Frequently used dopaminergic agents include levodopa (a dopamine precursor), amantadine, and bromocriptine. Benztropine is a common anticholinergic agent. For drug use–related parkinsonism, discontinue the causative drug.

Amyotrophic Lateral Sclerosis

Amyotrophic lateral sclerosis (ALS), also known as Lou Gehrig's disease, is a disease of motor neurons involving a progressive loss of anterior horn cell function. Most cases of ALS are idiopathic, but 5% have a genetic, autosomal dominant transmission. Middle-aged men are most commonly affected.

The initial presentation involves lower motor neuron dysfunction, with hand or foot weakness and atrophy. Progression to other muscles is asymmetric, and there are no sensory abnormalities. Later, muscle spasticity with increased deep tendon and extensor plantar reflexes reflect upper motor neuron involvement. Dysarthria and dysphagia, secondary to brainstem involvement, may also be present. Half of ALS patients die within 3 years of onset, and only a small minority live more than 10 years.

The clinical presentation is diagnostic. Electromyography may be helpful in demonstrating motor neuron abnormalities.

No effective treatment is known.

Tay-Sachs Disease

Tay-Sachs disease is an autosomal recessive disorder that is most common in Eastern European Jews and French Canadians. It involves the absence of hexosaminidase A, which is needed for metabolism of lipid gangliosides, so gangliosides accumulate within the brain.

Infants have early and progressive developmental delay, paralysis, blindness, and dementia. Cherry-red spots may be observed on the retina. Death occurs by age 4.

Decreased hexosaminidase A activity can be detected in the serum.

No treatment exists for the affected infant.

Genetic screening identifies carriers of the Tay-Sachs gene, who should undergo counseling prior to pregnancy. Prenatal diagnosis of infants is also possible, and prospective parents may choose to terminate affected pregnancies.

Demyelinating Disorders

Multiple Sclerosis

Multiple sclerosis (MS) is a progressive demyelinating disease that affects the brain, spinal cord, and optic nerve. The cause is unknown, but immune-mediated and viral etiologies are both popular theories. Women are more commonly affected than men, with peak ages of onset between 20 and 40 years old. Although the patient's life span is not reduced, permanent disability is common.

Initial presentations are diverse, including unilateral optic neuritis, diplopia, focal parasthesias, focal weakness or unsteadiness, and bladder dysfunction. The disease progresses slowly with periods of remissions and exacerbations. Infection or childbirth may trigger relapses. Eventually the patient may develop optic atrophy, nystagmus, dysarthria, upper motor neuron deficits, cerebellar dysfunction, and sensory abnormalities. About half of patients are significantly disabled 10 years after symptoms begin.

Gradual and variable onset of CNS symptoms suggests multiple sclerosis. CSF is abnormal in most patients, with mildly increased protein, mild lymphocytosis, and oligoclonal bands. MRI shows multiple plaques in the white matter.

No treatment prevents progression of the disease, but avoiding stress and fatigue seems to help. Corticosteroids may decrease the duration of the exacerbations.

Guillain-Barré Syndrome

Guillain-Barré syndrome is a polyneuropathy of unknown cause that can follow minor viral infections, inoculations, or surgeries. It is presumed to be immune-mediated and is the most common acquired demyelinating disorder.

Patients present with progressive, bilateral weakness in the legs. Weakness is typically proximal and can extend to the upper body and arms. Sensory deficits may be associated, and deep tendon reflexes are abnormal. Autonomic dysfunction may occur, including instability of temperature and blood pressure. Involvement of the respiratory muscles or the pharynx can be lethal. The disease generally stabilizes within 1 month of onset. Most patients recover completely, but some retain neurologic defects.

Diagnosis is largely clinical. CSF shows increased protein, with normal pressure, glucose, and cell number.

Plasmapheresis accelerates recovery. Corticosteroids are contraindicated, as they may exacerbate symptoms. Because of the risks of respiratory and vascular collapse, patients should be closely monitored.

Developmental Disorders

Cerebral Palsy

Cerebral palsy (CP) is primarily a disease of movement that results from CNS damage before the age of 5. Risk factors include in utero complications, intrauterine growth retardation (IUGR), prematurity, neonatal jaundice, birth trauma, and asphyxia.

Most patients have spastic syndromes, with any or all limbs affected. Affected limbs show increased deep tendon reflexes, increased tone, weakness, and underdevelopment. Toe-walking and a scissors gait are characteristic. Some patients develop syndromes involving choreoathetoid movement of the extremities or trunk, and these patients often have severe dysarthria. A minority of patients have ataxic syndromes due to cerebellar damage. Some affected children have normal intelligence, while others are mentally disabled. Hyperactivity and short attention spans are common. Seizures are present in one-fourth of patients with CP.

CP is hard to identify early in infancy, but the clinical syndrome in a child at risk becomes apparent over time.

Cerebral palsy has no cure, but early intervention can maximize future independence. Physical therapy, speech training, bracing, orthopedic surgery, and occupational therapy may all be useful. Special schooling is needed only with severe mental or physical deficits.

Dyslexia

Dyslexia is a congenital disorder that causes difficulty in reading despite normal intelligence.

Early signs include word-finding problems, difficulty in word substitutions, and delayed ability to name objects. Visual confusion and reversal of letters are common by elementary school.

Children who do not read at their expected level should be evaluated for language and auditory processing, reading ability, and decoding skills.

Training to improve skills for comprehension and pronunciation may be helpful. Indirect treatments, such as perceptual training and drug therapy, are not indicated.

Neuromuscular Disorders

Myasthenia Gravis

Myasthenia gravis involves a slowly progressive muscle weakness. Autoimmune antibodies against the acetylcholine receptor at the neuromuscular junction impair normal neuromuscular transmission. Myasthenia gravis is more common in women and occurs with greatest frequency between the ages of 20 and 40.

Episodic weakness and easy muscle fatigability may involve all muscles, particularly those innervated by the cranial nerves. The most common presentations involve ptosis, diplopia, dysarthria, and enhanced muscle fatigue with exercise. Respiratory compromise may cause death.

Most patients have acetylcholine-receptor antibodies present in their serum. Chest x-ray or CT may show a thymoma, which is a frequently associated finding. Diagnosis is confirmed when administration of an exogenous anticholinesterase, such as edrophonium or neostigmine, leads to increased levels of acetylcholine at the neuromuscular junction and provides transient relief of symptoms.

Anticholinesterase drugs such as neostigmine provide symptomatic benefit. Thymectomy in patients under 60 usually leads to improvement. Corticosteroids or azathioprine are used in patients unresponsive to other treatments.

Muscular Dystrophy

Progressive muscular weakness and atrophy, together called muscular dystrophy, may occur in a number of inherited disorders. Duchenne's muscular dystrophy (DMD) is the most common type. It is an X-linked, recessive disease caused by a mutation in the dystrophin gene.

By age 5, patients present with toe-walking, a waddling gait, and difficulty running. The proximal legs are affected first, and then the proximal arms become involved. Pseudohypertrophy of the calves, due to fatty infiltration of the muscle, is a classic sign in DMD. By age 11, patients are usually no longer able to walk, and IQ testing eventually shows mental retardation. Heart involvement, scoliosis, and flexion contractures follow as the disease progresses. Death usually occurs by 20 years of age.

The clinical presentation is suggestive. Muscle necrosis and variation in muscle fiber size can be seen on muscle biopsy, and dystrophin is absent from the muscle specimen. Serum creatine kinase (CK) levels are elevated even before the onset of symptoms.

No treatment exists. Exercise is encouraged and corrective surgery is helpful. Physical therapy and braces can prevent or treat contractures.

Symptoms, Signs, and III-Defined Conditions

Peripheral Neuropathy

Dysfunction of the peripheral nerves may involve motor, sensory, and/or autonomic fibers. **Mononeuropathy** refers to involvement of a single nerve. Mononeuropathies are most commonly caused by trauma, particularly when entrapment or compression is involved. Leprosy can also cause a form of mononeuropathy. **Multiple mononeuropathy** refers to involvement of more than one nerve asymmetrically and in separate areas. Multiple mononeuropathies arise in collagen vascular disorders, such as systemic lupus erythematosus (SLE) and rheumatoid arthritis (RA); in metabolic diseases, such as diabetes mellitus; and in infectious diseases, such as HIV or Lyme disease.

Polyneuropathy is the involvement of many nerves simultaneously and in the same region. It usually develops slowly, affecting the distal lower extremities first. The disorder most often arises in the setting of metabolic disorders or nutritional deficiencies, such as deficiency of vitamins B_1 or B_{12}, but it may also arise with malignancy and toxins, such as phenytoin, heavy metals, and industrial solvents.

Clinical manifestations typically include muscle weakness and atrophy, decreased deep tendon reflexes, sensory loss, and vasomotor symptoms.

Electromyography (EMG) and nerve conduction velocity studies are useful in confirming neuropathy. General work-up for etiology includes a CBC, urine levels, and thyroid function tests, as well as a thorough history and exam.

Treatment of the systemic disorders will permit a slow recovery. Apposition of transected nerves is important in cases of trauma. Surgical decompression or corticosteroids can be useful in entrapment neuropathies.

Coma

Coma is a state of unresponsiveness from which the patient cannot be aroused. It arises from dysfunction of both cerebral hemispheres or of the brainstem reticular activating system. It can develop in the context of mass lesions, metabolic encephalopathy, or seizures.

The patient does not respond to verbal command or mechanical stimulation, although flexor or extensor posturing in response to mechanical stimulation may be present.

Coma of acute onset is typical of a subarachnoid hemorrhage or a brainstem stroke. A progression to coma over minutes or hours occurs with intracerebral hemorrhage. Onset over days to a week suggests chronic subdural hematoma, tumor, or abscess. A coma that develops without focal signs of lateralization and that follows symptoms of delirium often results from metabolic causes.

Pupil size can suggest the presence and location of an intracerebral mass. Pupils are slightly smaller than their normal 3- to 4-mm diameter during early transtentorial herniation with thalamic involvement. Dilated pupils (5–7 mm) unreactive to light suggest damage at or below the midbrain. Pinpoint pupils of 1-mm diameter suggest a pontine lesion, opioid overdose, or some other exogenous toxin. In metabolic coma, pupil constriction remains intact, even when extraocular movements are impaired.

Motor response to pain also indicates the level of brain dysfunction. Localizing responses to pain occur in superficial coma. The decorticate response, with flexion at the elbow and leg extension, suggests a thalamic lesion of compression. The decerebrate response, characterized by elbow and leg extension, suggests a midbrain lesion (Fig. 15-3). No response to pain occurs in patients with pontine or medullary compromise.

Emergency management of the comatose patient involves the "ABCs," with maintenance of *airway* patency, *breathing*, and *circulation*. Blood must be analyzed for infection and metabolic abnormalities. Glucose, thiamine, and naloxone may be administered intravenously to treat several possible causes of coma. Diazepam is given if seizures are present. The underlying cause of the coma should be rapidly identified and treated.

Confusion

Confusional states are less acute in onset and less severe in intensity than delirium. They are common in the hospitalized elderly. Confusion often arises in systemic organ failure, overmedication, febrile infections, and nutritional deficiencies.

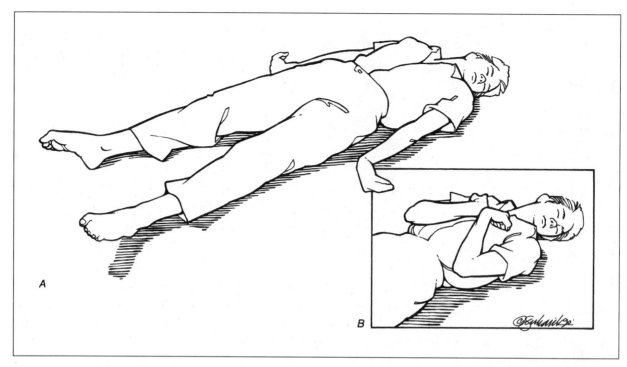

Fig. 15-3. A. Decerebrate posture. B. Decorticate posture. (From N Caroline. *Emergency Care in the Streets*, Fifth Edition. Boston: Little, Brown, 1995.)

Drowsiness, apathy, disorientation, decreased concentration, and other mental status abnormalities are common. Physiologic tremor and asterixis may also be present.

Diagnosis is by presentation.

Correct the underlying problem. Medication dosages may need to be decreased, and unnecessary agents should be discontinued.

Syncope

Syncope (fainting) is an acute and transient loss of consciousness. Cardiac etiologies may lead to syncope if reduced cardiac output causes insufficient cerebral blood flow. In these patients, syncope is generally related to exertion. Other causes include arrhythmia, obstruction of cardiac outflow, hypovolemia, peripheral vasodilation, and decreased venous return. Orthostatic hypotension and vasovagal syncope do not cause symptoms if the patient is lying down. Seizures, pulmonary embolism, and metabolic abnormalities may all cause noncardiogenic syncope.

Ataxia

Ataxia involves a lack of coordination caused by cerebellar, vestibular, or sensory dysfunction. It may present with abnormalities of gait, speech, or eye movement. Cerebellar ataxia presents with irregular voluntary movement. These patients have decreased muscle tone, decreased coordination, intention tremor, nystagmus, gaze paresis, and abnormal smooth pursuit and saccades.

Vestibular ataxia presents as a lack of limb coordination that resolves while the patient is lying down. These patients may have a unilateral nystagmus and may complain of vertigo. Sensory ataxia derives from lesions of the proprioceptive pathway. Lesions of the posterior columns and polyneuropathies tend to affect the legs symmetrically. Joint position and vibration sense are impaired.

Gait Abnormality

Normal gait requires intact coordination of the motor, vestibular, and proprioceptive pathways. Lesions at any level will produce characteristic abnormalities. A few examples are given below:

- **Cerebellar lesions** cause a truncal ataxia, with a broad-based, unsteady, and irregular gait. Turning is impaired.
- In **corticospinal disorders** such as hemiparesis, the affected leg circumducts as it steps forward and may also drag somewhat, leading to asymmetric shoe wear. A scissors-like gait is typical of bilateral involvement.
- **Extrapyramidal lesions**, such as those seen in Parkinson's disease, have a characteristic festinating gait. Patients assume a flexed posture and walk in small but rapid steps, without arm swinging.
- **Motor system lesions** (lesions of anterior horn cells, peripheral motor nerves, and skeletal muscle) cause footdrop if the anterior tibial muscle is involved. Calf muscle involvement prevents patients from being able to walk on their toes. Pelvic muscle involvement may cause a waddling gait.
- Patients with **sensory deficits** walk with their feet markedly raised in a "steppage gait." They also have difficulty walking with closed eyes.

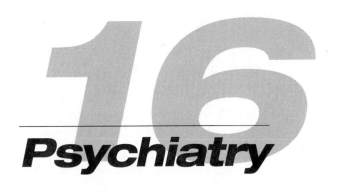

Psychiatry

Basic Principles of Care

Principles of Diagnosis

Psychiatric and medical disorders are classified on a multi-axis scheme. Axis I is reserved for diagnosed clinical psychiatric disorders, and axis II is used for personality disorders. Although the two may be related, there are different criteria for clinical and personality disorders. Axis III is used for any coexisting medical condition.

Diagnosis of psychiatric disorders is based on fulfilling specific sets of criteria, which involve the presence of signs or symptoms of the disorder for a specified period of time. Most diagnostic criteria also require that the disorder cause severe stress or deficits in functioning. In this chapter, impairment of function is not included in the diagnosis section for each disorder, but unless otherwise noted, it must always be present to establish the diagnosis.

Chronic Care

Many psychiatric disorders can be fully controlled with appropriate long-term care. The medications used in this field, however, can have significant side effects that increase over time. The effects of chronic medication use must be monitored, and adjustments in dose or changes in the type of medication may be necessary. In addition, many of the side effects can be treated—for example, antipsychotic medications cause chronic extrapyramidal side effects (e.g., parkinsonian effects, tardive dyskinesia, dystonia), which can be treated with anticholinergics. When possible, medications should be tapered slowly, and the patient should be carefully monitored to ensure that reintroduction of a medication is not needed.

Emergency and Acute Care

Suicidal Ideation

Suicidal thoughts or actions are a serious problem, and many suicides may be preventable if properly addressed. Hospitalization may not be required in patients who agree to call their physicians if their suicidal ideation worsens. In this case, the physician must be available to the patient at any time. Environmental stresses should be addressed, support should be offered, and alternatives to suicide should be discussed. However, hospitalization is necessary if any question about the patient's suicidal potential remains. Involuntary hospitalization is clearly permitted for patients who may pose a danger to themselves. Medications, therapy, and electroconvulsive therapy (ECT) should then be initiated as needed.

Homicidal Ideation

The possibility of causing danger to others is another clear indication for involuntary hospitalization. The patient may be restrained or sedated if necessary. Treatment directed at any underlying disorder should be initiated.

Neuroleptic Malignant Syndrome

Neuroleptic malignant syndrome is a serious complication of antipsychotic medications that occurs within 1–3 days of starting medication and may last up to 2 weeks. Men have this reaction more frequently than women. The pathology is not understood. Mortality is as high as 25%.

Extremely high fever and muscular rigidity develop in addition to agitation, tachycardia, elevated blood pressure, tremor, incontinence, and an altered level of consciousness that may progress to coma.

The presentation, in the context of a new antipsychotic medication, is usually sufficient for diagnosis. Lab evaluation indicates muscle damage, with high creatine phosphokinase (CPK). Myoglobin may also be elevated and the high level can result in renal failure.

Treatment involves immediate cessation of the antipsychotic agent, cooling of the patient, and maintaining acceptable vital signs and urinary function. Dantrolene, a skeletal muscle relaxant, can relieve the muscle rigidity and improve the patient's prognosis.

Disorders Diagnosed in Childhood

Mental Retardation

Low mental functioning, with an IQ of 70 or less, is also associated with defects in adaptive functioning (i.e., the ability of a person to adapt to the surrounding environment). Early alterations in embryonic development are the most common cause. Other mental disorders are diagnosed in these patients at 3–4 times the rate of the general population and are often caused by the same factor that caused the mental retardation. Retardation is graded as mild, moderate, severe, profound, or unspecified, with about 85% of cases considered mild.

The infant is significantly delayed in reaching social and developmental milestones. Physical exam has related findings only in certain syndromes, such as Down's syndrome.

IQ can be assessed by several standardized intelligence tests. Adaptive functioning can be assessed by questioning the patient's caregivers, as well as by several available scales for adaptive functioning. The defects must begin before age 18 for this diagnosis to apply.

Appropriate environments for patients with mental retardation depend on the severity of the disorder. Patients with mild retardation and good support may live in the community, but more severe disease generally requires more supervised settings.

Communication Disorders

Communication disorders include a variety of defects in speech and language. The disorder may interfere with social communication. Standardized tests are available to evaluate the defects. Speech therapy may be helpful. Up to 80% of patients who stutter recover spontaneously.

Learning Disorders

Academic functioning below what would be appropriate for the patient's age, IQ, and education is the primary feature of learning disorders, which include disorders of reading, mathematics, and written expression. Associated medical conditions, such as fetal alcohol syndrome or lead poisoning, may be present.

Poor academic achievement may be accompanied by low self-esteem and problems in social skills. Patients have a high drop-out rate from school. Patients may also have attention deficit disorder or major depressive disorder.

The patient's scores on certain standardized tests are at least two standard deviations lower than expected on the basis of general intelligence. Vision and hearing problems must be ruled out.

When learning disorders are identified early, intervention with direct and individualized instruction can improve functioning significantly.

Attention Deficit/Hyperactivity Disorder

Attention deficit/hyperactivity disorder (ADHD) is a disorder of inattention and hyperactivity that is four times more prevalent in males than females. It is most often diagnosed in elementary school-aged children, and symptoms tend to remit as the patient matures. Some patients continue to have symptoms, particularly low self-esteem and academic failure, into adolescence and adulthood. Personality disorders may arise in adults.

Lack of attention in school work and play is often manifested as the inability to finish a task. Patients may be easily distracted or forgetful. Hyperactivity may involve fidgetiness, excessive talkativity, or feelings of restlessness. Impulsivity is also a hallmark of ADHD, characterized by impatience, interrupting, and involvement in potentially dangerous activities.

The patient's symptoms must begin before age 7 and must be present in at least two separate settings.

Psychostimulant medications and behavioral therapies can control the disorder. Methylphenidate (Ritalin) is most effective, but side effects include insomnia, depression, headaches, stomachaches, and high blood pressure. Growth reduction may occur with high doses.

Conduct Disorder

Conduct disorder consists of disruptive behavior patterns that violate basic societal norms. It is more common in boys than girls.

Patients act aggressively, fight often, use weapons, act cruelly, or are sexually aggressive. Destruction of others' property and theft are also common.

The above behavior patterns must persist for at least 1 year. The four subtypes include:
1. Aggressive behavior toward others or toward animals.
2. Nonaggressive behavior with resulting property damage.
3. Theft or deceit.
4. Serious violations of societal rules.

Psychotherapy, family therapy, and special schooling. Children with this disorder are at increased risk for developing antisocial personality disorder and substance abuse as adults.

Oppositional Defiant Disorder

Oppositional defiant disorder is a disruptive behavior disorder characterized by negativity, hostility, and defiance. Before puberty, the diagnosis is more common in boys, but girls and boys have equal rates of developing this disorder after puberty.

Children lose their temper often, argue with authority figures, actively annoy others, blame others for mistakes, and are frequently angry, annoyed, or vindictive.

Patients must show the above behaviors persistently for at least 6 months.

Psychotherapy, family therapy, and special schooling.

Tic Disorders

A tic is an involuntary but sometimes suppressible motor movement or vocalization that is sudden, repeated, and stereotypical for the individual. **Tourette's disorder** is a tic disorder that involves multiple, severe tics, both motor and vocal, that change over time. **Coprolalia**, a complex tic involving involuntary utterance of obscenities, is seen in less than 10% of Tourette's patients, contrary to popular perceptions of this disorder. Patients have periods of remission, and symptoms lessen throughout adolescence and adulthood, but the disease usually lasts a lifetime. A genetic predisposition to Tourette's disorder has an autosomal dominant pattern of inheritance.

Simple motor tics are eye blinking, grimacing, or shrugging, whereas complex motor tics can be gestures, jumping, or twirling when walking. Simple vocal tics such as throat clearing or barking are common. Complex vocal tics include repeated phrases, coprolalia, and echolalia (i.e., echoing another person's words). Stress tends to worsen tic disorders, and sleep or involvement in an activity generally diminish tic activity.

Diagnosis requires frequent tics for at least 1 year, beginning before age 18.

Haloperidol or pimozide.

Separation Anxiety Disorder

In separation anxiety disorder, patients are extremely anxious about being away from home or loved ones. The disorder usually develops before adolescence and may follow a traumatic event.

Patients may be homesick and extremely worried that something bad may happen to them or to their loved ones when they are away. Children often cling to parents and refuse to attend activities away from home. They often have difficulty sleeping and may have nightmares.

Excessive anxiety for at least 4 weeks.

Separation anxiety disorder resolves within several years. Counseling may be useful.

Enuresis

Enuresis is an elimination disorder that involves a pattern of urinating in inappropriate places. It is usually involuntary, and coexisting mental disorders may be present in a minority of patients.

Enuresis may be diurnal, nocturnal, or both. It may result in low self-esteem or limitation of the child's activities.

Inappropriate urination must occur at least twice weekly for longer than 3 months or must cause significant problems in social or academic functioning. The child must be at least 5 years old. Physiologic causes should be ruled out.

Motivational counseling, behavioral modification, enuresis alarms, or imipramine are commonly used.

Encopresis

Encopresis is an elimination disorder that involves the passage of feces in inappropriate places. Elimination is generally involuntary. It may involve constipation with overflow incontinence, resistance to toilet training, or a disruptive behavior disorder.

In addition to inappropriate passage of feces, the child may suffer from embarrassment and avoidance of social situations. If constipation is present, the patient may have continuous fecal leakage and anal fissures.

The child must be at least 4 years old with episodes of encopresis at least once a month for 3 months.

Complete bowel evacuation should be followed by establishment of regular bowel movements. Giving the patient mineral oil, roughage, and laxatives and encouraging regular visits to the toilet may help.

Pervasive Developmental Disorders

Pervasive developmental disorders involve severe difficulties in many areas of development, including social skills, communication, and behavior. These pervasive deficits are usually evident early in life, and patients often have concurrent mental retardation or other medical problems. This group includes:

- **Autistic disorder** (see below).
- **Rett's disorder** is seen only in females and involves the development of severe deficits after a 5-month normal period. Head growth slows, acquired hand skills disintegrate, and stereotyped hand movements develop. Social involvement also decreases over time but may improve again later. Deficient language skills and mental retardation are often severe.
- **Childhood disintegrative disorder** is a rare disorder in which the child has at least 2 years of normal development before deficits develop in language, social involvement, bowel or bladder control, and motor skills. Patients often have concurrent, severe mental retardation.
- **Asperger's disorder** consists of severe social impairment and stereotyped behaviors that occur without cognitive or language deficits.

SIGNS & SYMPTOMS

In addition to the above findings, nonspecific neurological symptoms may be present, including abnormal EEGs and increased frequency of seizure disorder.

DIAGNOSIS

These are clinical diagnoses based on the constellation of features discussed above.

TREATMENT

Behavioral therapy may be useful, although prognosis is poor.

Autistic Disorder

Autistic disorder involves deficits in communication, social involvement, and participation in activities, often coexistent with mental retardation or uneven intellectual ability. Males are affected 4–5 times more frequently than females. Patients may develop schizophrenia or seizure disorder as they age.

SIGNS & SYMPTOMS

Language is delayed or altogether absent. Nonverbal communication is impaired, peer relationships are deficient, and social skills are poorly developed. Patients may be unaware of others around them. Stereotyped behaviors and activities are present, often with an insistence on regular routine. Patients may be impulsive, hyperactive, or aggressive, with inappropriate emotional responses. Nonspecific neurologic signs and symptoms may be present, in addition to seizure disorder.

DIAGNOSIS

Signs and symptoms begin when the child is less than 3 years old, and a normal period rarely precedes onset.

TREATMENT

Behavior therapy and speech therapy may help, although no truly effective treatment is known. Butyrophenones may somewhat reduce aggressive or self-destructive patterns.

Mood Disorders

Major Depressive Disorder

Major depressive disorder is a mood disturbance characterized by at least one major depressive episode (described in box), without a history of manic episodes. Mean age of onset is in the 40s. About half of patients have subsequent episodes later in their lives. When disease is recurrent, remissions may last for years, but intervals tend to be shorter later in life. Patients have a high death rate, and many commit suicide.

Women have a lifetime prevalence of up to 25%, while men have a prevalence of around 10%. Risk is not associated with socioeconomic status, education level, or ethnicity. There is a familial tendency toward major depressive disorder, as well as increased rates of alcohol dependence and attention deficit/hyperactivity disorder among first-degree relatives.

SIGNS & SYMPTOMS

Symptoms are described in detail in the box on major depressive episodes. No physical findings are associated.

DIAGNOSIS

The criteria for a major depressive episode must be met.

TREATMENT

A combination of psychosocial therapy and pharmacotherapy is most effective. Several effective antidepressant medications are available:

- Tricyclic antidepressants (TCAs) require 3–4 weeks for effect and may induce a manic episode. Side effects include sedation and anticholinergic effects (e.g., dry mouth, constipation, blurred vision, urinary retention). Overdose causes cardiac effects, which may be lethal.
- Monoamine oxidase inhibitors (MAOIs) also require several weeks for effect. They are particularly useful for patients with atypical depression. Foods containing tyramine (red wine, cheese) must be avoided, as they can precipitate a hypertensive crisis.
- Serotonin reuptake inhibitors, such as Prozac, are widely prescribed. They take effect within 1–3 weeks. Side effects include GI complaints, headaches, and impotence. Overdose is not lethal.
- Atypical antidepressants, such as bupropion, are newer and increasingly used. Anticholinergic side effects are absent, and overdose is not lethal.

Electroconvulsive therapy (ECT) is used for refractory or very severe disease, or in patients who cannot tolerate medications. ECT is very effective when used properly and has few side effects (e.g., short-term memory disturbances).

Major Depressive Episode

A major depressive episode is a component of several mood disorders. It is defined as a period of more than 2 weeks of either excessive sadness, anhedonia (inability to experience pleasure), or irritability. In addition, at least four of the following must be present: vegetative symptoms (change in appetite, weight, sleep, and psychomotor activity), low energy level, indecisiveness or lack of concentration, a sense of guilt or worthlessness, and suicidal ideation. Insomnia is much more typical than hypersomnia, and abnormal sleep EEGs are common. Significant distress or impaired functioning must also result from the mood disturbance.

If untreated, a major depressive episode often lasts more than 6 months, after which individuals generally recover completely. About 25% continue to have a lesser degree of symptoms. Women often note a worsening of symptoms during the premenstrual period. Neurotransmitters that may be contributory include norepinephrine, acetylcholine, serotonin, dopamine, and gamma-aminobutyric acid (GABA).

Seasonal Affective Disorder

Actually a subtype of major depressive disorder, seasonal affective disorder (SAD) involves depressive episodes that occur in winter, with improvement in spring and summer. Abnormal melatonin secretion may be responsible. Phototherapy or sleep deprivation therapy is useful in treatment.

Dysthymic Disorder

Dysthymic disorder is characterized by a persistent feeling of depression that does not meet the criteria for major depressive disorder but lasts more than 2 years. Each year, about 10% of patients with dysthymic disorder develop major depressive disorder. Many patients also have evidence of personality disorders. Men and women are equally likely to have dysthymic disorder.

SIGNS & SYMPTOMS

In addition to depressed mood, patients experience changes in appetite and sleep, decreased energy, inability to concentrate, hopeless feelings, and low self-esteem. Vegetative symptoms are less common than in major depressive disorder.

DIAGNOSIS

The patient must have a depressed mood more days than not for 2 years and at least two of the associated symptoms.

TREATMENT

Combination psychotherapy and cognitive therapy. Medications may be used for persistent symptoms.

Manic Episode

For at least 1 week, an individual experiences an abnormally euphoric, expansive, or irritable mood. At least three associated features must be present, which may include grandiosity, decreased need for sleep, increased pressure or volume of speech, flight of ideas, increased distractibility, psychomotor agitation, increased goal-directed activity, and an increase in pleasurable activities that could have a high cost (e.g., extravagant shopping). Grandiose delusions and psychotic features may occur. Social, academic, or occupational functioning is impaired, and hospitalization is often necessary. Such a constellation of symptoms resulting from medication or ECT does not constitute a manic episode. If criteria of a major depressive episode are also present, the term "mixed episode" is used.

Bipolar Disorder

Bipolar I disorder is characterized by manic or mixed episodes, and it may also involve one or more major depressive episodes. Bipolar II disorder involves major depressive episodes with at least one instance of a hypomanic episode. Hypomania has basically the same set of criteria as a manic episode, except that severe impairment and psychotic features may not be present.

Bipolar disorder is generally a recurrent disease, and each patient has an individual pattern of cycling. The natural history of the disease shows about four episodes in a 10-year period, although a minority of patients are "rapid cyclers" with more than four episodes in a year. The frequency increases as the patient ages. Most patients function normally between episodes, although about 25% continue to have deficits.

Men and women have equal rates of bipolar disorder. Episodes may develop in women during a postpartum period. There is a familial tendency toward mood disorders, which has been shown in twin and adoption studies.

SIGNS & SYMPTOMS

The features of a manic episode are present in bipolar I disorder. History of a major depressive episode and a hypomanic episode are present in bipolar II disorder. In addition, 10–15% of patients commit suicide, and truancy and violence against others are not uncommon.

DIAGNOSIS

The criteria discussed above must be met, with concurrent impairment in social or work performance for bipolar I disorder. Onset typically occurs in the 30s. In patients over 40, organic etiologies must be thoroughly excluded.

TREATMENT

Psychotherapy and cognitive therapy in combination with lithium are often effective. Lithium may cause GI distress, weight gain, fatigue, and tremor. Toxicity causes vomiting, diarrhea, ataxia, and confusion, leading to seizures and coma. Lithium prophylaxis is indicated in severe disease, and levels should be monitored carefully. Patients may also require antipsychotic medications.

Mood Disorder Due to a General Medical Condition

A pervasive mood disturbance can be caused by biological changes from another medical disease, but the disorder is not associated with the stress of having a medical condition. Atypical features of a mood disorder, such as later-than-expected age of onset, may help to establish the diagnosis. Common etiologies include degenerative neurological conditions, cerebrovascular disease, endocrine or metabolic conditions, cancer, and autoimmune disease. Risk of suicide is particularly high when the patient suffers from an incurable and painful condition.

Anxiety Disorders

Panic Disorder

In panic disorder, patients experience recurrent, uncued panic attacks (see box) and suffer from constant worry about having another attack. Panic disorder may coexist with agoraphobia, which is an extreme fear of any situation in which escape or help may not be immediately available.

The course of panic disorder varies greatly. It is generally chronic but episodic. Patients may have attacks regularly or in sporadic bursts with long asymptomatic periods. Some patients also have "limited symptom" attacks, in which criteria for a full panic attack are not met. Panic disorder generally begins in late adolescence or early adulthood.

During an attack, the patient may have elevated heart rate and blood pressure. Studies suggest that mitral valve prolapse or thyroid disorders may be more prevalent among panic disorder patients. Avoidance of crowded or restricted situations, such as elevators or airplanes, may result from agoraphobia. Patients also may have generalized anxiety, worry, or low self-esteem. Major depressive disorder occurs in more than 50% of patients.

Recurrent attacks must involve at least four of the related symptoms and be associated with at least 1 month of related anxiety. The diagnosis of panic disorder is classified as either with or without agoraphobia.

TCAs or MAOIs with behavioral or psychotherapy.

Panic Attacks

Panic attacks are a feature of several anxiety disorders. Unexpected, or "uncued," panic attacks are often involved in panic disorder, whereas situationally bound, or "cued," panic attacks are generally related to phobias. An attack is defined as a period of extreme fear or anxiety, often with a feeling of impending danger and a need to escape. Four of 13 associated symptoms must be present, including palpitations, sweating, trembling, shortness of breath, a sense of choking, chest discomfort, nausea, dizziness, derealization or depersonalization, fear of losing control, fear of dying, paresthesias, and chills or hot flushes.

Specific Phobia

Previously called simple phobia, specific phobia is the extreme fear of a specific object or situation. The fear may concern being injured, losing control, or even fainting. Most phobias have a childhood onset, and traumatic events or panic attacks may predispose one to developing a phobia. Females are diagnosed with this disorder more frequently than males.

The phobic item immediately provokes a panic attack or manifestation of excessive anxiety. The level of severity is related to the proximity of the phobic object and to the patient's capacity to escape. Instead of the usual increase in autonomic function, patients may have a vasovagal response, particularly with phobias to blood, injection, and injury. Patients try to avoid the phobic object, and this avoidance or worry can cause significant impairment in social or occupational functioning. Adult patients generally have some insight as to the unwarranted nature of their fears.

An excessive fear of a particular object results in anxiety and avoidance. Subtypes of phobias include animal, natural environment, blood-injection injury, and situational.

Behavioral therapy.

Social Phobia

Excessive fear of social or performance settings is accompanied by extreme anxiety when the patient is exposed to these situations. Generalized social phobia involves fear in most social interactions, and patients often have very severe impairments in their daily lives. Social phobia usually begins in the mid-teens and may follow an embarrassing incident. It lasts throughout the patient's life, with exacerbations at times of stress.

The anxiety response may be a panic attack or severe anxiety, with such symptoms as palpitations, sweating, shaking, and confusion. Patients avoid the phobic situations and dread being embarrassed. Patients often have low self-esteem and may be underachievers. Anxiety may be evident with even minimal contact, and other anxiety or mood disorders are often present. Adults have insight that their fear is unwarranted, but children usually do not.

A patient with extreme, persistent fear of social or performance situations has an anxiety response in these public settings.

Behavioral therapy. If unsuccessful, MAOIs may be used.

Post-Traumatic Stress Disorder

The typical symptoms of post-traumatic stress disorder (PTSD) develop after experiencing or witnessing a traumatic event. The syndrome generally, but not always, develops within 3 months of the event. Half of patients recover completely within 3 more months, whereas others have symptoms for over a year. PTSD may coexist with other anxiety disorders or with depression. Social supports and personal history can affect the development of PTSD, although it can occur in patients without any apparent predisposition.

Dreams, memories, and "flashbacks" of the trauma are prominent. The resulting psychological distress is severe. Certain situations trigger the distress and memories, and patients try to avoid these settings. Patients may be amnestic of the trauma. They may feel detached, unemotional, or as if they are unable to experience pleasure. Some have a persistent sense of doom. Survivor guilt, self-destructive behavior, somatization, and social withdrawal are common. Anxiety or arousal is constant. Increased autonomic arousal may be noted on exam, with rapid heart rate and increased sweating.

A patient must have had a very stressing experience and must have experienced severe fear, helplessness, or horror. Re-experiencing the event and avoidance of associated stimuli must be present, with concurrent increased arousal. These symptoms must last at least 1 month for an acute diagnosis and last more than 3 months for a diagnosis of chronic PTSD.

Imipramine (a TCA) and phenalzine (an MAOI) are most often used. Psychotherapy is also effective.

Acute Stress Disorder

Anxiety or other characteristic symptoms develop within 1 month of a traumatic event. During the event, the patient experiences a sense of detachment or numbed emotion, a lack of awareness, derealization or depersonalization, or dissociative amnesia.

Dissociative symptoms follow the trauma, with numbed emotions, anhedonia, or guilt. As in PTSD, the patient later re-experiences the event and avoids related stimuli. On physical exam, injury resulting from the recent trauma may be evident.

Symptoms must last at least 2 days and less than 4 weeks, after which the diagnosis of PTSD applies.

Supportive therapy may be helpful.

Generalized Anxiety Disorder

In generalized anxiety disorder, patients experience persistent anxiety and apprehension that they cannot control. Anxiety may concern normal daily events, and the worry is excessive relative to likely possible outcomes. Many patients are nervous or overly worried prior to the development of this disorder. Patients present in childhood, adolescence, or early adulthood, and symptoms continue throughout their lives. Generalized anxiety disorder is somewhat more prevalent in women than in men.

In addition to anxiety, the patient may experience restlessness, lack of concentration, easy fatigability, difficulty sleeping, irritability, and muscle tension or other musculoskeletal problems. Some somatic complaints or stress-related conditions may be present.

Anxiety and worry persist at least 6 months with at least 3 of the above symptoms.

Psychotherapy and anxiolytics (benzodiazepines and buspirone) may be helpful.

Obsessive-Compulsive Disorder

The severe, recurrent obsessions or compulsions that characterize obsessive-compulsive disorder cause the patient significant distress and may require excessive time to complete. An **obsession** is a recurrent thought, feeling, idea, or image that is unpleasant and intrusive but cannot be controlled by the patient. The patient realizes its inappropriateness and experiences severe anxiety; therefore, the obsessions are considered "ego-dystonic." Common obsessions concern contamination, order, frightening images or doubts, or disturbing sexual images. Patients try to suppress, ignore, or counteract their obsessions. A **compulsion** is a repeated mental or motor behavior performed to lessen anxiety, usually following an obsessive thought. These acts are either very excessive or clearly unable to accomplish the desired goal. Common compulsions are repetitive checking, washing, counting, and stereotyped ordering.

Obsessive-compulsive disorder begins early, at an average age of 20 years old. Men and women have equal rates of this diagnosis. Most patients have exacerbations at stressful times. There is a high rate of concordance with Tourette's syndrome and other tic disorders.

Patients may avoid settings that evoke obsessions or compulsions. Sleep disturbances, alcohol use, and feelings of guilt are common. Skin problems from cleaning compulsions may be found on physical exam.

Obsessions and compulsions must require excessive time or cause severe distress. Adult patients must at some point have some insight, realizing that the behaviors are unusual.

Clomipramine, possibly with behavioral therapy. Most patients improve, although one-third later develop major depression.

Anxiety Due to a General Medical Condition

In this disorder, excessive anxiety is directly caused by another medical disorder. Common conditions include endocrine, cardiovascular, respiratory, metabolic, and neurological diseases, and this condition is present on history and physical exam. Symptoms of many anxiety disorders may be present, including generalized anxiety, panic attacks, obsessions, or compulsions. This diagnosis is supported by an appropriate temporal relation between the medical condition and the anxiety disorder.

Schizophrenia and Other Psychotic Disorders

Schizophrenia

Schizophrenia is a devastating psychotic disorder with a poor prognosis. Onset is from the late teens to the early 30s, and it has a chronic course. The actual cause is unknown, although dopamine hyperactivity has been implicated. A genetic predisposition seems to exist as well, and first-degree relatives of schizophrenic patients have 10 times the rate of disease as the general population. Schizophrenia affects all socioeconomic and ethnic groups, although the incidence is somewhat higher in large cities. The disproportionate number of poor and homeless people with schizophrenia is probably due to "downward drift," as these patients function poorly in society. Overall, schizophrenic patients have a high mortality rate, and 50% attempt suicide.

Prognosis is best with a late, sudden onset in a patient with good premorbid functioning, especially when an obvious event precipitates the onset of symptoms. Patients with a family history of mood disorders and those who have primarily affective or positive symptoms (see below) tend to do better. Also, married patients with good support systems have a better prognosis. History of perinatal trauma, family history of schizophrenia, personal history of aggressive behavior, presence of negative symptoms (see below), and neurological signs and symptoms are considered poor prognostic features.

Onset may be abrupt, but most patients have a prodrome of increasingly bizarre behavior. Two categories of symptoms are present: positive symptoms (delusions, hallucinations, disorganized speech, and disorganized or catatonic behavior) and negative symptoms (flat affect, apathy, anhedonia, inattentiveness). There are several subtypes of schizophrenia:

- The paranoid type has relatively intact cognition and affect, but delusions and hallucinations are prominent. Delusions are often, but not necessarily, persecutory or grandiose.
- The disorganized type involves inappropriate and fragmented speech, behavior, and affect.
- Patients with the catatonic type have a prominent psychomotor disturbance, such as very decreased activity, excessive activity, mutism, echolalia (repetition of others' speech), echopraxia (repetition of others' movements), or extreme negative symptoms.
- Residual type is used to describe patients with an asymptomatic period following an episode of diagnosed schizophrenia.

DIAGNOSIS

Some prodrome or symptoms must be present for at least 6 months, including 1 month with at least two of the above symptoms. If delusions are bizarre, only this symptom need be present for diagnosis.

TREATMENT

Antipsychotics (also called neuroleptics or major tranquilizers) are used, including dopamine-receptor antagonists and clozapine. All medications require a trial period of at least 4–6 weeks. Hospitalization may be needed for stabilization of severe disease or for patient safety. Psychosocial therapy should be integrated into a comprehensive treatment plan.

Side effects of dopamine-receptor antagonists include orthostatic hypotension, peripheral anticholinergic effects (dry mouth, blurry vision, constipation, urinary retention, mydriasis), and increased prolactin secretion (causing breast enlargement, galactorrhea, and impotence in men; amenorrhea and anorgasmia in women). Parkinsonian symptoms may begin in 3 months, and **tardive dyskinesia** (usually stereotypical oral movements such as chewing) may develop after at least 6 months of use. Clozapine is a newer drug, and it is usually used as a second-line treatment. Two adverse effects are agranulocytosis (rare) and seizures.

Schizophreniform Disorder

The same constellation of symptoms are present in schizophreniform disorder as in schizophrenia, but the disorder has not lasted 6 months and impaired functioning is not consistent. If the patient has active symptoms for less than 6 months, schizophreniform disorder is applied as a provisional diagnosis, because the criteria for schizophrenia may be met in the future. Antipsychotic medications or ECT are used, and hospitalization may be needed for effective monitoring and treatment.

Schizoaffective Disorder

When the patient has a mood disorder and separate psychotic symptoms, the term schizoaffective disorder applies. The patient must experience delusions or hallucinations for at least 2 weeks without concurrent mood symptoms in order to establish the presence of separate psychotic features. Mania or depression may be present, and antimanic or antidepressant medications are the first line of treatment. Antipsychotics are used only if needed for acute management. Hospitalization and psychosocial approaches are appropriate as well.

Delusional Disorder

Delusional disorder involves the presence of one or more nonbizarre delusions in a patient without markedly impaired functioning.

The delusion may be grandiose, jealous, erotomanic (when the patient believes that a certain individual, who may be entirely unconnected with the patient, is in love with him or her), persecutory, or somatic. Ideas of reference, in which random events are interpreted as having personal significance, are common. Auditory or visual hallucinations may be present, but they are not prominent. Tactile or olfactory hallucinations, on the other hand, may be prominent and may be related to the delusion. Otherwise, psychosocial functioning and behavior are not severely impaired.

Symptoms last at least 1 month. If delusions are bizarre, the diagnosis of schizophrenia or schizophreniform disorder applies.

Antipsychotic medications with hospitalization and psychotherapy. Half of patients recover completely.

Brief Psychotic Disorder

Formerly called brief reactive psychosis, patients with brief psychotic disorder have an abrupt onset of psychotic features followed by complete recovery.

Positive symptoms of delusions, hallucination, and disorganized speech or behavior are present. Functional impairment may be extreme.

Symptoms are present for more than 1 day and less than 1 month. Diagnosis is specified as "with marked stressor," "without marked stressor," or "with postpartum onset."

Hospitalization, low-dose antipsychotics, and psychotherapy.

Shared Psychotic Disorder (Folie à Deux)

Shared psychotic disorder occurs when a patient becomes involved in the delusions of another, already psychotic person. The inducer, or primary case, is typically the dominant person in a close relationship. The inducer often has schizophrenia, and the delusion may be bizarre. If the relationship between the two is interrupted, the patient's delusional belief will diminish. Significant support is needed for this separation. Antipsychotics may be used, and family therapy is critical.

Psychotic Disorder Due to a General Medical Condition

In this disorder, prominent delusions or hallucinations are directly caused by another medical disorder. Common conditions include neurological diseases (e.g., neoplasms, cerebrovascular disease, and migraines), endocrine or metabolic diseases, electrolyte imbalance, and renal disease. A general medical condition is present on history and physical exam. This diagnosis is supported by an appropriate temporal relation between the medical condition and the psychotic disorder, or by atypical features such as olfactory hallucinations.

Substance-Related Disorders

Substance Intoxication

Reversible symptoms result from the use of a psychoactive substance due to its direct physiological effects on the central nervous system. Initial episodes of substance use and intoxication usually start in the patient's teens and may develop into problems of abuse and dependence.

Behavioral changes are significantly maladaptive and may involve aggressive behavior, impaired judgment or cognition, mood lability, and impaired occupational or academic functioning. Symptoms are specific to the substance used. Intoxication tends to be more immediate and intense with agents that are inhaled or injected because they have more rapid increases in blood levels.

The above symptoms follow substance use and are not related to a medical disorder. This diagnosis does not apply to nicotine.

Treatment is discussed under individual substances below.

Substance Abuse

A self-destructive pattern of substance use continues despite negative consequences.

Physical danger or harm, recurrent academic or occupational problems, legal problems, and impaired functioning in home or social environments may all result from substance use.

Repetitive problems occur over 1 year, but criteria for substance dependence are not met. This diagnosis does not apply to caffeine or nicotine.

Discussed under specific substances, below.

Substance Dependence

Dependent patients continue to use a substance in spite of significant problems related to substance use. Inhaled and injected agents, other rapidly acting agents, and substances with a short duration of action are more likely to cause dependence. Even with teenage substance use and intoxication, dependence does not usually develop until the patient is 20–40 years old.

Tolerance and/or withdrawal develop, and the patient may use the substance in order to ease symptoms of withdrawal. Patients often experience a strong "craving" for the substance. Compulsive use is often present, including use of the substance in greater amounts than intended and excessive time spent in the acquisition or use of the substance. Other aspects of compulsive use include reduction in other activities in favor of substance use and continued use of the substance even when psychological or physical problems develop.

All substances except caffeine may cause dependence. Three or more of the above symptoms are present over 1 year.

Discussed in separate sections concerning each substance, below.

Substance Withdrawal

Decreasing or stopping the prolonged use of a substance causes symptoms of withdrawal specific to that substance.

Behavioral, physiological, and cognitive changes are maladaptive and cause severe distress.

This diagnosis is generally associated with substance dependence.

Discussed in separate sections concerning each substance, below.

Substance-Induced Mental Disorders

Delirium, persisting dementia, persisting amnestic disorder, psychotic disorder, mood disorder, anxiety disorder, sexual dysfunction, and sleep disorder may all result from substance use. Any substance may be responsible, including illicit drugs, alcohol, medications, toxins, and even ECT or light therapy. These disorders may develop during or after intoxication and withdrawal, but the symptoms must be more severe than expected from intoxication or withdrawal alone. A history of substance use must precede the onset of symptoms, and symptoms usually do not last more than 4 weeks after the acute intoxication or withdrawal. Atypical features help to establish this diagnosis, such as age of onset that differs from what is typically seen in other mental disorders.

Alcohol-Related Disorders

While the majority of Americans have used alcohol at some time in their lives, and many have experienced negative consequences, most do not go on to develop alcohol abuse or dependence. Those who develop alcohol dependence often abuse other substances as well, and some have concurrent mood or anxiety disorders or schizophrenia. Alcohol-abusing and -dependent patients have increased rates of accidents, suicide, and criminal acts. Use correlates with unemployment, low socioeconomic status, and lack of education.

Men develop alcohol dependence at a rate five times greater than women. Caucasians and African-Americans have equal rates of this disorder, and Latino men have somewhat higher rates. A genetic predisposition is evident, with 3–4 times the prevalence in first-degree relatives of patients with alcohol dependence.

SIGNS & SYMPTOMS

Alcohol intoxication involves slurred speech, decreased coordination, unsteadiness, nystagmus, and attention or memory deficits, and it may progress to stupor and coma. Many Asians do not have the enzyme aldehyde dehydrogenase and cannot metabolize alcohol properly. After intake, they experience flushing and palpitations.

Alcohol withdrawal begins about 12 hours after last intake. Withdrawal involves increased autonomic activity (rapid pulse, diaphoresis), nausea and vomiting, hand tremor, difficulty sleeping, psychomotor agitation, anxiety, and even seizures. Perceptual disturbances, such as transient hallucinations or illusions, are common. Grand mal seizures, delirium, and extreme autonomic activity can be life-threatening but occur in only a small minority of patients. Alcohol withdrawal delirium, known as delirium tremens or "DTs," may reflect the presence of a related medical disorder. Symptoms of withdrawal peak within 2 days and improve by 5 days, but some residual effects can last up to 6 months.

Physical effects of chronic alcohol intake include GI ulcers and bleeding, liver cirrhosis, pancreatitis, and peripheral neuropathy. Cerebellar degeneration occurs, as does Wernicke-Korsakoff syndrome, an alcohol-induced persisting amnestic disorder. Head and neck cancers are more common among heavy alcohol users.

DIAGNOSIS

Previously discussed criteria for intoxication, abuse, dependence and withdrawal apply.

Alcohol intake eases symptoms of withdrawal but clearly does not address issues of abuse and dependence. Supportive measures, supplemental nutrition, benzodiazepines, and occasionally anticonvulsants are used in the management of withdrawal. Rehabilitation should address problems with alcohol use and any concurrent medical conditions. Treatment of dependence and abuse has success rates of up to 65% for 1-year abstinence.

Caffeine-Related Disorders

Caffeine, a commonly used substance, may cause intoxication, but (fortunately) it does not cause clinical dependence. Effects include insomnia, restlessness, flushing, diuresis, twitches, nervousness, rambling thoughts and speech, tachycardia, and psychomotor agitation. Symptoms last 6–16 hours.

Cannabis-Related Disorders

Marijuana and hashish from cannabis leaves cause psychoactive effects due to tetrahydrocannabinol (THC). Synthetic THC is used medically to relieve nausea from chemotherapy and anorexia from AIDS. In addition to feelings of elation, intoxication causes increased appetite, conjunctival injection, dry mouth, and tachycardia. Cannabis use and dependence, but not withdrawal, may develop. One-third of Americans have used cannabis, but only 4% meet criteria for dependence or abuse.

Nicotine-Related Disorders

All forms of tobacco use can contribute to dependence and withdrawal. The incidence of smoking is declining, with rates between 20–30% in the general population, although it is much higher among psychiatric patients.

Withdrawal includes depression, insomnia, irritability, anxiety, bradycardia, increased appetite, and difficulty with concentration. Other medical findings are discussed in more detail in Chap. 3.

The diagnostic criteria for dependence and withdrawal apply.

Options for cessation include support groups, hypnosis, aversive therapy, nicotine gum, nicotine patches, and medications (clonidine or doxepin). Less than 25% of smokers are able to quit on their first attempt. Desire for a cigarette may last more than 6 months after quitting.

Cocaine-Related Disorders

Cocaine can be snorted, smoked, or injected. "Crack" cocaine is a smoked form of cocaine that has extremely rapid onset. Because cocaine use causes strong feelings of euphoria, dependence can develop quickly. A short half-life requires frequent "dosing," and a great deal of money may be spent to buy cocaine in a short period of time, leading to theft, prostitution, and drug dealing.

Intoxication produces euphoria, hyperactivity, anxiety, grandiosity, and impaired judgment. Tachycardia, pupillary dilation, nausea and vomiting, psychomotor agitation, and chest pain or cardiac arrhythmias are possible physical manifestations. Withdrawal symptoms include dysphoric mood, fatigue, unpleasant dreams, insomnia or hypersomnia, and psychomotor retardation.

The above symptoms of intoxication, in addition to criteria for dependence and withdrawal.

Hospitalization is often necessary to remove the patient from the drug source. Psychological intervention and medical treatment with bromocriptine and desipramine may be useful.

Amphetamine-Related Disorders

Amphetamine and amphetamine-related compounds are generally purchased illegally but may be prescribed for obesity, ADHD, and narcolepsy.

Intoxication involves rapid heart rate, dilated pupils, high blood pressure, nausea and vomiting, psychomotor agitation, and sweating or chills. Respiratory depression, arrhythmias, seizures, and coma may result. Within several hours to days after intoxication, patients develop dysphoria, fatigue, insomnia or hypersomnia, increased appetite, psychomotor retardation, and vivid dreams.

The above symptoms of intoxication, in addition to criteria for dependence and withdrawal.

Supportive treatment and an antipsychotic may be used to manage withdrawal.

Opioid-Related Disorders

The term opioid includes morphine, heroin, codeine, hydromorphone, methadone, and other synthetics. Opioid use is associated with drug-related crimes, antisocial personality disorder, and posttraumatic stress disorder.

In addition to euphoria, intoxicated patients have slurred speech, pupillary constriction, deficits in attention and memory, and stupor or coma. Withdrawal causes dysphoria, tearing, runny nose, muscle aches, nausea and vomiting, pupillary dilation, diarrhea, yawning, insomnia, and fever.

The above symptoms for intoxication, in addition to criteria for dependence and withdrawal.

Methadone is a synthetic opioid used to stabilize dependent patients. It is then tapered down and withdrawn. Opioid antagonists, such as naloxone, are used to treat overdose. Therapeutic communities are the best option for rehabilitation, although dropout and relapse rates are high.

Sleep Disorders

Stages of Sleep

Sleep can be categorized into rapid eye movement (REM) sleep and four stages of non-REM sleep. Relaxed wakefulness, with alpha waves on the EEG, precedes stage 1, or light sleep. Half of our sleeping time is spent in stage 2 sleep, in which K complexes and sleep spindles appear on the EEG. Together, stages 3 and 4 comprise "slow-wave" sleep, with an increasing appearance of delta waves as the patient falls into deeper sleep. Children have more slow-wave sleep than adults do. Dreams occur during REM sleep, which accounts for about one-fourth of sleep time. Brain and physiologic activity are similar to activity during wakefulness, but muscle activity is inhibited. These stages cycle in 90-minute intervals throughout the night, with more REM sleep and less slow-wave sleep occurring as the night progresses.

Insomnia

Insomnia refers to disturbances in initiating or maintaining sleep. Negative conditioning may occur, in that patients are so accustomed to having difficulties falling asleep that they expect and reinforce these problems. Mood and anxiety disorders are commonly associated. Polysomnography tests (sleep studies) often show increased stage 1 sleep and insufficient slow-wave sleep. Women and the elderly have higher incidences of this common disorder. Insomnia usually begins suddenly during a time of stress, but it may persist after the stressful episode ends. Untreated, the disorder typically worsens for a few months, then stabilizes, sometimes persisting for years.

Insomnia is best treated by improving sleep hygiene. Any drugs with CNS effects (e.g., caffeine, alcohol) should be avoided, regular waking and eating times should be maintained, and means of relaxation are recommended. If unsuccessful, benzodiazepines, chloral hydrate, or other sedatives may be useful.

Sleep Apnea Syndrome

Sleep apnea syndrome is characterized by periodic cessations of breathing (apnea) during sleep that result in reduced oxygenation of the blood and arousal from sleep. The obstructive form is seen most often in obese middle-aged men and in young children with tonsillar enlargement. Typical age at presentation is 40–60 years old.

Patients present with excessive daytime somnolence because the abnormal ventilation causes frequent arousals and disrupted sleep patterns during the night. Personality changes, memory problems, and sexual dysfunction are also common complaints. Bed partners often report loud, crescendo snoring.

Apneic episodes are evident on polysomnography, and time spent in slow-wave and REM sleep is diminished. Blood gas measurements reveal hypoxia during the apneic episodes.

Continuous positive airway pressure (CPAP) is provided with a nasal mask and machine that can be used at home. Weight loss is helpful. Nasal or palatal surgery may be necessary.

Narcolepsy

Narcolepsy is a disorder of REM sleep. Onset may be in childhood, with clinical presentation during adolescence.

Sudden bouts of daytime sleep and cataplexy (sudden loss of muscle strength triggered by emotional reactions) are typical symptoms. Attacks last 10 minutes to 1 hour and may occur several times a day. Intense dreams and temporary paralysis may occur during transitions between wakefulness and sleep.

Polysomnography shows that REM sleep is inappropriately present at sleep onset.

Scheduled naps may improve symptoms dramatically. Medical treatment involves amphetamines.

Circadian Rhythm Sleep Disorder

Circadian rhythm sleep disorder occurs when the patient's internal clock does not match that of occupational or societal requirements. Patients may be sleepy during the day and wakeful at night. Jet lag and shift work may be contributory.

Parasomnias

Parasomnias generally occur in children and involve unusual phenomena during sleep, most often during slow-wave sleep. Treatment is rarely required and these disorders tend to resolve, but diazepam can lessen symptoms somewhat.

- In nightmare disorder, patients have terrifying dreams that awaken them to an alert state. The dreams usually occur during REM sleep in the second half of the night. Onset is between 3 and 6 years old.
- Sleep terror disorder involves sudden awakenings from slow-wave sleep. This usually occurs early in the night and is accompanied by a scream or cry. Up to 10 minutes of panicked behavior and difficulty waking follow. Children with this disorder do not have an increased incidence of other mental disorders, but adults with this disorder may have an associated anxiety or personality disorder. Symptoms typically begin in 4- to 12-year-old children and remit during adolescence.
- Sleepwalking disorder may include a variety of complex behaviors and occurs during slow-wave sleep. The individual is unresponsive, unable to be awakened, and later cannot recall the event. Sleepwalking in children usually begins around 4 years of age, peaks at 12, and resolves by 15. Sleepwalking in children is not associated with other disorders, but adults may have mood, anxiety, and personality disorders.

Somatoform and Factitious Disorders

Somatization Disorder

The multiple, recurring somatic problems experienced in somatization disorder cannot be explained by the presence of a general medical condition. Complaints usually involve clinically significant pain with serious impairment. Frequent medical visits, diagnostic procedures, and unnecessary surgeries may result. These symptoms are not produced intentionally. Somatization disorder patients do not have a higher mortality rate than the general population. This disorder was referred to as hysteria or Briquet's syndrome prior to the DSM-IV.

SIGNS & SYMPTOMS

In addition to pain, patients may have nausea, bloating, diarrhea, vomiting, and vague neurological complaints. Women often have menstrual irregularities, and men may complain of sexual dysfunction.

DIAGNOSIS

Significant somatic complaints begin before age 30 and last several years. Four different sites of pain must be involved. Lab tests do not support the physical symptoms.

Psychotherapy.

Conversion Disorder

"Conversion" historically reflects the redirection of an unconscious psychological conflict into somatic symptoms, and the symptoms reported may reflect local or cultural ideas of expressions of distress.

Physical complaints affecting voluntary motor or sensory function seem to suggest a neurologic disorder. Symptoms are exacerbated by stress, implicating psychological factors, but they are not intentional or factitious.

Motor problems of imbalance, weakness, aphonia (loss of voice), and swallowing difficulties are common. Sensory symptoms may involve decreased sensation, vision, or hearing. Symptoms may be inconsistent, physiologically implausible, and not supported by physical exam or lab findings.

Motor or sensory deficits cause significant impairment in functioning without a medical explanation. This diagnosis should be considered tentative early on, because medical diagnoses may become clear years later.

Psychotherapy and reassurance.

Hypochondriasis

Patients with hypochondriasis misinterpret minor physical symptoms and develop excessive fears about having serious disease. They often have a history of childhood illness or serious disease in close family members. Women and men have equal rates of this disorder, usually with onset in middle age. The course is typically chronic except in children, who often recover completely.

Symptoms are multiple, and typically involve GI or cardiac function. Physical exam and lab evaluation do not show signs of a serious medical disorder, but the patient's concern is not eased. Symptoms continue to cause significant stress or impaired functioning.

The above constellation of symptoms must persist for at least 6 months.

Regular visits to the doctor may reassure the patient. Otherwise, these patients are typically unwilling to undergo psychotherapy and no effective treatment is known.

Factitious Disorder

Patients with factitious disorder intentionally produce physical or psychiatric complaints. Unlike malingering, in which feigning illness allows realization of an external goal such as monetary gain, factitious disorder is a means for the patient to assume a "sick role." This disorder is more common in men than women.

Feigned or exaggerated complaints may be complicated by self-inflicted injury. Abuse of prescription medications, particularly analgesics and sedatives, is common.

Feigned disease in the absence of external gain are categorized as either predominantly psychological symptoms or predominantly physical symptoms.

No effective treatment is known. Try to avoid unnecessary diagnostic procedures.

Sexual and Gender Identity Disorders

Sexual Dysfunctions

Sexual dysfunctions include decreased sexual desire and decreased physical responsiveness in the sexual response cycle. Disorders may result from psychogenic problems or biological ones. Stress, emotional imbalance, fears, and ignorance may all be involved. Endocrine disorders, including hyperthyroidism, diabetes mellitus, and primary hyperprolactinemia, may affect a woman's ability to achieve orgasm. Surgical procedures, such as prostatectomy, and some medications, such as fluoxetine, may inhibit male orgasms.

The sexual response cycle is described in four stages: desire, excitement, orgasm, and resolution. Symptoms involving any of these stages may be present and may be generalized or situational, total or partial, and lifelong or acquired.

Symptoms must cause severe distress or impaired functioning. Physical disorders must be ruled out.

Couples therapy, hypnotherapy, and behavioral therapy are the most appropriate responses. Antianxiety agents may be useful, and testosterone is occasionally used to increase libido.

Paraphilias

Patients with paraphilias experience recurrent sexual fantasies or arousal that involve inanimate objects, children or unconsenting adults, or suffering of self or partner. These uncommon disorders occur primarily in men and begin before age 18. Severity peaks around age 20 and then declines somewhat. Patients often have several paraphilias.

Symptoms depend on the type of paraphilia:
- **Pedophilia**, the most common paraphilia, involves sexual acts with a young child by a patient at least 5 years older.
- Patients with **exhibitionism** expose their genitals to strangers and may masturbate while exposed.
- **Fetishism** involves arousal from the use of inanimate objects, such as women's clothing.
- Patients with **frotteurism** are aroused by sexual touching of an unconsenting adult.
- Sexual **masochism** is characterized by arousal from acts of humiliation or physical aggression against oneself.
- Sexual **sadism** involves arousal by humiliating or being physically aggressive towards others.
- **Transvestic fetishism** involves arousal from cross-dressing.
- Patients with **voyeurism** are aroused by "peeping" at unknowing victims who are undressing or are involved in sexual activity.

The above symptoms must last at least 6 months.

Psychotherapy and behavioral therapy. Antiandrogens seem to be helpful with some hypersexual paraphilias.

Gender Identity Disorders

Discomfort about one's gender and a persistent desire to be the other gender are characteristic of gender identity disorder.

Boys often dress in women's clothing and are involved in "traditionally female pastimes." Girls show an aversion to feminine things, may urinate standing up, and plan to grow a penis or develop into a man. Peer conflicts are common. As adults these patients may be heterosexual or homosexual or may attempt to live as a member of the other sex.

A strong identity with the other sex causes distress or impaired functioning. The diagnosis of gender identity disorder may be made in children or in adults.

Play therapy is used in children, but this has not been shown to have any beneficial effects. Psychotherapy and surgical sex change are used as treatment for adults.

Other Common Psychiatric Disorders

Adjustment Disorder

Within 3 months of an episode of emotional stress, a patient develops emotional or behavioral changes that result in severe distress or impaired functioning. The symptoms must resolve within 6 months except when the stressor continues. Acute and chronic adjustment disorder are more prevalent in poor urban communities, where violence and poverty are constant stressors. This diagnosis does not apply to normal bereavement, which often follows the death of a loved one.

Dissociative Disorder

Dissociative disorders are characterized by a sudden disruption in the normal integration of cognitive functions, including identity, state of consciousness, memory, and perception. These disorders are generally, but not always, transient and reversible. Dissociation, repression, and denial are the major defense mechanisms used. There are four major dissociative disorders:

1. **Dissociative amnesia,** the most common, involves a deficit in recall of significant personal information, usually regarding a traumatic event. Depression, suicidal ideation, depersonalization, and spontaneous age regression may occur. Spontaneous recovery is usually abrupt and complete. Barbiturates may precipitate the recovery of memory. A recent increase in this diagnosis for patients with early childhood abuse has been disputed as being due to patient suggestibility.
2. **Dissociative fugue** involves amnesia about the past in a patient who has unexpectedly traveled away from home. Heavy use of alcohol, mood disorders, and personality disorders may be predisposing factors. Episodes may last months, with spontaneous but not always complete recovery.
3. **Depersonalization disorder** involves constant or recurrent feelings of ego-dystonic detachment from the patient's internal identity. A perception of being estranged and mechanical is accompanied by insight and intact reality testing. As depersonalization is not an uncommon experience, this diagnosis can be made only in the presence of severe distress or impaired functioning. Stress and physical or mental illness may precede or exacerbate this disorder.

4. **Dissociative identity disorder**, previously called multiple personality disorder, occurs when patients have at least two distinct personalities. The personalities alternate in controlling behavior, and deficits in memory result. Different personalities may even have different physiological traits, including visual acuity or response to insulin. Abuse in childhood, usually sexual, precipitates the development of this chronic disorder. Hypnosis or an amobarbital interview may elicit hidden personalities. Hypnotherapy and psychotherapy are used for treatment.

Delirium

Delirium may be an organic mental syndrome, a manifestation of medical illness, or a result of substance intoxication. It reflects widespread brain dysfunction that is most often reversible.

Decreased attention, disorganized thinking, and some change in level of consciousness, orientation, memory, or perception are present.

The above symptoms develop over hours to days and fluctuate. An underlying cause should be established; if one cannot be found, the diagnosis is an organic mental syndrome.

Identify and treat the underlying cause.

Dementia

Cognitive and intellectual deficits without any change in consciousness cause severely impaired functioning in dementia. Two major causes of dementia include degenerative dementia of the Alzheimer's type and multi-infarct dementia, which are addressed in detail in Chap. 15.

Impaired memory, cognition, and judgment are present, in addition to some deficits in language, motor skills, or sensory function. Personality changes may occur.

The above symptoms establish the diagnosis, and an underlying disorder should be sought.

The underlying disorder should be treated. Symptomatic and psychosocial support are helpful.

Personality Disorders

When an individual's character traits deviate significantly from cultural norms, a diagnosis of personality disorder may apply. For diagnosis, the personality disorder must be evident in at least two areas of cognition, affect, interpersonal relations, or impulse control. It is pervasive and constant, causing serious distress or impaired functioning. The maladaptive patterns begin in adolescence or early adulthood. Some personality disorders lessen with time, while others continue throughout the patient's life. Personality disorders are axis II diagnoses that fall into three clusters, discussed below.

Cluster A Personality Disorders

Patients are eccentric or somewhat bizarre:

1. **Paranoid personality disorder:** Patients have a pervasive pattern of interpreting actions and events as malevolent or demeaning. They are suspicious of the motives of others and fear exploitation or deceit, and they scrutinize peers closely. Other criteria for diagnosis include reluctance to share personal information, frequent misinterpretation of benign comments, unwillingness to forgive others, frequent angry reactions, and pathologic jealousy. In addition to these diagnostic criteria, alcohol and substance use are common, brief psychotic episodes are not unusual, and patients often develop major depressive disorder, agoraphobia, and obsessive-compulsive disorder.

2. **Schizoid personality disorder:** These patients are unable to form close relationships with others and have very restricted emotions. Patients do not attempt to achieve intimacy, prefer to be alone, have no close friends, show little interest in sexual activity, and do not enjoy most activities. Approval or disapproval from others is unimportant, and patients often appear without emotion. Major depressive disorder may develop, or schizoid personality disorder may precede the development of delusional disorder or schizophrenia.

3. **Schizotypal personality disorder:** In addition to difficulty maintaining close relationships, patients have odd or distorted behavior, cognition, or perception. Suspiciousness and ideas of reference are common, as are interests in superstitions or the paranormal. Distorted perceptions, eccentric speech, inappropriate affect and behavior, lack of close relationships, and social anxiety are other features of this disorder. Increased psychotic features may result in diagnosis of a psychotic disorder, and many have episodes of major depressive disorder.

Cluster B Personality Disorders

This group involves dramatic or overemotional personality traits:

1. **Antisocial personality disorder:** Previously termed psychopaths or sociopaths, these individuals demonstrate disregard for social norms and the interests of others. They break laws, act aggressively or deceitfully, and lack remorse for their actions. Other diagnostic features include failure to plan, reckless patterns of behavior, and lack of respon-

sibility. Conduct disorder may be present prior to age 18. Several disorders, such as anxiety and depressive disorders, substance use, and somatization disorder, are associated. The majority of these patients are male.

2. **Borderline personality disorder**: Patients experience unstable relationships, self-esteem, and emotions. They desperately fear being abandoned. Impulsivity, suicidal thoughts and actions, mood lability, uncontrolled anger, and feelings of boredom or emptiness are common features. Transient paranoid or dissociative symptoms may occur. Associated diagnoses include mood disorders, substance use, bulimia, PTSD, and ADHD. About 75% of patients are women.

3. **Histrionic personality disorder**: Labile emotions and attention-seeking patterns of behavior characterize this disorder. Patients want to be the center of attention and often use seductive behaviors or physical appearance to achieve this goal. Shallow or labile emotions, dramatic speech and behavior, easily influenced opinions, and inappropriately perceived intimacy are present. Major depressive disorder, somatization, and conversion disorder are common.

4. **Narcissistic personality disorder**: These self-centered patients have grandiose self-images, frequent fantasies of love and success, and a sense of entitlement. They expect admiration from others because they believe themselves to be superior. They lack empathy and may exploit, snub, or envy others. The majority of patients are men. Anorexia nervosa, substance use, and mood disorders may occur.

Cluster C Personality Disorders

Anxiety and fear characterize these disorders:

1. **Avoidant personality disorder**: Patients avoid social situations for fear of rejection, and they make friends only when they are certain of being accepted. Fears of embarrassment lead to a reluctance to be open or to try new activities, a pattern of misinterpreting comments as critical, and the development of low self-esteem and feelings of inadequacy. Mood and anxiety disorders are common.

2. **Dependent personality disorder**: These needy patients require support and advice for everyday decisions and allow others to be responsible for their life choices. Conflict or disagreement is very difficult, as is personal motivation or initiative. Patients feel unable to care for themselves, so they fear being alone and seek close relationships. Patients constantly try to have others nurture them. Mood and anxiety disorders are common. Men and women have equal rates of this diagnosis.

3. **Obsessive-compulsive personality disorder**: These perfectionistic and controlling patients may be overconscientious to the point of missing deadlines. Their extreme devotion to work is accompanied by extreme preoccupation with petty details and rules and an inability to delegate tasks to others. Patients are inflexible and stubborn, miserly, and often unable to discard old, unwanted objects. These patients do not typically meet criteria for obsessive-compulsive disorder. Mood and anxiety disorders are common. Men have this diagnosis more frequently than women.

17

Preventive Medicine and Public Health

Infancy and Childhood

Normal Infant and Childhood Growth and Development

Growth and development in infants and children are rapidly occurring and constantly changing processes. Major developmental landmarks are listed in Table 17-1. Although specific ages are mentioned below, keep in mind that these are guidelines that may vary from child to child. Slow development in any area may be hereditary; only *significant* delays in growth and development are likely to become cause for concern.

Newborns generally lose about 10% of their body weight in the first few days of life, but they should gain it back within 10 days. Babies gain about 30 g (1 oz) per day for the first few months. Prior to **6 months**, nutrition is the primary factor in infant weight. After 6 months, genetic factors predominate, so growth percentiles can change significantly. By **1 year**, infants weigh about three times their birth weight and are 1.5 times as tall. At **age 2**, the child is about half its final adult height (strange but true!). After age 2, children stabilize to a growth rate of about 2–3 kg per year and 5–8 cm per year.

Child-Parent Interaction

As a child grows, the parent must adapt to the child's changing requirements. When the child is an infant, the parent must respond to nonverbal communication of the child's needs. Over time, the infant forms an attachment to the primary caregiver. According to Ainsworth, this attachment can be **secure** (the infant feels secure enough to explore the environment but keeps the parent within close distance and periodically returns for security), **anxious-resistant** (the child is afraid to explore and is clingy and agitated), or **anxious-avoidant** (the child explores the world with independence and does not look back to the parent for security, believing the parent will not be there for support). The anxious-avoidant child tends to be very accident-prone. As a toddler begins to develop his or her own identity, the parent must encourage the child's individuation and exploration, while enforcing enough limitations to keep the child safe. In early childhood, the child begins to assume a role in the social structure, and the parent should gradually allow the child to accept more responsibility. In middle childhood, the child can exert more self-control and think more logically. The parent should respond by using reason in rule-setting. In adolescence, the child moves toward even greater independence. This may cause conflict in the parent-child relationship until a new balance of mutual tolerance and respect is achieved.

Physician-Child-Parent Communication

When dealing with pediatric patients, physicians often have to participate in three-way communication and address issues concerning both the parent's and the child's interests. The following suggestions for communication may be helpful.

Table 17-1. Childhood developmental landmarks

Age	Gross motor	Fine motor	Language	Personal	Cognitive/social
2 mos	Lifts head to 45 degrees	Eyes follow to midline	Vocalizes	Smiles	State of half-waking consciousness
4 mos	Lifts head to 90 degrees	Eyes follow past midline	Laughs	Regards own hand	Slight awareness of caregiver
6 mos	Rolls over	Grasps rattle	Turns to voice	Feeds self	Separates world into "Mom" and "not Mom"
12 mos	Sits without support Pulls to stand	Pincer grasp	Babbles	Indicates wants	Stranger anxiety
18 mos	Walks well	Makes tower of two blocks	Says three words	Uses spoon and cup	Temper tantrums Desires comfort but not help Bridges gap by bringing objects to caregiver
2 yrs	Runs Climbs steps	Makes tower of four blocks	Combines words	Removes clothes	Develops concept of object permanence
4 yrs	Balances on one foot for 2 seconds	Copies a circle	Explains pictures Speech can be understood	Dresses self	Magical thinking Egocentric (only aware of own viewpoint) Symbolic play
6 yrs	Balances on one foot for 6 seconds	Draws a person with six parts	Defines words Knows opposites	Prepares cereal	Logical thinking begins Understands conservation of mass and volume

- Young children may be most comfortable undergoing examination while on a parent's lap. Ask older children, preferably when the parent is not around, if they would like to have a parent present in the room during the examination. For preteens and teens, try to see the patient without the parent, so that you will have adequate privacy to address such issues as sexual behavior, drug and alcohol use, and depression or suicidality.
- Children and teens may feel intimidated by an excessively authoritarian manner. Try to communicate with them on an equal basis when possible, while maintaining your professional demeanor.
- Beware of counter-transference on your part. This means that you shouldn't over-identify with either the child ("The parents are being too strict and are the enemy") or with the parents ("This child's actions are bad and should be controlled").

Well-Child Care

Regular screening is an important part of well-child care. Table 17-2 shows general guidelines for when screening exams should be performed. A shaded box indicates that screening tests should be performed at the corresponding ages.

Adolescence

Puberty

As we all know, adolescence is a time of many physical, social, and psychological changes. Early adolescence begins with the onset of puberty, usually between ages 10 and 13. At this age, the child may begin to have questions about the normalcy of his or her body. As adolescence progresses, sexual drives emerge, usually at ages 14–16. The teen's peer group becomes increasingly important and influential, and the teen explores his or her ability to be sexually attractive to others. Conflicts with authority over independence frequently arise. During late adolescence, ages 17–21, teens become more comfortable with their maturation and their relationships and more able to discuss roles and goals. At this point, the development of both concrete and abstract thought processes is complete.

As teens grapple with emotional and social issues, their difficulties in adaptation may be expressed in potentially damaging ways. Major causes of mortality in this age group include **accidents, suicide,** and **homicide.** Alcohol is often involved. Mortality rates for boys are about twice that of girls. Other important issues include the following:
- **Risk-taking behaviors,** such as drug and alcohol use, are common. Alcohol use has been reported in more than 90% of teens. Tobacco use (66%) and drug use (43%) are also common. Health education is sometimes ineffective, since many teens have a feeling of immortality ("It can't happen to me").
- **Psychiatric disturbances,** such as depression and suicide, may become more frequent. More than 30% of adolescent girls and 15% of adolescent boys are reported to have symptoms of major depression. Homosexual teens are more likely to attempt suicide than their heterosexual peers, perhaps because of fears of social rejection. Clinical suspicion of depression should be explored, and the physician should ask about suicidal ideation in a

Table 17-2. Pediatric screening schedule

Age (yrs)	B	1	2	3	4	5	6	7	8	9	10	11	12	13	14	15	16	17	18
Head Size	■	■	■																
Height	■	■	■	■	■	■	■		■		■		■		■		■		■
Weight	■	■	■	■	■	■	■		■		■		■		■		■		■
BP				■	■	■	■		■		■		■		■		■		■
Anemia	■								■										■
Lead		■	■																
Urinalysis	■	■				■			■										
TB (PPD)		■			■										■				
Hearing					■	■							■		■				■
Vision	■			■	■	■	■		■		■		■		■		■		■
Eye				■															
Dental				■	■	■	■		■		■		■		■		■		■

(shading indicates ages at which screening should be done)

straightforward manner. Contrary to a common fear, teens whose doctors discuss this topic are not more likely to commit suicide because "the doctor gave me the idea."

- **Eating disorders**, such as bulimia and anorexia, become more prevalent. Female adolescents are at special risk of developing distorted body images and eating disorders; more than 20% of teenage girls have manifestations of either anorexia or bulimia. In a clinical setting, physicians should openly discuss physical development with adolescents and reassure their anxieties about normalcy.

Adolescent Nutrition and Growth

Physical changes occur rapidly during adolescence. Body composition changes, with increased muscle mass and subcutaneous fat. The heart and lungs grow, and males experience an increase in blood volume and hematocrit. Neuroendocrine changes along the hypothalamic-pituitary axis alter gonadotropin function and concentrations of steroid hormones. A secondary growth spurt, which occurs during adolescence, accounts for about 25% of final adult height.

Reproductive growth in adolescents is generally classified by the Tanner stages, which provide a range of ages at which normal changes may occur. The age at which these changes occur varies widely among individuals, and adolescent patients should be reassured that earlier or later development may still be normal.

Tanner Stages: Female

- **Stage I**: Ages 0–15
  Preadolescent breast stage, with no pubic hair (Fig. 17-1).
- **Stage II**: Ages 8–15
  Thelarche (breast budding) with enlargement of areola.
  Small amount of pubic hair near the labia.
  Growth spurt often follows stage II.
- **Stage III**: Ages 10–15
  Breast and areolar enlargement with no contour separation of the areola.
  Increased amount of darker pubic hair.
  Menarche (onset of menses) occurs at this stage in about 25% of girls.
- **Stage IV**: Ages 10–17
  Further breast and nipple enlargement with some contour separation of the areola.
  Increased pubic hair, with adult quality but not distribution.
  The majority of girls experience menarche in this stage.
- **Stage V**: Ages 12–18
  Complete breast enlargement with no contour separation of the areola.
  Pubic hair of adult quality and distribution.

Tanner Stages: Male

- **Stage I**: Ages 0–15 (Fig. 17-2)
  Preadolescent testes (<2.5 cm), penis, and pubic hair.
- **Stage II**: Ages 10–15
  Testicular enlargement with increased pigmentation of scrotum.

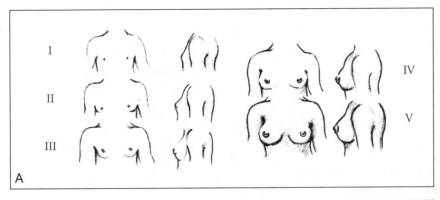

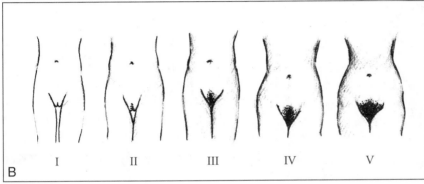

Fig. 17-1. A. The Tanner stages of breast development. B. The Tanner stages for the female development of pubic hair. (Adapted from G Ross, R Vande Wiele. The Ovaries. In R Williams [ed], *Textbook of Endocrinology* [5th ed]. Philadelphia: Saunders, 1974; and from WA Marshall, JM Tanner. Variations in pattern of pubertal changes in girls. *Arch Dis Child* 44:291,1969.)

Small amount of penile growth.
Variable amount of soft pubic hair.
- **Stage III**: Ages 11–16
  Continued enlargement of testes.
  "Growth spurt" of penis.
  Increased amount of curling pubic hair.
- **Stage IV**: Ages 12–17
  Further enlargement of testes and penis.
  Increased pubic hair, with adult quality but not distribution.
  Axillary and facial hair development.
  Growth spurt in height for the majority of males.
- **Stage V**: Ages 13–18
  Adult-size testes and penis.
  Pubic hair of adult quality and distribution.
  Increased body hair and muscle enlargement.

Physician-Patient Communication in Adolescence

Adolescents may be hesitant to discuss personal issues with physicians because they may fear that their parents will be getting a "report" from you. The physician is justified in maintaining confidentiality with teenage patients in most situations, especially with regard to sexual behavior and drug use. However, if life-threatening behavior is suspected, a physician may intervene and discuss the situation with the patient's parents or guardian.

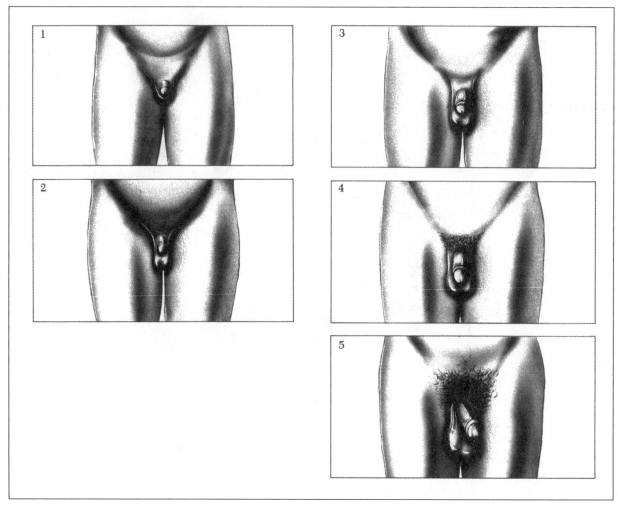

Fig. 17-2. The Tanner stages of male genital development. (From JP Bellack, BJ Edlund. *Nursing Assessment and Diagnosis.* Boston: Jones and Bartlett, 1992.)

Normal Adulthood and Aging

Well-Adult Care

Table 17-3 provides a brief summary of recommended adult screening and preventive care requirements. These guidelines apply only to adults with no history of related diseases and no family history for these diseases; patients at higher risk may require more frequent screening.

Stress Management

Stress has been implicated in the development of many medical conditions, including hypertension and heart disease. Holmes and Rahe studied stress and developed a scale of life event stressors, which shows that both positive and negative events can cause stress. The ten most stressful events are:

Table 17-3. Adult preventive health measures

Procedure	Frequency	After age
Blood pressure	Every 2 years	18
Cholesterol	Every 5 years	18
Tetanus immunization	Every 10 years	18
Pap smear	Every year	18
	Every 3 years	(after 2 normal smears)
Breast examination (by provider)	Every year	40
Mammography	Baseline (debated)	35
	Every 1–2 years	40
	Every year	50
Hemoccult stool test	Every year	50
Sigmoidoscopy	Every 3–5 years	50
Digital rectal exam	Every year	40
Influenza vaccination	Every year	65
Pneumococcal vaccination	Once	65

Source: Adapted from the U.S. Preventive Services Task Force Guidelines

- Death of a spouse or child
- Divorce
- Marital separation
- Institutional detention (e.g., jail)
- Death of close family member
- Major personal injury or illness
- Marriage
- Loss of job
- Marital reconciliation
- Retirement
- Taking the Step 2 exam

Stress management techniques include:

- Counseling
- Social support
- Biofeedback
- Hypnosis
- Relaxation techniques
- Antianxiety medications
- Health-promoting strategies, including a healthy diet, exercise, and recreational activities.

Normal Aging

Some decrease in physical and mental ability is a natural part of aging; however, clinicians should rule out treatable illnesses before accepting a decrease in function in an older patient. More than 80% of persons over age 65 have one or more chronic illness, and the average number of prescription drugs taken ranges from three to five. In fact, drug interactions account for more than 10% of hospital admissions in this age group. Assessment of the activities of daily living (ADL) (e.g., bathing, eating, dressing) may provide more specific information on functional status.

Some decrease in memory and intellectual capability is normal, but it is incorrect to assume that senility is a normal part of aging. Clinicians should investigate other causes, such as depression. Decreasing mental function due to "old age" should be a diagnosis of exclusion. Only 5% of patients over age 65 have significant dementia; this increases to about 10% in patients over age 80. Comparatively, up to 40% have significant depression.

Psychosocial Adaptations of Aging

Most older persons attempt to maintain their previous level of social activity. Isolation, loss of family and friends, health problems, and changes in living situation can all lead to depression. Depression in the elderly is associated with insomnia and loss of appetite, as well as memory impairment. The elderly also have a high incidence of suicide. Unmarried, widowed, and divorced patients are at greater risk of developing depression than married patients. In a clinical setting, physicians should assess the full range of issues in the elderly, including physical, psychological, and social functioning. Possible approaches to increasing socialization and combating depression include therapy, senior day-care centers, volunteering, and support groups.

Nutrition with Aging

Aging is associated with a lower caloric requirement, due to decreased muscle mass, although this may depend on the patient's activity level. Some elderly persons may be malnourished due to difficulties in obtaining and preparing food, cost, difficulty with teeth or dentures, and depression. Reductions in fluid intake may make elderly patients prone to dehydration. Dehydration is one of the most common causes of acute confusional states in the elderly.

Death and Dying

The emotional states that people experience when informed of a terminal illness have been described in detail by Elizabeth Kübler-Ross. A brief overview of the five stages is presented below:

- **Denial** is the phase in which the patient may be in a state of shock and reject the diagnosis or the presence of physical impairment.
- The next stage is one of **anger**. The patient may be upset and frustrated and ask, "Why me?"
- The patient may **bargain**, making promises of good behavior and charity to family, physician, or God in exchange for a cure.

- Patients often experience some amount of **depression**; however, serious depression should not be accepted as a normal response and should receive appropriate psychiatric treatment. Mild depression, which may include insomnia, hopelessness, and suicidal ideation, is a normal part of accepting death.
- Ultimately, patients reach the stage of **acceptance**, realizing that death is inevitable and coming to terms with their prognosis.

Medical Ethics

Competency and Decision-Making Capacity

A competent patient is capable of making his or her own decisions about care. Competent patients may refuse medical interventions at any time, not solely in the case of terminal illness. The basis of competency is the idea of patient **autonomy**, the fact that we respect the patient's self-determination and individual right to make decisions about his or her care. Exceptions may be made in some cases of communicable disease, when patients must be treated or quarantined. Issues regarding pregnant women, whose decisions may threaten the life of the fetus, are currently under debate, and legal precedents in these cases have been contradictory.

How do we assess that a person has "decision-making capacity"?

- The mental status exam is used to ensure that decisions are not a product of delusional beliefs or hallucinations.
- The patient must understand the situation enough to give informed consent.
- The patient's decision should be relatively stable over time and consistent with the patient's values and goals.

In general, decisions concerning children should be made with the child's best interests in mind, and with the child's preferences taken into consideration. Parents are presumed to be the appropriate decision-makers for their children, except in emergencies (when physicians may provide care without explicit parental instruction) or when parents themselves lack decision-making capacity. The courts may overrule the parents' decision if it is not felt to be in the best interest of the child, but most physicians prefer not to resort to this option unless it is absolutely necessary.

Full Disclosure

In general, the physician has the responsibility to inform the patient about his or her condition in a manner the patient can understand. When family members ask that a patient not be told about a diagnosis or test results, the physician should ask about their specific fears and concerns. Ascertain if it is the family's wish or the patient's wish, and focus on how to tell the patient in an appropriate way, not whether you should tell the patient. One approach is to say to the patient, "Many patients want to know their test results, whereas others do not. Would you like to know?" Also, try to be aware of cultural issues regarding the disclosure of diagnoses.

Informed Consent

Informed consent is a process through which decision-making power is shared between doctor and patient. The required components are as follows:

- The pertinent information is discussed with the patient, including the nature of the proposed interventions, the risks, the benefits, any available alternative treatments, and the expected consequences of receiving no medical treatment.
- The patient decides whether or not to proceed with the treatment plan.
- There is no coercion from any party.

Informed consent is not required when the patient lacks decision-making capacity. In this case, an appropriate surrogate must make decisions. In an emergency, there is a **doctrine of implied consent**, and the physician is permitted to intervene in a manner presumed to be in the best interests of the patient.

Involuntary Confinement

Involuntary confinement involves hospitalization or detainment of a patient against the patient's wishes. It may be invoked when the patient is thought to pose an immediate danger to himself or herself or to others. Confinement may also be enforced if the patient is unable to care for himself or herself (e.g., by providing food, clothing, and shelter).

Confidentiality

Confidentiality, the idea that all communication between a patient and physician is private, is integral to the patient-doctor relationship. The rules of confidentiality do not apply if:

- The patient waives confidentiality and allows the doctor to discuss the condition with the family, partner, or other persons.
- There is serious potential harm to the patient or a third party (such as suicidal or homicidal plans).

Public Reporting

Reporting of a medical impairment to public officials may be required for the following conditions, but this varies from state to state:

- Impaired drivers (e.g., those prone to loss of consciousness).
- Elder and child abuse.
- Some infectious diseases (see Surveillance and Reporting in Chap. 9).
- HIV infection (in some states).

If possible, discuss the fact that you will be breaching confidentiality with the patient before you report the illness!

Advance Directives

Advance directives allow patients to indicate their preferences for medical interventions and appoint a surrogate if they lose their decision-making capacity. Directives can take the form of an oral or written statement. In "living wills" (not available in all states), the patient can ask that life-sustaining treatment be withheld in specified circumstances. Patients may also have a "durable power of attorney," which appoints a particular person to act as a surrogate (i.e., an agent or proxy) to make decisions if decision-making capacity is lost.

Do Not Resuscitate Orders

"Do not resuscitate" (DNR) orders or "no code" orders are written to withhold CPR if cardiac arrest occurs. (Even with CPR, more than 85% of patients requiring intervention do not survive.) The physician should discuss CPR preferences with the patient and ensure that the patient understands all options. The patient may choose to request limited DNR orders, which allow CPR for a specified period of time or allow only certain parts of the code. DNR orders are appropriate if:

- The patient refuses CPR.
- The patient does not have decision-making capacity, and the surrogate refuses CPR on the patient's behalf.
- CPR is futile. There is currently much debate on the exact definition of "futility," but the general meaning implies that the overall long-term status of the patient would not be improved with emergent resuscitation, as is often the case with end-stage terminal illness.

Life Support

Patients on life support may have left instructions regarding their desire for such medical care or may have previously appointed a surrogate to make these decisions. Without such instructions—although it is still legally challenged from state to state—physicians generally allow the discontinuation of a respirator. Discontinuation of nutrition and hydration, however, has been seen in many cases as "morally different" from the discontinuation of respiration. Patients may be able to reject nutrition and hydration if they are able to make that decision, but discontinuing this support in an unconscious patient generally depends on the patient's previously stated wishes or the decision of the surrogate.

Diagnosing Death

Believe it or not, this is more confusing than you might think. There are several different and competing definitions used to diagnose death. "Heart death" is defined as the moment at which a spontaneous heartbeat cannot be restored. Usually, however, "brain death" is considered better grounds for a determination of death. Brain death is generally defined as an irreversible coma with no brain stem reflexes present (e.g., absent pupillary, corneal, vestibular, gag, and respiratory reflexes) for at least 6 hours. It may also involve the absence of EEG tracings for a specified amount of time, but this has been challenged by people who have recovered from drug overdoses who had previously shown flat EEGs. In any case, cessation of spontaneous respiration is not generally considered enough to diagnose death in a medical setting.

Autopsy

Autopsy is the postmortem examination of a body, usually to determine the cause of death. Autopsies may be mandatory when intentional death is suspected, but if this is not the case, consent must be obtained from the patient's surrogate. Families may request autopsies, and some find that the objective information is helpful during the grieving process.

Organ Donation

The Uniform Anatomical Gift Act, adopted in all 50 states, allows any competent adult to allow or forbid use of his or her organs through a written statement (usually a donor card). If no donor card has been provided, a surrogate may make the decision. However, if a donor card exists, physicians may procure organs over the objection of the family, although this is rarely done in practice for fear of lawsuits. In 1986, the U.S. government enacted a law requiring all hospitals that receive Medicare payments (essentially all of them) to perform a "required request" for organs, in which the family of a deceased patient is asked to donate the patient's organs.

Euthanasia and Assisted Suicide

Euthanasia is the act of taking the life of a patient in order to avoid the prolongation of pain and suffering. Assisted suicide is the act of providing the means for a patient to commit suicide. Assisted suicide and euthanasia are currently illegal in the United States. Although a few states have successfully passed euthanasia and assisted suicide initiatives, these laws are still being challenged in court.

What if a patient requests assisted suicide? Here are some recommendations:

- Don't impose your own values or become judgmental of the patient.
- Try to find out reasons for the request (e.g., inadequate pain control, fears).
- Try to relieve the patient's distress, if possible.
- Reaffirm the patient's control over medical decisions.

Suicide

About 30,000 suicides occur every year in the United States. For every "successful" suicide, there are about 10 attempted suicides. Risk factors for suicide include:

- Age >45
- Alcoholism
- Rage and violent behavior
- Prior suicide attempts
- Male sex
- Depression
- Unemployment or retirement
- Being single, widowed, or divorced
- Experiencing a recent loss or separation

Abortion

In the United States, about one induced abortion occurs for every five live births. The U.S. Supreme Court has upheld that abortion cannot be denied to women in the first 3 months of pregnancy. Methods of abortion induction include suction curettage, surgical curettage, dilation and evacuation, and intra-amniotic instillation. In France, the abortion drug RU486, which acts as a progestin analogue, is commonly used; RU486 is not legal in the United States, although testing has begun in some large cities. Methotrexate and misopristol have recently been proposed as abortifacients and may be used more frequently in the future.

Maternal-Fetal Conflict

Maternal-fetal conflict arises during pregnancy when a treatment or request that benefits one party may be harmful to the other. Two common issues are surgical interventions and maternal behavior that may be toxic to the fetus.

Surgical intervention (e.g., cesarean section) against the mother's will is extremely controversial. Some courts have upheld that forcing a women to undergo a C-section (and forcing a Jehovah's Witness to accept a blood transfusion during the procedure) is acceptable if the child's life would otherwise be lost. However, other courts have disagreed, stating that it is a violation of patient autonomy. Judges generally rule in favor of the intervention (especially after it has already been performed).

Another recent area of controversy is the maternal use of known fetotoxic substances, such as drugs and alcohol. Most cases are tried under child abuse laws without success, since most child abuse laws do not include "prenatal conduct or omissions." Some states are adopting more specific laws in the hope of prosecuting these cases successfully.

Research Issues

Clinical Trials

Clinical trials are used to test the effectiveness of a new drug or treatment for a particular condition. Subjects are randomly divided into a treatment group (which receives the intervention) and a control group (which does not receive the intervention). If an effective treatment is already available, the new treatment may be compared with the current standard of care; otherwise, the control group should receive a placebo, an inert substance that is similar in appearance to the treatment. After a period of time, the treatment outcomes of the two groups are compared. To decrease the bias, it is important to carry out these trials in a blinded fashion, so that neither the patients nor the clinicians know which patients are receiving treatment.

Community Intervention Trials

Community intervention trials are experiments in which a community is the unit of intervention. For example, fluoridated water may be supplied to one community and the average number of dental caries per child compared with a community that does not receive fluoridated water. In structuring these interventions, it is important to ensure that the members of the community will not be exposed to any significant risk of illness. Animal testing may be required before testing in humans.

Cohort Studies

Cohort studies begin by classifying a group of individuals by exposure status. Studies that follow a group over time to identify those who develop disease are **prospective cohort studies**. Exposure and disease have both already occurred in **retrospective cohort studies**. For example, work records from shipyards in World War II describe exposure to asbestos. Death records of men who worked in the shipyards can be used to assess the number of cancer deaths. The advantages of cohort studies include the ability to calculate the **relative risk** and the ability to study more than one effect of an exposure. **Recall bias** is minimized in prospective studies, because exposure status is established before the disease develops. Disadvantages include the need to study large numbers of people to ensure an adequate number of subjects with a disease. It is virtually impossible to use a cohort to study a rare disease, because any given population will have very few cases. Other disadvantages include time (it may take years to get enough data to analyze) and expense.

Case-Control Studies

Case-control studies compare a group of individuals who have a particular disease (cases), to a group of individuals without the disease (controls). The frequency of various exposures are assessed in the two groups. From this information, the **odds ratio** can be calculated, which is an approximation of the relative risk. Case-control studies are relatively quick and inexpensive and may not require many subjects. Case-control studies are ideal for studying diseases that are rare or have long latent periods. Disadvantages include the need to rely on a subject's recall to assess exposure and the inability to calculate rates of disease incidence.

Case Series

A case series is a report of the characteristics of a group of individuals with a particular disease. A case series may raise hypotheses about risk factors for a disease but cannot be used to test these hypotheses.

Cross-Sectional Study

Cross-sectional studies assess risk factors and disease status in a group of people at one point in time. They are useful for correlating disease prevalence with exposure prevalence, but no conclusive statement can be made about whether a risk factor precedes the onset of a disease.

Research Design

Subject Selection

If a study's results are to be generalizable to the population of interest, the subjects in the study must be representative of that population. Any systematic variation from the population (e.g., being more or less ill, more willing to volunteer, of a different socioeconomic status) may introduce bias that will reduce the validity of the study. A randomly selected population is usually ideal.

Sample Size

If the sample size of a study is too small, an observed difference between the exposed and unexposed may not be statistically significant. Standard formulas for sample size determination allow for choice of a proper sample.

Consent

In a research context, a subject must be clearly informed about the interventions and possible consequences, and the subject must give definite agreement and permission.

Placebos

Placebos are substances that have no known pharmacologic activity. However, many patients experience improvement of symptoms after receiving placebo medications, due to psychological interactions in the perceptions of symptoms and pain. Whenever the efficacy of a medication is tested, results should be compared to a control group receiving placebos, unless the current existence of a helpful treatment makes the use of placebos unethical.

Conflict of Interest

Conflicts of interest occur when what is best for the patient is not best for the experiment. For example, an investigator may have to choose between keeping a subject in the experiment or treating his or her newly diagnosed diabetes. The patient's best interests are always considered most important.

Vulnerable Populations

Research protocols using populations that are unable to give informed consent (e.g., children or the mentally ill) or that may be subject to coercion (e.g., prison inmates) should be carefully monitored.

Statistics

Measures of Central Tendency

The **mean** (or average) is calculated by adding all observations and dividing by the number of observations.

Example: Data set {1, 3, 5, 5, 6}

Mean = $\dfrac{(1 + 3 + 5 + 5 + 6)}{5} = \dfrac{20}{5} = 4$

The **median** is the "middle" observation, obtained by ordering all data and finding the center value. (With an even number of observations, the middle two values are averaged to obtain the median value.) The median is not affected by extreme values, as is the mean.

Example: Data set {1, 3, 5, 5, 6}
Median = centermost value = 5

The **mode** refers to the most frequent observation. Some data sets may have more than one mode ("bimodal") or may have no mode (i.e., all observations are different).

Example: Data set {1, 3, 5, 5, 6}
The mode = most common value = 5

Measures of Variability

Measures of variability describe the spread of data from the center values. The common measures are range, variance, and standard deviation.

The **range** is simply the difference between the maximum and the minimum values.

Data set: {1, 3, 5, 5, 6}
Range = maximum value − minimum value = 6 − 1 = 5

The **variance** (known as s^2) is obtained by adding the squares of each point's deviation from the mean, and dividing by sample size minus one.

Data set: {1, 3, 5, 5, 6}

Variance = $\dfrac{(1 − 4)^2 + (3 − 4)^2 + (5 − 4)^2 + (5 − 4)^2 + (6 − 4)^2}{(5 − 1)} = \dfrac{16}{4} = 4$

The **standard deviation** is the square root of the variance. The units of standard deviation are the same as the original units of measurement.

Data set: {1, 3, 5, 5, 6}
Standard deviation = $\sqrt{4} = 2$

Gaussian (bell-shaped) distributions have a mean = median = mode. Approximately 67% of the population falls within one standard deviation of the mean, 96% of the population falls within two standard deviations, and 99% of the population falls within 2.5 standard deviations (Fig. 17-3).

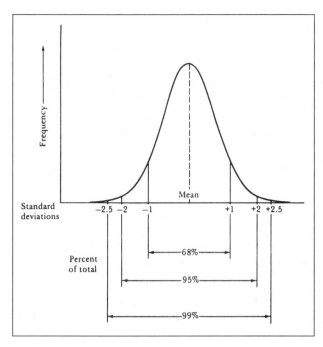

Fig. 17-3. Percentage of measurements within various standard deviations of the mean. (From CH Hennekens, JE Buring. *Epidemiology in Medicine*. Boston: Little, Brown, 1987.)

Probability and Distribution

Probability distributions allow us to evaluate the likelihood of a particular event by its location on a graph. When graph values are high, the events are more probable, whereas low graph values correspond to less probable events. Many biological variables (e.g., albumin, height) follow "bell-shaped" or "normal" distributions. If the "tail" of the curve is on the right side (toward higher x values), the curve is said to be **skewed right**, whereas a curve with a "tail" to the left is **skewed left** (Figs. 17-4 through 17-6).

Incidence and Prevalence

Incidence = Number of **newly** reported cases of a disease
Total population

Prevalence = Number of **existing** cases of a disease at a given time
Total population at that time

Prevalence depends on the incidence and the natural history of the disease. If patients survive a long time after diagnosis, prevalence will be higher than incidence.

Disease Frequency

Disease frequency = Number of people with disease
Population at risk

Remember to think about which individuals are at risk! For example, pregnancy (which is not technically a disease) only affects reproductive-aged women, generally accepted as ages 15–44.

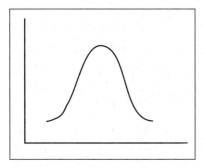

Fig. 17-4. Normal distribution.

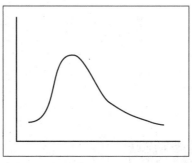

Fig. 17-5. Distribution with right skew.

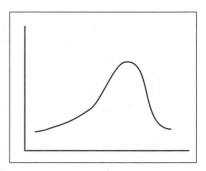

Fig. 17-6. Distribution with left skew.

Case Fatality Rate

Case fatality rate = $\dfrac{\text{People who die from the disease in a given time period}}{\text{Number of people with disease}}$

This is sometimes mistakenly used as a measure of risk. However, the case fatality rate will tell you only what percentage of people who have the disease die, not the risk faced by the general population.

Relative Risk

Relative risk (RR) is the risk of developing a particular disease for people with a known exposure, compared to the risk of developing the same disease without the exposure. A relative risk greater than one implies a **positive association** between the exposure and the disease, while a relative risk less than one implies a **negative association**. A relative risk of 1 shows **no association** between the exposure and the disease, with an equal risk of the disease in both populations (Table 17-4).

Relative risk can be calculated only from **cohort** studies.

$RR = \dfrac{a/(a+b)}{c/(c+d)} = \dfrac{\text{Disease in exposed population}}{\text{Disease in unexposed population}}$

Odds Ratio

Odds ratio (OR) is the odds of developing a disease among exposed individuals, compared to the odds of getting the disease among the unexposed. It is also used to measure the strength of association between a particular exposure and disease. This estimate of relative risk can be calculated from **case-control trials**.

$OR = \dfrac{a/c}{b/d} = \dfrac{ad}{bc}$

Standardized Mortality Rate

Mortality rates are the number of people dying per year within a certain population. Mortality rates are often used to assess differing risks for populations living in different areas.

Table 17-4. Calculating relative risk and odds ratio

		Disease		
		Present	Absent	
Exposure	Present	a	b	a + b
	Absent	c	d	c + d
		a + c	b + d	a + b + c + d = N

If, however, the age distributions of the two populations are different, then we might expect the mortality rate to be different. Adjusting the mortality rate according to the age distribution results in standardized mortality rates, which can then be compared to assess risk.

Attributable Risk

Attributable risk, or risk difference, is the difference in rates of disease between exposed and unexposed populations. It is an estimate of the percentage of disease attributable to a certain risk factor. For example, if nonsmokers have a lung cancer rate of 5 per 100,000 and smokers have a lung cancer rate of 180 per 100,000, the attributable risk is 180 − 5 = 175 per 100,000. Thus, for a population of 100,000, 175 lung cancer deaths would be "attributable" to smoking.

Sensitivity

The sensitivity of a test is the probability that results will be positive in patients who actually have the disease. It reflects the test's ability to diagnose accurately all cases of the disease. If a person is disease-free but has a positive test result, the result is termed **false-positive** (Table 17-5).

$$\text{Sensitivity} = \frac{a}{a + c}$$

Specificity

The specificity of a test is the probability that the test results will be negative in those without the disease. If a person has the disease but has a negative test result, the result is termed **false-negative**.

$$\text{Specificity} = \frac{d}{b + d}$$

Table 17-5. Calculating sensitivity, specificity, negative predictive value, and positive predictive value

	Disease		
	Present	Absent	
Positive	a	b	a + b
Negative	c	d	c + d
	a + c	b + d	a + b + c + d = N

Test results

Positive Predictive Value

The positive predictive value (PPV) of a test is the probability that an individual who gets a positive test result actually has the disease.

$$PPV = \frac{a}{a + b}$$

Negative Predictive Value

The negative predictive value (NPV) of a test is the probability that an individual who gets a negative test result does not have the disease.

$$NPV = \frac{d}{c + d}$$

Decision Analysis

Decision analysis is a process in which quantitative methods are applied to a medical problem in an attempt to determine the best option. This technique involves the use of decision trees and estimation of probabilities for each possible outcome.

Accurate vs. Precise Measurements

An accurate measurement provides true information that matches a particular standard (Fig. 17-7). For example, if a patient weighs 140 lbs, and a weighing scale provides the same information, the measurement is accurate. A precise measurement refers to the size of units used for measurement. For example, a weighing scale may provide the information that a patient weighs 145.75 lbs, which is a precise measurement. However, if the patient in reality weighs 140 lbs, this precise measurement is also inaccurate!

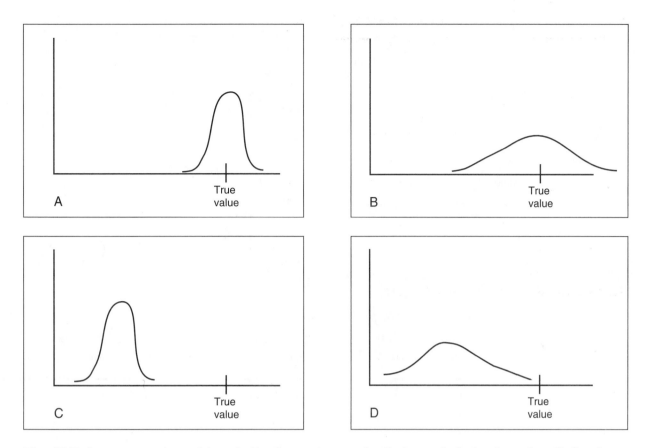

Fig. 17-7. Accuracy and precision. A. Precise and accurate. B. Accurate but not precise. C. Precise but not accurate. D. Not precise or accurate.

Valid vs. Reliable Measurements

A valid measurement is one that provides true and genuine information about the subject being measured. For example, blood pressure is a valid measure of risk of cardiovascular disease. A reliable measurement is reproducible, so it will result in similar results if repeated. Blood pressure measurements may not be reliable from one measure to the next, depending on changes in the patient's position or stress level.

Hypothesis Generation and Test Statistics

Hypotheses are generated from clinical observation and descriptive epidemiology (case reports, case series, cross-sectional surveys). They are tested by conducting analytic studies (case-control, cohort, intervention) and assessing the statistical significance of the results by using test statistics (Chi-square, Z-tests, t-tests). In general, the null hypothesis (H_o) states that there is no association between the exposure and the disease, while the alternate hypothesis (H_1) states that an association is present.

The p-value is the probability of getting the results of a study by chance alone, if the null hypothesis is true. By convention, the null hypothesis is rejected (i.e., there is a dif-

Table 17-6. Possible errors in hypothesis testing

		Actual case	
		H_0 is true	H_0 is false (H_1 is true)
Decision based on study	Accept H_0	Correct decision	Type II error
	Reject H_0 (assume H_1 is true)	Type I error	Correct decision
	Total	1	1

ference between the two groups) when the likelihood of a particular result occurring by chance alone is less than 5% (p <.05). A **type I error** occurs when the null hypothesis is rejected even though it is true (Table 17-6). A **type II error** occurs when the null hypothesis is not rejected even though it is false. **Statistical power** is defined as the probability of rejecting the null hypothesis when it is false. An investigator can reduce the chances of type I and type II errors by increasing sample size.

Confidence Intervals

A confidence interval provides the range of values that is statistically consistent with a particular study's data. If the 95% confidence interval for an odds ratio or relative risk estimate spans 1.0, then the data do not support the hypothesis that the factor in question is associated with an increased risk of disease. This is the same as having a p >.05, and the null hypothesis is not rejected.

18

Injury and Poisoning

Levels of Prevention

- Primary prevention: Actions that decrease the incidence of a health problem (e.g., prenatal care, immunization).
- Secondary prevention: Intervention at an early stage of a health problem in order to limit its further development (e.g., diabetes screening, Pap smears).
- Tertiary prevention: Intervention to treat the health problem itself and to prevent further morbidity or mortality (e.g., coronary artery bypass graft).

Accidental Injury and Death

Death from accidental injury accounts for a significant proportion of the mortality in younger age groups. After about age 45, chronic diseases such as cancer and cardiovascular disorders become more important causes of mortality (Table 18-1).

By far the largest cause of accidental death is motor vehicle accidents, which account for almost half of all childhood injuries. However, the incidence of childhood automobile deaths is declining, due to regulations requiring car seat and seat belt use. Motor vehicle accidents often involve alcohol and are particularly common in adolescents. Suicide and homicide are also seen primarily in teens, while falls, drowning, and fires are more common in younger age groups. Fires are often associated with households using alcohol and cigarettes, which are a common cause of residential fires (Table 18-2).

Drowning

About 2,000 people under age 20 drown each year in the United States. The distribution of drowning deaths is bimodal, with the first group consisting of children under age 5 and the second group consisting of male teenagers.

Infants under the age of 2 are at risk for drowning in bathtubs and buckets, and children between the ages of 2 and 5 are at greatest risk of drowning in swimming pools. Often, the child may have escaped supervision for only a few minutes. Mandatory pool fencing is being considered in some states, as this measure reduces the drowning rate by more than 80%. CPR instruction has also been suggested for all pool owners.

Teenage drowning victims are most often boys. The accident usually occurs in a large body of water, such as a lake or river, and alcohol is frequently involved.

Aspiration

Most cases of foreign body aspiration occur in children ages 6 months to 3 years. Common high-risk objects include small toys, hard candy, peanuts, and pieces of hot dogs.

Table 18-1. Contribution of accidental injury to overall mortality rate by age group

Age group (years)	Percentage of deaths caused by injury
1–4	44
5–14	52
15–24	63
25–44	40
45–64	6
65+	2

Table 18-2. Leading causes of deaths from injury

1. Motor vehicle accidents
2. Suicide
3. Homicide
4. Falls
5. Drowning/suffocation
6. Fires

The common triad of symptoms is choking, coughing, and wheezing.

Diagnosis may be difficult, since parents may not notice that aspiration has occurred. Plain chest x-ray may suggest the site of the foreign body. Because of the position of the bronchi, most aspirated objects fall into the right middle lobe.

Diagnosis and removal may require bronchoscopy. Sequelae of foreign-body aspiration include atelectasis, lung abscess formation, and pneumonia.

Parents should be counseled on the risks of giving small objects to children in this age group.

Poisoning

Unintentional poisoning occurs most often in children under 6 years of age who ingest common household products, such as analgesics and cosmetics. Iron poisoning from vitamin overdose is a particular hazard, since many parents are under the mistaken impression that vitamins are harmless and therefore do not seek timely medical attention. Prevention measures include child-proof cupboard latches and childproof medication bottles.

Table 18-3. Common poisons and their antidotes

Poison	Antidote
Aspirin	Dialysis
Acetaminophen	*N*-acetylcysteine
Digitalis	Lidocaine, antidigitalis antibodies
Insecticides (organophosphates, anticholinesterases)	Atropine, pralidoxime
Methanol (wood alcohol)	Ethanol
Ethylene glycol (antifreeze)	Ethanol
Carbon monoxide	Oxygen
Narcotics/opioids	Naloxone
Iron	Deferoxamine
Copper, arsenic, and lead	Penicillamine
Cyanide	Sodium nitrite, sodium thiosulfate

Emergency treatment is essential and depends on the poison ingested. Parents with small children should always have syrup of ipecac and activated charcoal readily available for use. These remedies should not be administered if the patient is unconscious or if the poison is corrosive. Ipecac induces vomiting, while activated charcoal helps to adsorb many poisons. Gastric lavage or dialysis may be necessary. Common antidotes to poisonous substances are listed in Table 18-3.

Burns

Burn injuries are generally classified by their extent and depth. The extent of the burn describes the amount of body surface area affected. In adults, the "rule of nines" divides the body surface into areas consisting of about 9% of the total area. In children, the surface of one side of the child's hand can be used to approximate 1% of body surface area. The "rule of nines" is shown in Fig. 18-1.

The depth of the burn is classified by degree. First-degree burns affect only the epidermis. They are red or gray and do not blister (due to lack of dermal injury). Second-degree burns appear hyperemic and generally blister due to partial-thickness injury to the dermis. Third-degree burns involve full-thickness injury to the dermis. They may appear leathery or pearly. These burns are numb to the touch due to destruction of nerve endings in the dermis.

Initial treatment of the patient includes airway management, cooling, and IV fluid resuscitation for burns of more than 25% of body surface area. The Parkland formula suggests giving lactated Ringer's solution at a rate of 3–4 ml per kg of body weight for each 1% of body surface burned. It should be administered over the first 24 hours, with half of the solution given in the first 8 hours. Complications of burns include paralytic ileus, which requires placement of a nasogastric tube to prevent aspiration, and stress gastritis, which requires treatment with intravenous H_2-antagonists.

Infections are a common and extremely serious complication of burn injuries. Burn patients are particularly at risk for infection with *Pseudomonas aeruginosa* and may develop sepsis. Systemic antibiotics are generally not effective in full-thickness burns due to lack of vascularity, so topical antibiotics, particularly silver sulfadiazine, are used. All patients

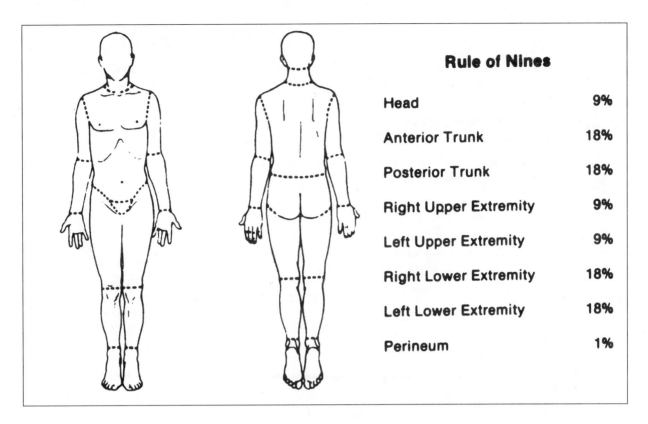

Rule of Nines

Head	9%
Anterior Trunk	18%
Posterior Trunk	18%
Right Upper Extremity	9%
Left Upper Extremity	9%
Right Lower Extremity	18%
Left Lower Extremity	18%
Perineum	1%

Fig. 18-1. Rule of nines. (From J Rippe, R Irwin, M Fink, F Cerra. *Intensive Care Medicine*, Third Edition. Boston: Little, Brown, 1996.)

should receive tetanus immunoglobulin as well as tetanus toxoid if they have not received a tetanus booster within 5 years. Large burn wounds require analgesia and debridement, as well as evaluation for possible skin grafting.

Burns are an important cause of injury and death in children, most commonly as a result of scalding injuries. Parents can adjust water heater thermostats to below 54ºC to minimize this risk. Cigarette use causes a large number of building fires. Smoke detectors and fire alarms should be installed and maintained in all buildings.

Electrical Injuries

The passage of high-voltage electricity through body tissue results in thermal injury. These injuries are sometimes known as "fourth-degree" burns to denote damage to the muscle and bone, often despite relatively normal skin appearance. Patients typically have a charred area of skin where the current entered the body, as well as an "exit wound" that resembles the explosive exit wound from a projectile injury. Cardiac arrest may occur, requiring CPR. Other complications include extensive nerve damage and the development of cataracts. Treatment of electrical burn patients is otherwise similar to that of other burn patients.

Prevention measures include installing grounding structures and disconnecting circuit breakers whenever work is done on electrical appliances. Injuries in children can be prevented by unplugging appliances not in use and installing safety guards in electrical outlets.

Common Injuries

Types of Fractures

Open (compound) fracture: A fracture with an associated open skin wound.
Closed (simple) fracture: A fracture with no associated open wound.
Greenstick fracture: An incomplete fracture that generally occurs in children (Fig. 18-2).
Spiral fracture: A fracture involving a twisting breakage of the bone
Comminuted fracture: A fracture with multiple bone fragments.

Fractures

The most common cause of paraplegia and quadriplegia is spinal cord injury from **vertebral fractures**, often after motor vehicle or diving accidents. Emergency treatment includes immobilization and ensuring an airway. C-spine protectors should be kept in place until cross-table neck films that show no evidence of injury have been obtained. Compression fractures of the vertebral bodies are also frequently seen in postmenopausal women, as a result of osteoporosis and degenerative joint disease.

Hip fractures are a major cause of disability and death in the elderly. Osteoporosis weakens bones, which can then be broken in a minor fall. More than 200,000 hip fractures occur in the United States annually, and 10–20% lead to death. Many of the survivors require long-term care. Avascular necrosis of the femoral head may occur if displacement of the femoral head compromises blood flow. Treatment includes immobilization, bed rest, and often surgery within hours of the injury. A prosthetic hip may be implanted to increase stability. Prevention includes safety measures to prevent falls, such as handrails in the tub and nonslip bath mats, as well as estrogen replacement therapy and calcium supplementation to prevent bone loss in women.

The presence of a **skull fracture** should be assumed until ruled out in any patient suffering significant head trauma. Clinical signs of skull fracture include Battle's sign (discoloration over the mastoid bone), blood drainage from the ears, bruising of the orbit, cranial nerve palsies, and CSF leakage from the ears and nose. Skull fractures may require surgical treatment.

Simple **rib fractures** are the most common thoracic injury and are typically caused by direct blows to the chest. The fifth through ninth ribs are most often injured, because the lower "floating" ribs are more flexible and resilient to trauma. Patients typically experience localized pain that worsens on deep breathing, and a pneumothorax may be present. Splinting the fracture may help control pain.

Colles' fracture, involving the breakage and displacement of the distal radius, is the most common wrist fracture. It typically results from an attempt to "break" a fall on an outstretched hand. This fracture is seen commonly in postmenopausal women.

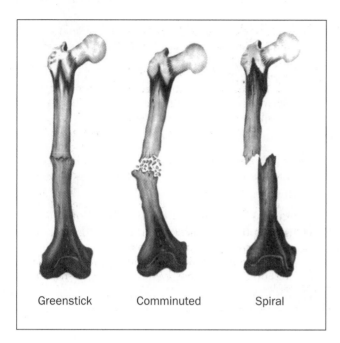

Fig. 18-2. Types of fractures. (Adapted from N Caroline. *Emergency Care in the Streets*, Fifth Edition. Boston: Little, Brown, 1995.)

Elbow fractures generally occur in children under age 10, following a fall on an outstretched hand with the elbow in extension. It can result in compression of the radial and median nerves or the brachial artery. Improper care can lead to the development of **Volkmann's ischemic contracture**, in which the fingers are permanently contracted.

Pelvic fractures occur primarily as a result of motor vehicle accidents. Bleeding is a common cause of death in these patients, as more than 30% of a patient's blood volume can be lost to the pelvic cavity. ABCs (airway, breathing, and circulation) should be established, and these patients should be managed as shock victims. Pelvic x-rays should be obtained in all cases of major trauma.

Tibial fractures frequently result from skiing injuries, although they occur in many other contexts. Patients with tibial fractures are at high risk for developing **compartment syndrome**, in which bleeding into the tight muscle compartments causes compression of the blood supply, leading to muscle ischemia. The "six Ps" of compartment syndrome are *p*ain, *p*allor, *p*ulselessness, *p*uffiness, *p*aresthesias, and *p*aresis (weakness) or *p*aralysis. Surgical opening of the compartment is necessary to prevent permanent muscle and nerve damage.

General Guidelines for the Treatment of Limb Fractures

- Splint fracture and elevate above the heart, if possible.
- Apply ice to reduce swelling.
- Perform a neurologic exam and check that both sensory and motor pathways are intact.
- Administer anesthesia and reduce fracture if necessary.
- Immobilize with a cast or splint.

Sprains

Sprains refer to injuries of the ligaments or other soft tissues surrounding a joint. Severe sprains may involve the complete separation of a ligament from the bone, resulting in joint instability. The most commonly affected joints are the ankle and the knee. Symptoms can range from slight loss of function to severe swelling and pain.

Treatment guidelines for the first 24–48 hours are remembered as "RICE":

- Rest: Immobilize the joint for 24–48 hours. Use crutches if some mobility is necessary.
- Ice: Apply cold packs immediately to reduce pain and swelling.
- Compression: Wrap with an elastic bandage to immobilize and compress the joint.
- Elevation: Keep afflicted limb propped up on pillow and above the heart whenever possible to help reduce swelling.

In addition, NSAIDs may be helpful for their analgesic and anti-inflammatory properties. After 2–3 days, the patient may begin weight-bearing on the joint as tolerated.

Dislocation

Dislocation refers to the disruption of joint placement, sometimes associated with tearing of the ligaments. Shoulders, elbows, fingers, hips, knees, and ankles are the most common sites of dislocation injury. They are often treated by manipulation and traction but may require surgery.

Hip dislocation commonly occurs as a result of motor vehicle accidents. If the knee hits the dashboard at high speed, posterior displacement of the femoral head from the acetabulum may result. This may damage the blood supply, causing avascular necrosis of the femoral head. Additionally, compression of the sciatic nerve may occur, leading to an abnormal gait and footdrop.

Sternoclavicular dislocation (posterior dislocation of the clavicle at the sternum) may be seen after strong pressure to the chest. It is a typical football injury. Symptoms include a sensation of choking and a sensory deficit of the ipsilateral upper extremity. Complications include damage to the mediastinal structures, including the trachea and the esophagus.

Injuries to the Head

- **Concussion** is a transient loss of consciousness resulting from trauma. Bruising of the brain may occur under the site of injury (**coup** injury) or on the contralateral side (**contrecoup** injury). As consciousness is regained, patients often experience confusion, headache, dizziness, and sometimes amnesia.
- Blunt **eye trauma** may cause periorbital ecchymosis ("black eye"), hemorrhage into the anterior chamber (hyphema), and edema. Fracture of the orbital bone is called a blowout fracture. Severe injury should be seen by a specialist, and daily ophthalmologic exams should be performed until the symptoms resolve. Aspirin or other anticoagulants are contraindicated.
- Following blunt **ear trauma**, an auricular hematoma ("cauliflower ear") may develop. It requires prompt drainage to prevent dissolution of the cartilage.

Lacerations

Treatment of lacerations generally requires local anesthetic, debridement, and suturing. Avoid vasoconstricting anesthetics, such as those containing epinephrine or cocaine, on the digits, nose, outer ear, and penis.

Gunshot Wounds

Bullet wounds produce damage by crushing the tissue in the bullet's path. Travel through the tissue results in the formation of a cylindrical "permanent cavity" of the same diameter as the bullet. Bullets may not travel in a straight line but may tumble or oscillate, resulting in a larger, permanent cavity. The size of entrance and exit wounds depends on the type of bullet used, but the exit wound is generally the larger one. Bits of hair and skin may accompany the bullet on its path, resulting in contamination of the wound.

Stab and Puncture Wounds

Stab and puncture wounds may not cause significant external injury, but internal injuries may be severe. If the knife or object remains in the wound, do not remove it, as this may cause hemorrhage and further damage. Instead, attempt to stabilize the item until it can be surgically removed.

Injuries to the Chest

Injuries to the thorax can result in hemothorax, pneumothorax, and aortic rupture, all of which may be rapidly fatal. Cardiac tamponade is another commonly seen injury, discussed in Chapter 2. Blunt trauma to the heart may also result in myocardial injury. Injuries below the level of the nipples are considered abdominal injuries as well, due to presence of the liver and the spleen directly under the diaphragm.

Injuries to the Abdomen

Penetrating abdominal injuries usually result in hemorrhage and perforation of the intestines. Blunt abdominal trauma may initially appear to have been harmless but often results in rupture of the spleen or liver; the large blood supplies to these organs may cause massive internal bleeding. A distended, tender abdomen following injury indicates internal bleeding, which can rapidly lead to shock.

Injuries to the Pelvis

Severe injuries to the pelvis often result in damage to the bladder and ureters. Trauma to the flanks may result in kidney damage and may be accompanied by a bluish skin discoloration (Grey Turner's sign), which indicates hemorrhage. As with the abdomen, blunt trauma may cause massive internal bleeding with few external indications.

Bites and Stings

- **Dog and cat bites** are quite common, especially in young children. Wound care includes high-volume, high-pressure saline irrigation, wound debridement, and tetanus prophylaxis. Rabies prophylaxis may also be necessary if the animal has not been vaccinated. Likely organisms from dog and cat bites include *Pasteurella multocida,* staphylococci, streptococci, and anaerobes. Antibiotic treatment is indicated.
- In the United States the most common poisonous **snake bites** come from pit vipers, such as rattlesnakes, water moccasins, and copperheads. Without treatment, swelling, pain, coagulopathy, and respiratory distress ensue, and death usually occurs within 6–8 hours. First aid includes splinting of the affected area and transporting the patient to a medical facility. Tourniquets, ice packs, and incision and suction by mouth are not recommended. Once hospitalized, specific antivenin is administered.
- The most clinically important **spider bites** are from black widow spiders and brown recluse spiders. Black widow bites cause vomiting, abdominal pain, and shock. These symptoms may mimic an acute abdomen, but they are generally not lethal. Calcium gluconate and methocarbamol are effective therapies, but local bite treatment is not useful. Brown recluse spider bites are slightly more dangerous. The bite develops into a black scab that is associated with rash, fever, vomiting, and jaundice. Fatal disseminated intravascular coagulation can occur. Treatment includes dexamethasone, dapsone, colchicine, and total excision of the lesion.
- Most **insect stings** result from bees, wasps, and ants. The resulting local pain, redness, and swelling are best treated with removal of insect tissue (the "stinger") and cool compresses. Rapid onset of urticaria, respiratory distress, and hypotension indicate the development of anaphylaxis, an allergic reaction in a sensitized individual. Immediate treatment for anaphylaxis consists of intubation and epinephrine injection, which may be followed by administration of bronchodilators and IV fluids. Patients who are known to be sting-allergic should carry antianaphylaxis kits.

Shock

The basic treatment of shock is the ABCs:

- **Airway:** Ensure that the patient has a patent airway, and intubate if necessary.
- **Breathing:** Use bag or ventilator.
- **Circulation:** Ensure adequate circulation. Treatment will depend on the type of shock (Table 18-4).

Intentional Injury

Child Abuse

More than 2.4 million reported incidents of child abuse occur annually. Child abuse may include physical and emotional abuse, sexual abuse, or neglect. Physicians must report sus-

Table 18-4. Characteristics of different types of shock

	Hypovolemic	Septic	Cardiogenic	Neurogenic
Etiologies	Hemorrhage	Infection	Arrhythmias	Spinal cord injury
	Burns	Gangrene	Myocardial infarction	
	Vomiting	Necrosis	Congestive heart	Drug overdose
	Diarrhea	Cardiovascular	failure	
		obstruction	Cardiovascular	
			compression	
Skin	Pale	Pale/pink*	Pale	Pink
Neck veins	Distended	Flat	Flat	Flat
Pulse	High	High	High	Normal/Low
Vascular resistance	High	High/low*	High	Low
Treatment	Rehydration	Ventilation	Medication	Ventilation
	Transfusions	Fluid	Pacemaker	Fluid
	Medications	Antibiotics	Naloxone	Drainage

*Septic shock varies depending on whether it is low-output or high-output septic shock.

pected abuse and may be held legally liable if they do not. Confidentiality of the physician's identity is maintained. The increase of mandatory reporting laws have made clinicians more aware of the signs of child abuse, although many cases are still missed.

The clinician should look for a history of multiple injuries, regardless of how "nice" the family may appear. Children should be interviewed alone, if possible. Also, evaluate whether the extent of trauma matches the injury history. Common child abuse injuries include burns, fractures, abdominal trauma, and head trauma.

On exam, the distribution of an injury often suggests whether it was intentional or not. For example, splash marks tend to accompany accidental scald burns, whereas clearly demarcated lines without splash marks indicate intentional injury. A small circular area that is spared also suggests intentional injury, if the abuser used that area to hold and "dunk" the child. Injuries to a child's front are generally accidental, whereas trauma to the back may be intentional. Signs of neglect include dehydration, poor weight gain, hypervigilance, and depression.

Clinicians should document all lesions, and any remarks by the child or parent that suggest abuse must be recorded verbatim. Photographs and x-rays are allowed in most states without parental permission if abuse is suspected. Reporting to the Department of Social Services should be done as soon as possible by phone, and a written report should be sent within 48 hours. If in doubt, it is always better to report suspected cases of abuse.

Sexual Abuse

Sexual abuse is any nonconsensual sexual activity and includes exposure, genital manipulation, oral sex, and intercourse. Physical contact is not required. A child victim cannot give informed consent and may not even understand that what is occurring is considered abusive.

Dysfunctional behavior in children, such as clinging, unusual fears about other people, and recurrent nightmares may reflect abuse. Chronically abused children often display poor self-esteem and depression.

In a clinical setting, questions should focus on living and caretaking arrangements and on possible touching or hurting of any body part. Proceed from head to toe; do not focus solely on the genital area. The physical exam should occur with another health care worker in the room, and the child should be reassured that he or she has not done anything wrong. A supine, frog-legged position is best for the genital exam, and any bruises, swelling, or lacerations should be noted. An enlarged horizontal diameter of the hymen may indicate that penetration has occurred, although a normal exam does not exclude abuse. The anal area, scrotal area, and penis must be examined. Gonorrhea and chlamydia cultures should be taken, and any unusual discharge must be investigated. Throat cultures should also be performed in cases of suspected oral sex. As with other forms of child abuse, all observations should be recorded clearly and reported to the Department of Social Services as soon as possible.

Spouse Abuse

Spouse abuse is the deliberate physical, sexual, or emotional assault by one romantic partner on another. Most commonly, men abuse their female partners; however, women may be batterers, and spousal abuse may occur in homosexual relationships as well. Other problems associated with spousal abuse include child abuse and alcoholism. As many as 10% of battered women attempt suicide.

Battering is the most common cause of injury for which women seek medical attention. Clinicians should be aware that patterns of repeated emergency room or clinic visits may be a sign of domestic violence. As with child abuse, the history may not match the severity of injury. In addition to complaints related to their injuries, victims of battering may manifest symptoms of depression, post-traumatic stress disorder, or pelvic disorders.

If spousal abuse is suspected, the patient should be interviewed alone and asked direct questions in a supportive manner. Plans for intervention are made according to the patient's wishes and may include safety plans, hotlines, shelters, or family therapy. The patient may choose not to take action. If so, clinicians should continue to provide support and information about possible alternatives.

Elder Abuse

Elder abuse is broadly defined as physical or emotional abuse and neglect of persons aged 65 or over, typically occurring in a domestic setting. A caretaker or family member is often the perpetrator, and patients are reluctant to report abuse for fear of losing their only support. As the American population ages, elder abuse is becoming an increasingly common problem.

Clinicians should be aware of unusual or frequent bruises, welts, and fractures. Evidence of poor nutrition, dehydration, social isolation, and depression should also arouse suspicion. Currently, all 50 states have mandatory reporting laws. Protective services may evaluate the patient's competence and make recommendations for alternate guardianship.

Rape

Rape is forced sexual assault. In the United States, roughly 1 in 10 women will be raped in her lifetime. Current estimates indicate that only 20% of rapes are reported to the authorities, and many rapes are perpetrated by an acquaintance or family friend.

Patients need emotional support as well as clinical attention. They should be treated respectfully and nonjudgmentally. History-taking should include details of the assault as well as activities such as bathing that may have been performed afterwards. Physical exam must document traumatic injuries anywhere on the body, including external and internal genital, anal, and oral areas. A Pap smear may show sperm, and vaginal fluid should be collected by cotton swab and placed on slides and in glass tubes. Wood's lamp examination of the patient's body is useful because seminal fluid will fluoresce. The pubic area should be combed, and material collected should be saved as possible evidence. Fingernail scrapings and pubic hair samples may also be useful. Any sites penetrated should be cultured for venereal diseases, including gonorrhea, syphilis, *Chlamydia*, and *Trichomonas*. VDRL tests are performed on blood. Follow-up exams should include HIV and pregnancy testing. Prophylactic protocols include penicillin, tetracycline, and tetanus immunization.

It is important to ensure that the patient has social support systems and follow-up exams, both for physical as well as psychological evaluation.

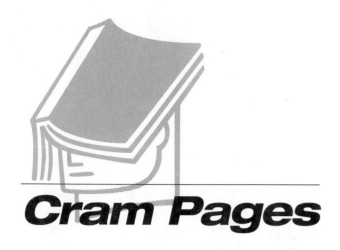

Cram Pages

This chapter contains charts of "word associations" that often appear on the Step 2 exam. For some, the association may not be completely obvious; we suggest that you refer back to earlier chapters or to more detailed medical texts if you are unfamiliar with the topic.

These pages are for you to tear out, write on, and "personalize" as much as you want, and we encourage you to add your own "cram facts." After the exam, write to us (using the form in the back of the book) with your favorite cram facts, and we'll try to include them in the next edition! Remember, if we use your input, you'll receive a $10 gift certificate toward any medical book published by Little, Brown and Company.

GASTROENTEROLOGY

Vitamins

Vitamin A	Night blindness
Vitamin D	Rickets Osteomalacia
Vitamin K	Clotting deficiency with long PT

Thiamin (B$_1$)	Beriberi
	    Peripheral neuropathy
	    Cardiomyopathy
	Wernicke-Korsakoff
	    Confabulation

Niacin	Pellagra
	    Diarrhea
	    Dermatitis/stomatitis
	    Dementia

Pyridoxine (B$_6$)	Neuropathy Cheilosis
Cobalamin (B$_{12}$)	Macrocytosis Pernicious anemia
Folate	Macrocytosis Common in alcoholics
Vitamin C	Scurvy Bleeding gums Connective tissue problems

Esophagus and Stomach Disorders

Tracheoesophageal fistula	Congenital defect Coughing and cyanosis when feeding
Achalasia	Dysphagia for solids *and* liquids Absent peristalsis and tight LES "Beak-like" esophagus on x-ray
Esophageal cancer: Risk factors	Smoking Alcohol use Gastroesophageal reflux Barrett's esophagus
Gastritis: Risk factors	NSAIDs Alcohol use *H. pylori*
Peptic ulcer disease	*H. pylori* infection Duodenal > gastric
Zollinger-Ellison syndrome	Gastrinoma Recurrent ulcers
Gastric cancer	Risk factor is *H. pylori* gastritis Virchow's (supraclavicular) node

Intestinal Disorders

Indirect inguinal hernias	Infants Persistent processus vaginalis
Direct inguinal hernias	Adults Weakness in Hesselbach's triangle
Ulcerative colitis	Colon and terminal ileum without skip lesions "Lead pipe" appearance on x-ray

Crohn's disease	Can affect entire GI tract
	Begins in terminal ileum
	Transmural
	Skip lesions
	"Cobblestoning"
Colon cancer	Right-sided lesion
	"Napkin ring" on x-ray
	Anemia
	Left-sided lesion
	"Apple core" on x-ray
	Pencil stools
Volvulus	Seen in newborns and elderly
	"Double bubble" sign on x-ray
	"Bird's beak" sign on barium enema

Gastroenteritis

Cholera	Fecal-oral transmission
	"Rice water" stools
***Shigella* dysentery**	Very small bacterial dose needed
	Blood and mucus in stools
Staphylococcal enteritis	Onset in 3–6 hours
	"Church picnic" epidemic
***Salmonella* enteritis**	Undercooked poultry
Viral enteritis	Norwalk
	Rotavirus in young children

Biliary System

Acute pancreatitis	Pain radiates to back
	Grey Turner's sign (blue flank)
	Cullen's sign (blue around umbilicus)
Chronic pancreatitis	Alcoholics
	Causes malabsorption and diabetes
Hepatitis A	Fecal-oral transmission
Hepatitis B	Bloodborne and sexually transmitted
	HBsAg in early infection
	HBc IgG present for life
Hepatitis C	Most common post-transfusion hepatitis
Cholelithiasis	"Female, fertile, fat, forty"
Cholangitis	Charcot's triad
	Biliary colic
	Jaundice
	Fever
Hepatocellular CA:	HBV
Risk factors	HCV
	Alcoholic cirrhosis
	Aflatoxins

Congenital Disorders

Pyloric stenosis	Projectile vomiting in neonates
	"String sign" on x-ray
Meconium ileus	Associated with cystic fibrosis
Hirschsprung's disease	No autonomic nerves in colon
	Obstipation
	Megacolon

CARDIOVASCULAR

Congenital Defects

Atrial septal defect	Widely split and fixed S2
Ventricular septal defect	Pansystolic murmur
Patent ductus arteriosus	Continuous "machinery" murmur
Tetralogy of Fallot	Ventricular septal defect Right ventricular hypertrophy Pulmonic stenosis Overriding aorta
Pulmonic stenosis	Early systolic click High-pitched systolic ejection murmur Soft or absent S2

Vascular Disorders

Coarctation of the aorta	Hypertension in arms but not legs Murmur heard on back
Bacterial endocarditis	New heart murmurs Splinter hemorrhages under fingernails Osler's nodes (nodules on digits) Roth's spots (retinal hemorrhages)
Aortic aneurysms	Abdominal 　　Pulsatile mass on exam 　　Atherosclerosis, smoking, hypertension Thoracic 　　Marfan's, syphilis

Peripheral vascular disease	Weak pulses
	Atrophic skin
	Little hair growth
	Nonhealing ulcers
Raynaud's phenomenon	Pallor, cyanosis, erythema of fingers
	Most cases idiopathic; others related to collagen vascular disease

Valvular Disorders

Mitral stenosis	Most caused by rheumatic fever
	Loud S1 and opening snap after S2
	Low-pitched diastolic rumble
Mitral regurgitation	Midsystolic click
	Harsh, blowing holosystolic murmur
Aortic stenosis	Angina
	Syncope
	Left-sided heart failure
	Crescendo-decrescendo systolic murmur radiating to carotids
Aortic regurgitation	Decrescendo murmur
	Widened pulse pressure
	"Water hammer" pulse
	"Pistol shot" over femoral artery

Arrhythmias

Atrial flutter	"Sawtooth" pattern on ECG
Atrial fibrillation	Absent P waves and irregular baseline on ECG
	Irregularly irregular pulse

Supraventricular tachycardia	Sudden attacks due to re-entrant rhythm
	P waves hidden in T waves on ECG
Ventricular tachycardia	3 or more consecutive PVCs
	Independent P waves on ECG
Ventricular fibrillation	No definable waves on ECG
	No pulse

Heart Disease

Left-sided failure	Dyspnea on exertion
	Orthopnea
	Paroxysmal nocturnal dyspnea
Right-sided failure	Neck vein distention
	Liver enlargement
	Edema
Heart failure signs	S3 due to rapid ventricular filling
	S4 due to noncompliant ventricle
Myocardial infarction	ST elevation, T wave inversion on ECG
	CPK-MB peaks after 12–40 hours
	LDH peaks after 3–6 days
Congestive cardiomyopathy	Alcohol use

Pericardial Disease

Acute pericarditis	Pansystolic "friction rub"
Chronic pericarditis	Causes right-sided heart failure
	Kussmaul's sign present

Pericardial effusion	Friction rub
	Distant heart sounds
	"Water bottle" appearance on x-ray
Cardiac tamponade	Pulsus paradoxus
	Kussmaul's sign absent

RESPIRATORY DISORDERS

Upper Respiratory Infections

Streptococcal pharyngitis	High fever
	Red pharynx with exudate
Peritonsillar abscess	Displaced uvula
	Painful swallowing
	Trismus (cannot open mouth)
Sinusitis	Yellow-green discharge
	Viral, *S. pneumoniae*, *H. influenzae*
Epiglottitis	*H. influenzae* type b
	Inspiratory stridor
	Dysphagia with drooling
	Must intubate
Laryngotracheitis (croup)	Parainfluenza virus
	Barking cough
	Stridor

Lower Respiratory Infections

Bronchiolitis	Respiratory syncytial virus

***S. pneumoniae* pneumonia**	Red-brown "rusty" sputum
	Lobar pneumonia
	Gram-positive diplococci
***H. influenzae* pneumonia**	COPD patients
	Small gram-negative rods
Viral pneumonia	Flu-like prodrome
	Patchy infiltrates on x-ray
***Klebsiella* pneumonia**	Alcoholics, aspiration
	"Currant jelly" sputum
	Encapsulated gram-negative rods
Staphylococcal pneumonia	Pink "salmon-colored" sputum
	Often nosocomial
	Gram-positive cocci in clusters
***Mycoplasma* pneumonia**	Young adults
	X-ray looks worse than patient does
***Pseudomonas* pneumonia**	Cystic fibrosis and immunocompromised patients
***Legionella* pneumonia**	CNS and GI symptoms
Tuberculosis	Fever
	Night sweats
	Weight loss
	Bloody sputum

Chronic Obstructive Pulmonary Disease

Emphysema	Destruction of alveolar walls
	Risk factors
	Smoking
	Alpha$_1$-antitrypsin deficiency

"Blue bloaters"	Bronchitis > emphysema
	Cyanosis
"Pink puffers"	Emphysema > bronchitis
	Underweight
Cystic fibrosis	Autosomal recessive
	COPD
	Pancreatic insufficiency
	High chloride in sweat

Interstitial Lung Disease

Sarcoidosis	Increased calcium
	"Ground glass" appearance on x-ray
Asbestosis	Increased risk of lung CA and mesothelioma
	Construction or shipyard workers
Silicosis	Increased risk of TB
	Metal mining

Other Lung Disorders

Pleural effusion	Transudates
	<3 g/dl protein
	Plasma/serum protein <0.5
	Plasma/serum LDH <0.6
	Caused by CHF, cirrhosis, nephrotic syndrome
	Exudates
	>3 g/dl protein
	Plasma/serum protein >0.5
	Plasma/serum LDH >0.6
	Caused by neoplasms and infection

Pulmonary edema	Pink, frothy sputum
	"Kerley B" lines on x-ray
Pulmonary embolism	Most arise from DVTs in leg
	$\dot{V}/\dot{Q}$ scan useful for diagnosis, angiography is gold standard
Respiratory distress syndrome	Usually <37 weeks gestation
	Test for lung maturity
	L/S ratio >2
	+ PG
	Beclomethasone hastens maturity
Pulmonary hypertension	Accentuated P2
	Cyanosis and clubbing

ENDOCRINOLOGY

Thyroid

Hypothyroidism	Weight gain
	Lethargy
	Coarse hair and dry skin
	Irregular menses
	Cold intolerance
	Myxedema
Hyperthyroidism	Weight loss despite good appetite
	Nervousness
	Sweating
	Tachycardia
	Heat intolerance
	Arrhythmias
Thyroid nodule: CA risk factors	Previous neck irradiation
	Hoarse voice
	"Cold" nodule on thyroid scan

Thyroid cancer	Papillary: Most common, best prognosis
	Follicular
	Anaplastic: Worse prognosis
	Medullary: Calcitonin-producing cells, MEN type II

Diabetes

Diabetes symptoms	Polyuria
	Polydipsia
	Polyphagia
Diabetic complications	Retinopathy
	Nephropathy
	Neuropathy
	Vascular disease

Parathyroid

Hypoparathyroidism	Tingling
	Tetany
	Chvostek's sign/Trousseau's sign
Hyperparathyroidism	"Bones, stones, abdominal groans, and psychic moans"

Pituitary/Hypothalamic Disorders

Diabetes insipidus	Lack of ADH
	Polyuria and polydipsia
SIADH	Tumor, trauma, pulmonary disease, drugs
	Hyponatremia
	Concentrated urine
	Treat by restricting water

Acromegaly	Bone and tissue enlargement
	Glucose intolerance
	Osteoarthritis

Adrenal

Addison's disease	Decreased cortisol
	Weight loss and fatigue
	Skin pigmentation
	Eosinophilia
Cushing's syndrome	Increased cortisol
	Buffalo hump, moon facies, central obesity
	Easy bruising and striae
	Osteoporosis
	Cushing's disease due to ACTH from pituitary adenoma
Pheochromocytoma	Episodic hypertension
	Diagnosis by urinary catecholamines

Lipid Metabolism

Familial hypercholesterolemia	Autosomal dominant
	Xanthomas and xanthelasmas
	MIs in 40s
Familial hypertriglyceridemia	Autosomal dominant
	Pancreatitis
	Milky serum
Familial combined hyperlipidemia	Autosomal dominant
	Increased cholesterol and/or triglycerides
	No xanthomas

Other Endocrine Disorders

MEN I	Parathyroid tumors
	Pituitary tumors
	Pancreatic tumors
MEN II	Pheochromocytoma
	Parathyroid tumors
	Thyroid tumors (medullary)
Hemochromatosis	Autosomal recessive
	Excessive iron accumulation
	Cirrhosis
	Diabetes
	Bronze skin
Wilson's disease	Autosomal recessive
	Excessive copper accumulation
	Ataxia and dementia
	Kayser-Fleischer rings on cornea

GENITOURINARY SYSTEM

Urinary System

Cystitis	Usually *E. coli*
	Frequency, urgency, dysuria
	Suprapubic pain
Bladder carcinoma: **Risk factors**	Smoking
	Schistosomiasis
	Analine dyes
Renal artery stenosis	Cause of secondary hypertension
	Fibromuscular dysplasia (young women)
	Atherosclerosis (older patients)

Uremic syndrome	CNS changes
	Asterixis
	Pericarditis
	Nausea and vomiting
	Yellow-brown skin
Glomerulonephritis	Hematuria
	Proteinuria
	RBC casts
Nephrotic syndrome	Proteinuria
	Edema
	Hypoalbuminemia
Acute tubular necrosis	Due to ischemia or toxins
	Resolves in several weeks
	May need dialysis
Polycystic kidney disease	Autosomal dominant
	Hematuria
	Hypertension
	UTIs
Alport's syndrome	X-linked
	Deafness and renal failure
Wilms' tumor	Children <4 years of age
	Hematuria
	Abdominal mass

Electrolyte Disorders

Hypernatremia	>155 mEq/liter
	Due to dehydration
	CNS depression

Hyponatremia	<135 mEq/liter
	Central pontine myelinolysis if corrected too fast
Hyperkalemia	>5.5 mEq/liter
	Muscular weakness
	Cardiac arrhythmias
Hypokalemia	<3.5 mEq/liter
	Muscular weakness
	Cardiac arrhythmias
	Respiratory failure

Male Reproductive System

Urethritis	Classified as "gonococcal" and "nongonococcal" (chlamydial)
	High rate of coinfection
	Ceftriaxone for gonorrhea
	Doxycycline for *Chlamydia*
Epididymitis	Induration and tenderness
	Support relieves pain
Torsion of the testes	Adolescent boys
	Swelling and tenderness
	Support does not relieve pain
	Emergent surgery required
Hydrocele	Painless lump
	Can be transilluminated
Varicocele	"Bag of worms"
	Associated with infertility
Seminoma	Painless lump
	Does not transilluminate
	Undescended testis at higher risk, even after surgical correction

Benign prostatic hypertrophy	Enlarged, rubbery prostate
	Urinary retention
Prostatic carcinoma	Firm, nodular, irregular prostate
	Bone metastases

GYNECOLOGY

Infections

Trichomonas vaginitis	Yellow-green, bubbly discharge
	"Strawberry patches" and petechiae
	Motile, flagellated organisms
	Metronidazole
Gardnerella vaginitis	Copious discharge with fishy odor
	"Clue cells" on microscopy
	Metronidazole
Venereal warts	HPV 6, 11
	Not associated with cervical cancer
Syphilis	Painless ulcer with rolled edges and punched-out base
	Penicillin
Pelvic inflammatory disease (PID)	Cervical motion tenderness
	Purulent discharge
	Associated with ectopic pregnancy and infertility
Candida	"Cottage cheese" discharge and red vulva
	Pseudohyphae on slide
	Associated with diabetes and antibiotics
Urinary tract infection (UTI)	Usually caused by *E. coli*
	Dysuria, frequency, urgency
	Trimethoprim-sulfamethoxazole
Toxic shock syndrome	*Staphylococcus aureus* exotoxin
	Rash
	High fever

Neoplasms

Vulvar cancer	Squamous cell
	Usually after menopause
	Pruritus
Cervical cancer	HPV 16, 18, 31
	Sexually transmitted
	Postcoital bleeding
Uterine myoma (fibroid)	Heavy, prolonged menses
	Anemia
Endometrial cancer:	Unopposed estrogen
Risk factors	Obesity
	Nulliparity
	Early menarche
	Late menopause
Breast fibroadenoma	Common in young women
	May recur
Breast cancer:	Family history
Risk factors	Nulliparity
	Early menarche
	Fibrocystic disease
Breast cancer	Painless lump
	Nipple retraction
	Most are in upper outer quadrant
	>90% are "invasive ductal" type

Other Gynecologic Conditions

Endometriosis	Ectopic endometrial tissue
	Dysmenorrhea
	Dyspareunia
	Infertility

Polycystic ovary syndrome (PCO)	High LH and low or normal FSH
	Hirsutism and obesity
	Menstrual irregularities
	Infertility
Menopause	High LH and FSH
	Hot flashes
	Atrophic vaginal epithelium

OBSTETRICS

Hydatidiform mole/ choriocarcinoma	Preeclampsia in first half of pregnancy
	Very high beta-HCG
	"Snowstorm" appearance on ultrasound
Ectopic pregnancy	Beta-HCG rises slowly
	Amenorrhea, spotting and pain
	Empty gestational sac on ultrasound
	Ampulla of fallopian tube is most common site
Labor: First stage	From regular, painful contractions to complete cervical dilation
Labor: Second stage	From cervical dilation to birth
Labor: Third stage	From birth to delivery of placenta
Fetal movements in labor	Descent
	Flexion
	Internal rotation
	Extension
	External rotation
Fetal cardiac monitoring: Early decelerations	Normal
	Occur with contractions

Fetal cardiac monitoring: Late decelerations	Occur >30 sec after contractions
	Indicates fetal hypoxia
	Deliver ASAP
Fetal cardiac monitoring: Variable decelerations	Variable onset
	Occur due to cord compression
	Change maternal position
Premature rupture of membranes (PROM)	Pooling of fluid in vagina
	Positive nitrazine test
	Positive ferning test
	Risk of endometritis
Alpha-fetoprotein	Increased levels
	Neural tube defects
	Abdominal wall defects
	Multiple gestation
	Fetal demise
	Decreased levels
	Down's syndrome
Amniocentesis	Performed weeks 16–20
	Recommended in women >35
Gestational diabetes	Macrosomia
	Respiratory distress syndrome
	Congenital abnormalities
Preeclampsia	Hypertension
	Proteinuria
	Edema
Polyhydramnios	Duodenal atresia
	Tracheoesophageal fistula
	Anencephaly
Oligohydramnios	Renal agenesis
	Pulmonary hypoplasia

PERINATAL DISORDERS

Congenital Infections

Congenital rubella	IUGR
	Cataracts
	Mental retardation and hearing loss
	Cardiac defects
	Purpura
Congenital CMV	IUGR
	Microcephaly
	Jaundice
	Petechiae
	"Blueberry corn muffin" appearance
Congenital syphilis	Jaundice
	Hepatosplenomegaly
	Rash on palms and soles
	"Snuffles"
Congenital toxoplasmosis	IUGR
	Seizures
	Jaundice
	Retinitis
Congenital varicella	Limb hypoplasia and scars
	Retinitis
	Cortical atrophy
Neonatal pneumonia	Group B *Streptococcus*
	E. coli
	Chlamydia
Neonatal meningitis	Group B *Streptococcus*
	E. coli
	Listeria

| **Neonatal *S. aureus*** | Epidemics in nurseries |
| | "Scalded skin syndrome" |

Other Perinatal Disorders

Fetal alcohol syndrome	IUGR
	Microcephaly
	Short palpebral fissures and philtrum
	Cardiac anomalies
Fetal narcotic exposure	Hypertonicity
	Sweating
	Stuffy nose
Fetal cocaine exposure	Limb reduction malformations
	Intestinal atresia
	Jitteriness and tremors
	Vomiting and diarrhea
Kernicterus	Jaundice
	Seizures and brain damage
	Bilirubin >15 mg/dl
"Gray baby" syndrome	Associated with chloramphenicol
	Due to decreased metabolism from immature liver

INFECTIOUS DISEASE

HIV/AIDS

| **HIV infection** | Flu-like illness |
| | Antibodies 1–6 months after infection |

AIDS-related infections: **Viruses**	Cytomegalovirus (CMV) Herpes simplex virus (HSV) Varicella-zoster virus (VZV) Epstein-Barr virus (EBV)
AIDS-related infections: **Bacteria**	*M. tuberculosis* *M. avium-intracellulare*
AIDS-related infections: **Fungi**	*Candida* *Coccidioides* *Histoplasma* *Cryptococcus*
AIDS-related infections: **Protozoa**	*Pneumocystic carinii* *Toxoplasma* *Cryptosporidium* *Giardia*

Congenital Immunodeficiency

DiGeorge's syndrome	Thymic aplasia Absent T cells "Poor George has no thymus"
Wiskcott-Aldrich **syndrome**	X-linked No antibodies against encapsulated bacteria
Chronic granulomatous **disease**	Autosomal recessive Recurrent bacterial and fungal infections
Chediak-Higashi **syndrome**	Autosomal recessive Recurrent streptococcal and staphylococcal infections
Bruton's disease	X-linked No B cells or antibodies

HEMATOLOGY

Anemia

Microcytic anemia (MCV <80)	Iron deficiency
	Chronic disease
	Lead poisoning
	Thalassemia
Normocytic anemia (MCV 80–100)	Hemolysis
	Chronic disease
	Bone marrow suppression (drugs, leukemia)
Macrocytic anemia (MCV >100)	B_{12} or folate deficiency
	Liver disease
	Hypothyroidism

Genetic Disorders

Alpha-thalassemia	Acanthocytes
	Target cells
	Very low MCV but mild anemia
Beta-thalassemia	Basophilic stippling
	Nucleated RBCs
	Very low MCV but mild anemia
Sickle cell anemia	*Salmonella* osteomyelitis
	S. pneumoniae sepsis
Hemophilia	X-linked factor VIII (A) or IX (B) deficiency
	Joint and soft-tissue bleeding
Von Willebrand's disease	Autosomal dominant deficiency of factors VIII and vWF
	Epistaxis
	Menorrhagia
	Bruising

Other Hematologic Disorders

Eosinophilia	"NAACP"
	*N*eoplasms
	*A*sthma/allergies
	*A*ddison's disease
	*C*onnective tissue disorders
	*P*arasites
Thrombotic thrombo-cytopenia purpura	Adults > kids
	Platelets consumed in clotting reactions
	Fluctuating neurologic deficits
Idiopathic thrombo-cytopenia purpura	Kids > adults
	Autoimmune destruction of platelets
	Purpura and petechiae
	Epistaxis and menorrhagia
Hemolytic-uremic syndrome	Usually caused by *E. coli* toxin
	RBC fragments on smear
Hodgkin's lymphoma	Painless cervical lymphadenopathy
	Reed-Sternberg cells
Burkitt's lymphoma	B cell lymphoma
	Associated with Epstein-Barr virus

DERMATOLOGY

Seborrheic dermatitis	Red skin with greasy scales
Psoriasis	Silvery-scaled plaques
	Pitted fingernails
Pilonidal cyst	Hair-lined tract in sacral area
Actinic keratoses	Firm, yellow scale
	Due to sun exposure
	May lead to squamous cell cancer

Skin cancer	Basal cell > squamous cell
	Associated with sun exposure
Malignant melanoma	Change in size, shape, color of mole
	Itching and ulceration

MUSCULOSKELETAL AND CONNECTIVE TISSUE DISORDERS

Osteoarthritis	Common in old age
	DIP and PIP joints
	Also affects hips, knees, spine
Rheumatoid arthritis	Symmetric
	PIP and MCP joints
	Subcutaneous nodules
	70% have positive rheumatoid factor
Gout	Affects big toe, pinna of ear
	Negatively birefringent crystals
Phocomelia	Hands and feet attached to trunk
	Associated with thalidomide
Slipped capital femoral epiphysis	Seen in overweight teenagers
Lyme disease	*Borrelia burgdorferi*
	Ixodes tick
	Arthralgias
	Rash with central clearing
	CNS changes 1 month after exposure
Osteoporosis: Risk factors	Postmenopause
	Caucasians and Asians
	Smoking
	Alcohol
	Corticosteroids

Systemic lupus erythematosus	Young African-American women
	Malar "butterfly" rash
	Arthralgias
	ANA is sensitive (most patients positive)
	Anti-dsDNA is specific (only positive in SLE)
Polymyositis and dermatomyositis	Violet discoloration of eyelids ("heliotrope" rash)
	Elevated muscle enzymes
Ankylosing spondylitis	"Bamboo spine" on x-ray
	Associated with HLA-B27
Shoulder-hand syndrome	Pain, stiffness, swelling in hand and shoulder
	Occurs 1 month after myocardial infarction
Bone metastases: Common primary sites	Breast
	Lung
	Prostate
	Kidney
	Thyroid
Paget's disease	Frontal "bossing" and shortened spine
	Elevated alkaline phosphatase
	"Cotton-wool" appearance on skull x-ray

PSYCHIATRY

Delirium	Decreased, fluctuating level of consciousness
	Often due to substance abuse or medical illness
	Reversible
Dementia	Decreased memory and cognition
	Irreversible
Schizophrenia	>6 months of delusions, hallucinations, disorganized behavior
	Genetic predisposition

Schizophreniform disorder	Symptoms of schizophrenia lasting <6 months
Schizoaffective disorder	Schizophrenia and a mood disorder
Schizoid personality	Unable to form close relationships Blunted or absent emotions
Somatization disorder	Multiple, vague, recurrent somatic problems May be related to personality disorder
Conversion disorder	Somatic expression of a specific psychological conflict
Factitious disorder	Feigned illness to assume sick role
Malingering	Feigned illness for external gain
Neuroleptic malignant syndrome	Occurs days after starting neuroleptics Hypertension and muscle rigidity Fever
Tardive dyskinesia	Stereotypical oral movements Associated with long-term neuroleptic use Irreversible

INJURY

Burns: Classification	1st-degree: Red-gray only 2nd-degree: Red with blistering 3rd-degree: Leathery, numb
Burns: Management	Remember "Rule of 9s" Fluid replacement at 3–4 ml/kg for each percent burned
Skull fractures	Battle's sign (discoloration over mastoid)
Colles' fracture	Distal radial fracture due to falling on outstretched hand

Compartment syndrome   Associated with tibial fractures

Pain

Pallor

Pulselessness

Puffiness

Paresthesias

Paresis

Index

Prescription for the Boards
USMLE Step 2

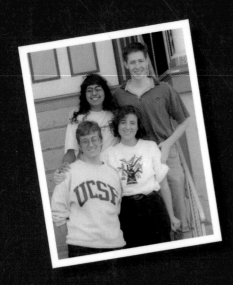

Radhika Sekhri Breaden

Cheryl Denenberg

Kate C. Feibusch

Stephen N. Gomperts

Written *by* students *for* students, this **Little, Brown Review Book** is a complete review of what you need to know to pass Step 2.

Addressing every subject listed in the USMLE test content outline, **Prescription for the Boards** is an ideal guide for exam preparation:

- An **overview of the exam** includes study tips and book reviews to help take the guesswork out of selecting review materials.

- A **summary of medical facts** presents a clear and brief description of each clinical entity, using consistent and clever icons to map out signs and symptoms, diagnosis, treatment, lab tests, and prevention.

- **"Cram pages"** provide word associations to help you remember large amounts of information.

Offering readable summaries of complex medical topics, **Prescription for the Boards** is ideal for medical students and foreign medical graduates who must take USMLE Step 2. Rely on this handy review to prepare months in advance for Step 2 *or* as a memory trigger in the days before the exam!

Also Available from Little, Brown:

The Washington Manual, Twenty-Eighth edition
Adler: *A Pocket Manual of Differential Diagnosis*
Alpers: *Manual of Nutritional Therapeutics*
Friedman: *Problem-Oriented Medical Diagnosis*
Platt: *Conversation Repair*
Smith: *The Patient's Story: Integrated Patient-Doctor Interviewing*
Wallach: *Interpretation of Diagnostic Tests*

Little, Brown and Company
Boston, Massachusetts 02108